AF680246

# Alzheimer's Disease: Diagnosis and Treatment

# Alzheimer's Disease: Diagnosis and Treatment

Editor: Sophia Hall

MURPHY & MOORE
www.murphy-moorepublishing.com

www.murphy-moorepublishing.com

MURPHY & MOORE

**Cataloging-in-Publication Data**

Alzheimer's disease : diagnosis and treatment / edited by Sophia Hall.
p. cm.
Includes bibliographical references and index.
ISBN 978-1-63987-041-7
1. Alzheimer's disease. 2. Alzheimer's disease--Diagnosis.
3. Alzheimer's disease--Treatment. I. Hall, Sophia.
RC523 .A49 2022
616.831--dc23

© Murphy & Moore Publishing, 2022

Murphy & Moore Publishing,
1 Rockefeller Plaza,
New York City, NY 10020, USA

ISBN 978-1-63987-041-7 (Hardback)

This book contains information obtained from authentic and highly regarded sources. Copyright for all individual chapters remain with the respective authors as indicated. All chapters are published with permission under the Creative Commons Attribution License or equivalent. A wide variety of references are listed. Permission and sources are indicated; for detailed attributions, please refer to the permissions page and list of contributors. Reasonable efforts have been made to publish reliable data and information, but the authors, editors and publisher cannot assume any responsibility for the validity of all materials or the consequences of their use.

**Trademark Notice:** Registered trademark of products or corporate names are used only for explanation and identification without intent to infringe.

# Contents

# Preface

The purpose of the book is to provide a glimpse into the dynamics and to present opinions and studies of some of the scientists engaged in the development of new ideas in the field from very different standpoints. This book will prove useful to students and researchers owing to its high content quality.

Alzheimer's disease is a disorder of the brain which impedes thinking skills and damages memory. It is considered to be progressive and irreversible. Some of the major features of Alzheimer's disease are amyloid plaques and neurofibrillary tangles in the brain. There is also a significant loss of connections between the brain's nerve cells. With the progress of the disease, other parts of the brain are affected and the brain tissue shrinks considerably. Some of the symptoms of this disease are memory issues, compromised reasoning and issues with vision. There is no known cure for this disease, however; there are numerous treatments available which can help in the management of symptoms. This book contains some path-breaking studies on Alzheimer's disease. It discusses the fundamentals as well as modern approaches of research within this field. This book will provide comprehensive knowledge to the readers.

At the end, I would like to appreciate all the efforts made by the authors in completing their chapters professionally. I express my deepest gratitude to all of them for contributing to this book by sharing their valuable works. A special thanks to my family and friends for their constant support in this journey.

**Editor**

# 1

# Pathophysiology of Late Onset Alzheimer Disease

Ahmet Turan Isik[1] and M. Refik Mas[2]
[1]*Bezmialem Vakif University, Faculty of Medicine, Department of Geriatric Medicine, Istanbul,*
[2]*9 Eylul University, Faculty of Medicine, Department of Internal Medicine, Izmir*
*Turkey*

## 1. Introduction

As the world population has aged, the number of people affected by Alzheimer Disease is rapidly increasing in the world. It is important for clinicians to recognize early signs and symptoms of dementia and to note potentially modifiable risk factors and early disease markers.

Accumulation of Aβ peptides may be the key event in pathogenesis of AD. The exact mechanism by which Aβ peptide deposition induces neurotoxicity is unclear, but it appears the oxidative stress plays an important role. Oxidative stress is extensive in AD and Aβ peptides stimulate oxidative stress by both direct and indirect mechanisms. Aβ peptides by themselves may act as enzymes and can bind to mitochondrial proteins resulting in the generation of free radicals. Furthermore, Aβ peptides generate oxidative stress via neuroinflammation. Considerable evidence has supported that neuroinflammation is associated with AD pathology. In addition, in AD, vascular injury and parenchymal inflammation perpetuate the cycle of protein aggregation and oxidation in the brain, and diffuse pathological changes include cerebral amyloid angiopathy, affecting more than 90% of patients with Alzheimer's disease, capillary abnormalities, disruption of the blood-brain barrier, and large-vessel. In addition, it was reported that clearance of Aβ along diseased perivascular channels and through the blood-brain barrier is impeded in AD atheroma and that deregulation of Aβ transport across the capillary blood–brain barrier is caused by the imbalanced expression of low-density lipoprotein receptor-related proteins and receptors for advanced glycation end products. Besides, insulin resistance and hyperinsulinemia are implicated in a number of pathophysiological processes related to AD. It was demonstrated that reduced brain insulin signaling is associated with increased tau phosphorylation and Aβ levels in a streptozotocin induced model of diabetes mellitus. Moreover, insulin promotes the release of intracellular Aβ in neuronal cultures and accelerates Aβ trafficking to the plasma membrane. In addition, impaired insulin or insulin like growth factor-1 (IGF-1) signaling can result in the hyper-phosphorylation of tau, which can cause cell death mediated by apoptosis, mitochondrial dysfunction or necrosis and promote oxidative stress, which contributes to the neurodegeneration cascade and leads to dementia-associated behavioral and cognitive deficits.

In shortly, the current pathophysiological approach to LOAD are based on a number of common mechanisms of neurodegeneration, such as accumulation of abnormal proteins, mitochondrial dysfunction and oxidative stress, impaired insulin signaling, calcium homeostasis dysregulation, early synaptic disconnection and late apoptotic cell death. Aging itself is associated with mild cognitive deterioration, probably due to subtle multifactorial changes resulting in a global decrease of a functional brain reserve.

## 2. Pathophysiology of late onset Alzheimer disease

As the world population has aged, dementia has become a common diagnosis in aging populations and the numbers will increase in the forthcoming years. Nowadays, the number of people affected by Alzheimer Disease (AD) is rapidly increasing in the world. AD is an age-related progressive neurodegenerative disorder presented by memory loss and severe cognitive decline (Isik & Bozoglu, 2010).

AD is characterized by extensive atrophy of the brain caused by a series neuropathologic change, including neuronal loss, intracellular neurofibrillary tangles (NFTs) made up of Tau protein, extracellular senile plaques formed by β-amyloid (Aβ) and synaptic loss (Ballatore et al., 2007 & Haass Selkoe, 2007). Amyloid plaques and NFT result from an aberration in deposition of the Aβ peptide and the hyperphosphorylated tau protein, respectively, and these depositions lead to neuronal loss and neurotoxicity in the brain affected by AD (Isik, 2010). However, plaques and NFTs are not unique to AD, as these same structural changes occur with normal aging and in many others neurodegenerative disorders (Jackson-Siegal, 2005). Great confusion existed as to whether the dementia often observed in normal aging and AD were the same or different entities. It took nearly a century to define that the plaques were composed primarily of a specific peptide initially named A4 and today referred to as Aβ and that tangles are composed primarily of hyperphosphorylated forms of tau, a microtubule-associated protein. Tau is a protein known to stabilize microtubules present primarily in axonal processes and involved in axonal transport of subcellular components. The abnormal phosphorylation of this microtubule-related protein leads to molecular protein structures called paired helical filaments (PHFs), which constitute the ultrastructural core of the microscopic structures recognized as NTFs. Most contemporary research on the molecular basis of the disease has focused chiefly on these two proteins, and the causality of the disease has been attributed to either or both of these proteins. For a while, the two camps of thought were humorously referred to as the Baptists (for Aβ) and the Taoists (for tau) (Cuello, 2007). A distinguishing feature of AD is that the plaques and NFTs are localized to areas in the brain corresponding to the clinical symptoms. Although the development of plaques and NFTs eventually leads to a noticeable clinical condition, the process is thought to start years before the initial onset of symptoms (Jackson-Siegal, 2005).

## 3. Risk factors

Great number of nongenetic risk factors have been identified or proposed for the sporadic form of the disease. Of these, unequivocally, aging is the most relevant. To define between the AD and aging, that AD might reflect a continuum of the brain aging can be proposed. In other words, given the opportunity, every individual should eventually succumb to AD. This view can be supported by the undeniable fact that aging is the most important of the nongenetic risk factors as shown by the ever growing incidence of AD with aging. On the other hand, the prevalent notion is that the incidence of AD is influenced by a multitude of risks factors in addition to aging, which might act in a cooperative manner. The extent of the life span could also be regulated by the genetic background interacting with environmental as well as lifestyle aspects. The role of genetics in determining the life span is complex and paradoxical. In short, the prevalent view is that for the sporadic form of AD, it is not necessarily all in the genes but rather interplay with the life experience of that particular individual. The molecular mechanisms of brain aging remain elusive. Several molecular events are suspects in the age-related downfall of brain function, which might be linked to the earlier appearance of AD. Some researchers have paid attention to low levels of vitamin B complex and the plasma elevation of homocysteine, as being responsible for age-related cognitive deficits and unleashing the AD pathology (Cuello, 2007). Furthermore, our results demonstrated that replacement and close follow up of vitamin B12 deficiency are crucial in the elderly population regardless of any disturbance in the hematological parameters (Bozoglu et al., 2010).

While early onset AD is almost genetically based, there are no specific gene mutations that are associated with inheritance of the disease in late onset AD (LOAD). The expression of the apolipoprotein E (ApoE) 4 allele is one of the risk factors identified for LOAD. In the central nervous system, ApoE is synthesized by astrocytes, microglia, and, to a lesser extent, by neurons. The role of ApoE in LOAD pathogenesis is not fully elucidated, but it has been suggested that ApoE is very important in trafficking of amyloid β (Aβ) peptide. In addition, apolipoprotein J (clusterin), an amyloid β-peptide chaperone, TOMM40, a transporter of proteins across the mitochondrial membrane, and Sortillin-related receptor, which functions to partition amyloid precursor protein away from β-secretase and γ-secretase, are recently discovered proteins encoded by the risk genes for LOAD. However, it was reported that higher plasma concentrations of clusterin correlate significantly with the presence and severity of AD but doesn't correlate with the risk for onset of the disease (Schrijvers et al, 2011).

In addition to nonmodifiable genetic risk factors, potentially modifiable factors, such as hypertension, diabetes mellitus, hyperlipidemia, hyperhomocysteinemia, coronary and peripheral artery diseases, alcohol, smoking, obesity, levels of physical or mental activity, levels of education, and environmental exposures have been investigated to identify risk factors for LOAD. Furthermore, it has been reported that risk index methods including these risk factors provide a practical, flexible, and objective framework for identifying the optimal combination of measures for identification of high-risk individuals for prevention and early intervention efforts. Despite the personal and social burden of LOAD, our understanding of the genetic predisposition to LOAD and the contribution of other risk factors remains limited. More importantly, there are few data to explain the overall risks and benefits of prevention strategies or their impact on risk modification (Isik, 2010; Querfurth & La Ferla, 2010).

## 4. Pathogenesis

The amyloid material was initially thought to be systemically derived from serum proteins and characterized as a short peptide (9). Aβ peptides are natural products of metabolism consisting of 36 to 43 amino acids. Monomers of Aβ40 are more prevalent than the aggregation-prone and damaging Aβ42 species. β-amyloid peptides originate from proteolysis of the amyloid precursor protein (APP) lodged in cell membranes by the sequential enzymatic actions of beta-site amyloid precursor protein–cleaving enzyme 1 (BACE-1), a β-secretase, and γ-secretase, a protein complex with presenilin 1 at its catalytic core (Cuello, 2007). In this process the release of Aβ peptides is achieved by the consecutive action of a β-secretase cleaving APP at the N-terminal site of the Aβ domain, followed by its cleavage at the γ-secretase site at the C-terminal end, thus generating Aβ fragments of diverse lengths, but typically of 40 and 42 amino acids in length. The longer peptide, Aβ 1-42, is more neurotoxic and more prone to aggregation and amyloidogenic. The β- and γ-secretases have been identified and cloned. Two proteins are currently recognized with β-secretase functions. They are named BACE 1 and 2, of which BACE 1 appears to be more important for the development of the AD pathology (Vassar & Citron, 2000). The β-secretases release a large peptide which in biochemical jargon is referred to as C99, containing both the Aβ motif and another motif defined as AICD (APP internal C-terminal domain). The γ-secretase site is more complex. Initially, it was proposed that presenilins (mutations of which were already known to cause familial forms of AD) were the actual γ-secretase. Today, there is consensus that the γ-secretase site is composed of an ensemble of proteins, some of which might be responsible for the modulation of the APP-catalytic activity preselinins 1 and 2. This complex has the peculiarity of being capable of a catalytic action in the fairly hydrophobic milieu of cell and organelle membranes (Cuello, 2007).The catalytic activity of the γ-secretase action is ultimately responsible for the liberation of the amyloidogenic Aβ peptide and the AICD fragment (Wolfe, 2006). AICD is suspected to either act as a transcription factor or be involved in cell signaling mechanisms in the CNS, however, its actual biological significance is still being debated (Cuello, 2007). Finally, an imbalance between production and clearance, and aggregation of peptides, causes Aβ to accumulate, and this excess may be the initiating factor in Alzheimer's disease. This idea, called the "amyloid hypothesis," is based on studies of genetic forms of AD, including Down's syndrome, and evidence that Aβ42 is toxic to cells (Querfurth & La Ferla, 2010).

Amyloid plaques, together with NFTs, occur in AD and other neurodegenerative disorders, in addition to normal aging (Guillozet et al., 2003). The number of NFTs is a pathologic marker of the severity of AD. The major component of the tangles is an abnormally hyperphosphorylated and aggregated form of tau. Normally an abundant soluble protein in axons, tau promotes assembly and stability of microtubules and vesicle transport. Hyperphosphorylated tau is insoluble, lacks affinity for microtubules, and self-associates into paired helical filament structures. Enzymes that add and those that remove phosphate residues regulate the extent of tau phosphorylation (8). These NFTs have a clear-cut temporal and topographic distribution across brain areas as the disease progresses. The best staging of such structures has been provided by Braak and Braak (Braak H& Braak E, 1998). Interestingly, the earliest Braak stage is the occurrence of NFTs in the entorhinal cortex in the absence of an obvious deposition of Aβ material in this brain region. This observation has been used as an argument to dissociate tau from Aβ pathology in AD. The causal relation between these two molecular pathologies remains uncertain (Cuello, 2007).

The amyloid cascade hypothesis posits that Aβ triggers Tau pathology, but the details of this relationship are still poorly understood. Accumulation of Aβ peptides may be the key event in the pathogenesis of AD and experimental models have suggested that exposure of neurons to Aβ is toxic and elicits abnormal changes in Tau (Garg et al., 2011). Although new imaging techniques and powerful animal models have helped understanding the time course and the mechanisms of the lesions, the relationship between Aβ accumulation and tau pathology is still badly understood and the mechanism of LOAD continues to be debated (4). In some studies, the changes in Tau were ascribed to a toxic Tau fragment of 17 kD generated by calpain cleavage and located in the N-terminal half of Tau, but other N-terminal parts of Tau were reported to be toxic as well. In these cases, the toxicity could be triggered by Aβ, but there was no apparent relationship to the aggregation of Tau. By contrast, studies on other cleavage reactions had shown that truncation of Tau in the C terminal domain by caspase-3 or by lysosomal proteases could generate Tau fragments with a high tendency for aggregation (Garg et al., 2011).

Data obtained by electron microscopy and immunocytochemical and biochemical analysis on synaptic marker proteins in AD biopsies and autopsies indicate that synaptic loss in the hippocampus and neocortex is an early event and the major structural correlate of cognitive dysfunction. From all cortical areas analyzed, the hippocampus appears to be the most severely affected by the loss of synaptic proteins, while the occipital cortex is affected least. Although the cause for this failure is still unknown, recent evidence indicates a link between plastic synaptic changes and control of differentiation and cell cycle-repression within a neuron (Arendt, 2009). In mild Alzheimer's disease, there is a reduction of about 25% in the presynaptic vesicle protein synaptophysin (Querfurth & La Ferla, 2010) and there is evidence that living neurons lose their synapses in AD. Furthermore, synaptic function is impaired in living neurons, as demonstrated by decrements in transcripts related to synaptic vesicle trafficking (Coleman & Yao, 2003).

The exact mechanism by which Aβ peptide deposition induces neurotoxicity is unclear, but it appears that oxidative stress plays an important role. Besides, Aβ is a potent mitochondrial poison, especially affecting the synaptic pool. In AD, exposure to Aβ inhibits key mitochondrial enzymes in the brain and in isolated mitochondria. Cytochrome c oxidase is specifically attacked. Consequently, electron transport, ATP production, oxygen consumption, and mitochondrial membrane potential all become impaired (Querfurth & La Ferla, 2010). Consequently, oxidative stress is extensive in AD, and Aβ peptides stimulate oxidative stress by both direct and indirect mechanisms. Aβ peptides by themselves may act as enzymes and can bind to mitochondrial proteins, resulting in the generation of free radicals (Lustbader et al., 2004; Newman et al., 2007) Aβ peptides also generate oxidative stress via neuroinflammation. Considerable evidence has supported the hypothesis that neuroinflammation is associated with AD pathology (Newman et al., 2007).

Interestingly, AD was speculated as the brain equivalent of non-insulin-dependent diabetes mellitus (Hoyer, 1998; Craft et al., 2000). It was demonstrated that reduced brain insulin signaling is associated with increased tau phosphorylation and Aβ levels in a Streptozotocin induced model of diabetes mellitus, and also insulin promotes the release of intracellular Aβ in neuronal cultures and accelerates Aβ trafficking to the plasma membrane. Similarly, Intravenous insulin infusion also raised plasma Aβ42 levels in patients with AD but not in normal adults, an effect that was exaggerated in patients with AD with higher body mass indexes. In addition, impaired insulin or IGF-1 signaling can result in the hyper-phosphorylation of tau, which can cause cell death mediated by apoptosis, mitochondrial dysfunction or necrosis and promote oxidative stress, which contributes to the neurodegeneration cascade, and leads to dementia-associated behavioral and cognitive deficits. For this reason, it seems that insulin resistance causes Tau phosphorylation and neurofibrillary tangle formation and increased beta amyloid aggregation in late onset AD (1). In a recent study, Zhao and Townsend are demonstrated that insulin resistance and Aβ disrupt common signal transduction cascades including the insulin receptor family/Phosphoinositide 3-kinase/Akt/Glycogen synthase kinase-3(GSK3) pathway. They reported that both disease processes contribute to overlapping pathology, thereby compounding disease symptoms and progression (Zhao & Townsend, 2009). Besides, Proctor and Gray reported that GSK3β over activity leads to an increase in levels of Aβ plaques and tau tangle (Weller et al., 2009).The age-associated decline in the metabolic rate and utilization of glucose by the frontal cortex imply that insulin resistance can cause executive dysfunctions in older people, not only global cognitive impairment. Insulin resistance may cause decreased cortical glucose utilization especially in hippocampus and entorhinal cortex and also increased oxidative stress with advanced glycation end-products. In humans, raising plasma insulin levels through intravenous infusion increased cerebrospinal fluid levels of the Aβ 42 peptide; this effect was exacerbated by age. That insulin may interfere with Aβ degradation via its regulation of the metalloprotease insulin-degrading enzyme (IDE) may also be an important mechanism in late-onset AD that the Aβ clearance rather than Aβ production may be of special importance. Actually, the Aβ-degrading capacity of IDE in the Alzheimer Disease brains is about 50% of that of control brains, but insulin degradation decreases by about 30% only. Decreased IDE mRNA and IDE activity have been found in the hippocampus of late-onset AD brains; however, in neurons adjacent to senile plaques, IDE is up-regulated (Isik & Bozoglu, 2010).

Furthermore, in AD, vascular injury and parenchymal inflammation perpetuate the cycle of protein aggregation and oxidation in the brain, and diffuse pathologic changes include cerebral amyloid angiopathy, affecting more than 90% of patients with AD, capillary abnormalities, disruption of the blood-brain barrier, and large-vessel channels (Querfurth & La Ferla, 2010; Price et al., 2001). It has also been reported that clearance of Aβ along diseased perivascular channels and through the blood-brain barrier is impeded in AD atheroma, (Deane & Zlokovic, 2007) and that deregulation of Aβ transport across the capillary blood–brain barrier is caused by the imbalanced expression of low-density lipoprotein receptor-related proteins and receptors for advanced glycation end products (Price et al., 2001; Proctor & Gray 2010).

The calcium hypothesis of AD proposes that activation of the amyloidogenic pathway remodels the neuronal Ca(2+) signalling pathways responsible for cognition by enhancing the entry of Ca(2+) and/or the release of internal Ca(2+) by ryanodine receptors or InsP(3) receptors. The specific proposal is that Ca(2+) signalling remodelling results in a persistent elevation in the level of Ca(2+) that constantly erases newly acquired memories by enhancing the mechanism of long-term depression. Neurons can still form memories through the process of long term potentiation, but this stored information is rapidly removed by the persistent activation of long-term depression. Further dysregulation in Ca(2+) signalling will then go on to induce the neurodegeneration that characterizes the later stages of dementia (Berridge, 2010).

Finally, the current pathophysiologic approach to LOAD is based on a number of common mechanisms of neurodegeneration, including accumulation of abnormal proteins, mitochondrial dysfunction, and oxidative stress, impaired insulin signaling, calcium homeostasis dysregulation, early synaptic disconnection, and late apoptotic cell death. Aging itself is associated with mild cognitive deterioration, probably due to subtle multifactorial changes resulting in a global decrease of functional brain reserve.

## 5. References

Arendt T (2009) Synaptic degeneration in Alzheimer's disease. Acta Neuropathol. 118:167-179.

Ballatore C, Lee VM & Trojanowski JQ (2007) Tau-mediated neurodegeneration in Alzheimer's disease and related disorders. Nat. Rev. Neurosci. 8: 663-672.

Berridge MJ (2010) Calcium Signalling and Alzheimer's Disease.Eur J Physiol. 459:441-449.

Braak H & Braak E (1998) Argyrophilic grain disease: Frequency of occurrence in different age categories and neuropathological diagnostic criteria. Journal of Neural Transmission. 105:801-819.

Bozoglu E, Isik AT, Doruk H, Kilic S (2010) The Effects of Early Vitamin B12 Replacement Therapy on The Cognitive and Functional Status of Elderly Subjects. Bulletin of Clinical Psychopharmacology. 20:115-119.

Craft S, Asthana S, Schellenberg G & et al. (2000) Insulin effects on glucose metabolism, memory, and plasma amyloid precursor protein in Alzheimer's disease differ according to apolipoprotein-E genotype. Ann NY Acad Sci. 903: 222-228.

Coleman PD & Yao PJ (2003) Synaptic slaughter in Alzheimer's disease. Neurobiol Aging. 24:1023–1027.

Cuello AC (2007) Overview of the Alzheimer's Disease Pathology and Potential Therapeutic Targets. Eds: Cuello AC. Pharmacological Mechanisms in Alzheimer's Therapeutics, Springer, Canada, 1-27.

Deane R & Zlokovic BV (2007) Role of the blood-brain barrier in the pathogenesis of Alzheimer's disease. Curr Alzheimer Res. 4:191–197.

Garg S, TimmT, Mandelkow E, Mandelkow E & Wang Y (2011) Cleavage of Tau by calpain in Alzheimer's disease: the quest for the toxic 17 kD fragment. Neurobiology of Aging. 32:1-14.

Glenner GG & Wong CW (1984) Alzheimer's disease and Down's syndrome: Sharing of a unique cerebrovascular amyloid fibril protein. Biochemical and Biophysical Research Communications. 12:1131-1135.

Guillozet AL, Weintraub S, Mash DC & Mesulam MM (2003) Neurofibrillary tangles, amyloid and memory in aging and mild cognitive impairment. Arch Neurol. 60:729-736.

Haass C & Selkoe DJ (2007) Soluble protein oligomers in neurodegeneration: lessons from the Alzheimer's amyloid beta-peptide. Nat. Rev.Mol. Cell Biol. 8, 101–112

Hoyer S (1998) Is sporadic Alzheimer disease the brain type of non-insulin dependent diabetes mellitus? A challenging hypothesis. J Neural Transm. 105: 415-422.

Isik AT (2010) Late onset Alzheimer's disease in older people. Clinical Interventions in Aging. 5:307-311.

Isik AT & Bozoglu E (2010) Chapter 20-Insulin resistance in Alzheimer disease: Eds: Aucoin L, Prideux T:Handbook of Type 1 Diabetes Mellitus: Etiology, Diagnosis, and Treatment, Nova Science, Hauppauge NY.

Jackson-Siegal J (2005) Our current understanding of the pathophysiology of Alzheimer's Disease. Adv Stud Pharm. 2(4):126-135.

Lustbader JW, Cirilli M & Lin C (2004) ABAD directly links Abeta to mitochondrial toxicity in Alzheimer's disease. Science. 304:448-452.

Newman M, Musgrave FI & Lardelli M (2007) Alzheimer disease: Amyloidogenesis,the presenilins and animal models. Biochimica Biophysica Acta. 1772:285-297.

Querfurth HW & La Ferla FM (2010) Mechanisms of Disease:Alzheimer's Disease. N Engl J Med. 362;4:329-344.

Price JM, Chi X, Hellermann G & Sutton ET (2001) Physiological levels of beta-amyloid induce cerebral vessel dysfunction and reduce endothelial nitric oxide production. Neurol Res. 23:506–512.

Proctor CJ & Gray DA (2010) GSK3 and p53 is there a link in Alzheimer's disease? Molecular Neurodegeneration. 5(7);1-15.

Schrijvers EM, Koudstaal PJ, Hofman A & Breteler MM (2011) Plasma clusterin and the risk of Alzheimer Disease. JAMA. 305:1322-1326.

Vassar R & Citron M (2000) Abeta-generating enzymes: Recent advances in beta and gamma-secretase research. Neuron. 27:419-422.

Weller RO, Boche D & Nicoll JAR (2009). Microvasculature changes and cerebral amyloid angiopathy in Alzheimer's disease and their potential impact on therapy. Acta Neuropathol. 118:87–102.

Wolfe MS (2006) The gamma-secretase complex: Membrane-embedded proteolytic ensemble. Biochemistry. 45:7931-7939.

Zhao WQ & Townsend M (2009) Insulin resistance and amyloidogenesis as common molecular foundation for type 2 diabetes and Alzheimer's disease. Biochimica et Biophysica Acta, 1792: 482-496.

# 2

# Role of Mitochondria in Alzheimer´s Disease

Genaro Genaro Gabriel Ortiz[1,2] et al. *
[1]*Lab. Estrés Oxidativo-Mitocondria & Enfermedad. Centro de Investigación Biomédica de Occidente (CIBO). Instituto mexicano del seguro Social (IMSS). Guadalajara, Jalisco,*
[2]*División de Ciencias de la Salud-Escuela de Medicina, Tecnológico de Monterrey, Campus Guadalajara. Zapopan, Jalisco,*
*México*

## 1. Introduction

Alzheimer's disease is the most common neurodegenerative disorder worldwide characterized by considerable atrophy and an enlargement and coarsening of the sulci, β-amyloid formation in neuritic plaques and brain vessels (amyloid angiopathy), neurofibrillary tangles, and neuronal loss, particularly in the limbic and association cortices. In addition, deficits in cholinergic transmission and associated loss of cholinergic cell bodies, granulovacuolar degeneration and rod-shaped eosinophilic inclusions (Hirano bodies) are common in Alzheimer's disease patients. Clinical symptoms are characterized by progressive worsening of memory, and cognitive impairment accompanied by one of the following symptoms: aphasia, apraxia, agnosia and disorders in the executive function (Selkoe, 2004).

The pathophysiological mechanisms that underlie the neurodegenerative characteristic of Alzheimer's disease are yet to be completely understood, although many factors in disease pathogenesis have been identified, and several theories are emerged. In the last years, mitochondrial dysfunction has been considered as a potential factor implicated at some stage of the pathogenic process (Anandatheerthavarada et al., 2003; Sullivan & Brown, 2005;

---

*Fermín Pacheco-Moisés[3], José de Jesús García-Trejo[4], Roció E. González-Castañeda[5], Miguel A. Macías-Islas[6], José A. Cruz-Ramos[1], Irma E. Velázquez-Brizuela[1], Elva D. Árias Merino[7] and Alfredo Célis de la Rosa[7]
[1]*Lab. Estrés Oxidativo-Mitocondria & Enfermedad. Centro de Investigación Biomédica de Occidente (CIBO). Instituto mexicano del seguro Social (IMSS). Guadalajara, Jalisco, Mexico*
[2]*División de Ciencias de la Salud-Escuela de Medicina, Tecnológico de Monterrey, Campus Guadalajara. Zapopan, Jalisco, México. Mexico*
[3]*Departamento de Química. Centro Universitario de Ciencias Exactas e Ingenierías. Universidad de Guadalajara. Guadalajara, Jalisco, Mexico*
[4]*Departamento de Biología. Facultad de Química. Universidad Nacional Autónoma de México, Mexico*
[5]*Departamento de Neurociencias. Centro Universitario de Ciencias de la Salud. Universidad de Guadalajara. Guadalajara, Jalisco, Mexico*
[6]*Departamento de Neurología. Unidad Médica de Alta Especialidad. Hospital de Especialidades-Centro Médico Nacional de Occidente. IMSS. Guadalajara, Jalisco, Mexico*
[7]*Departamento de Salud Pública. Centro Universitario de Ciencias de la Salud. Universidad de Guadalajara. Guadalajara, Jalisco, Mexico*

Atamna & Frey, 2007: Wang et al., 2008). As essential role players in cellular metabolism, mitochondria are pertinent to cell survival and thus any deviation from their operation is undoubtedly serious. Almost all aspects of mitochondrial function are altered in Alzheimer neurons; particularly it has been reported defects in oxidative phosphorylation (Chandrasekaran et al., 1996; Manczak et al., 2004; Schagger & Ohm, 1995) and both inherited and somatic mitochondrial DNA mutations in certain AD cases (Coskun et al., 2004; Qiu et al., 2001). In addition, changes in the redox status and membrane fluidity have been largely documented in brain and platelets (Mecocci et al., 1996; Zubenko et al., 1999; Mosconi et al., 2008; Ortiz et al., 2008; Su et al., 2008). The extent to which these changes in mitochondrial function represent primary or secondary components of the pathophysiological process are essential in order to understand the basic pathways that lead to the progress of disease. At this regard it has been shown that neurons are particularly vulnerable to any abnormalities of mitochondrial functioning, due to their large energy demand for their survival and specialized function. In this review we will describe the body of evidence supporting the role of mitochondria in the pathogenesis of Alzheimer's disease and discuss mitochondrial alterations in platelets from AD patients, particularly, mitochondrial enzymatic activities and membrane fluidity.

## 2. Mitochondrial function

### 2.1 ATP synthesis

Mitochondria are the major site of adenosine triphosphate (ATP) synthesis in most cells by the processes of oxidative phosphorylation. Mitochondria also mediate amino acid biosynthesis, fatty acid oxidation, steroid metabolism, calcium homeostasis, and reactive oxygen species production and detoxification. They synthesize amino acids, pyrimidines, lipids, heme, hormones and other metabolites. Each mitochondrion consists of four main compartments, including the outer membrane, the inner membrane, the inter-membranous space, and the matrix. The outer membrane encloses the entire organelle and is relatively porous, allowing the passage of small molecules. The inner mitochondrial membrane is characterized by a series of complex folds and tubules called cristae, which contain a variety of the enzymes, including those responsible for making ATP, is largely impermeant and forms the major barrier between the cytosol and the mitochondrial matrix. The space between the two membranes is referred to as the intermembrane space. The five complexes of the respiratory chain, complex I (NADH ubiquinone oxidoreductase), complex II (succinate ubiquinone oxidoreductase), complex III (ubiquinone-cytochrome c reductase), complex IV (cytochrome oxidase), and complex V (ATP synthase) are embedded in the inner mitochondrial membrane. The transfer of electrons along the respiratory chain provides the energy to pump protons from the matrix into the intermembrane space, generating the electrochemical gradient required to drive ATP synthesis (Hatefi, 1986).

ATP synthase is an enzyme that works as a rotary motor to carry out ATP synthesis by using $Mg^{2+}$-ADP complex, inorganic phosphate and a proton electrochemical gradient across energy-transducing membranes. It is composed by two main sectors: F0, a membrane-embedded proton-translocating sector that contains up to 10 different subunits and F1, a soluble catalytic sector comprising five different subunits that is bound through two stalks to F0. The coupling between F1 and F0 is critical for efficient ATP synthesis to occur and a large body of evidence shows that F1 andF0 are structurally and functionally coupled through two stalks. The central stalk forms part of the rotor of the enzyme, and the peripheral stalk is part of the stator that anchors the catalytic sites of F1 to the membrane. The central rotor actually gyrates relative to a stator that holds the catalytic subunits; this rotation induces the alternating binding, catalysis, and product release from three catalytic sites of F1 (Noji & Yoshida, 2001).

Because of thermodynamic and mechanical reversibility, the ATP synthase also hydrolyzes ATP under conditions of partial or total collapse of the proton gradient in all energy-transducing systems. Thus, different subunits and mechanisms have emerged in nature to control the intrinsic rotation of the enzyme to favor the ATP synthase activity over its opposite and commonly wasteful ATPase turnover. A key regulatory subunit of ATP synthase is the mitochondrial inhibitor protein (IF1). Since its first isolation in 1963 (Pullman & Monroy, 1963), this protein was shown to inhibit the hydrolytic activity of the catalytic F1 sector. This protein is therefore crucial to prevent the hydrolysis of newly synthesized ATP in conditions of low membrane potential in mitochondria. Upon membrane energization, IF1 is believed to be relocated from its inhibitory site into an unknown position within (Dreyfus et al., 1981; Sanchez-Bustamante et al., 1982) or outside the F1F0 complex (Schwerzmann & Pedersen 1981; Power et al., 1983), therefore allowing ATP synthesis to occur. In de-energized or uncoupled conditions, IF1 is productively associated with the enzyme, inhibiting the ATPase turnover of the F1I or F1F0I complexes. However, this protein allows the rotational ATP synthesis turnover during energization of mitochondrial membranes. Therefore, IF1 is an important physiological regulator of the functioning of the ATP synthase. Recently, it has been shown that IF1 also contributes to stabilize dimeric and oligomeric forms of the mitochondrial ATP synthase that promote formation of mitochondrial cristae (Minauro-Sanmiguel et al., 2005; García et al., 2006; Campanella et al., 2008), thus adding a further key role of IF1 and dimeric F1F0 in the whole mitochondrial biogenesis (reviewed in García-Trejo & Morales-Ríos, 2008).

### 2.2 Mitochondrial dynamics

Mitochondrial dynamics implies that mitochondria continuously undergo fission and fusion to generate smaller organelles or elongated, tubular structures, respectively. Thus, mitochondria are not static organelles, but are dynamic bodies that constantly divide and fuse within the cell as the environment demands (Chan, 2006). These processes can facilitate formation of new mitochondria, repair of defective mitochondrial DNA through mixing, and redistribution of mitochondria to sites requiring high-energy production (Frederick & Shaw, 2007; Knott et al., 2008). Both processes effectively lower the percentage of defective mitochondria in the cell and ensure stability in cellular proliferation; indeed, metabolism, energy production, calcium signaling, reactive oxidative species production, apoptosis and senescence all depend on the balance of fission and fusion. Conversely, dynamic distortion (i.e., excessive fragmentation/elongation) results in inefficiencies in cell functioning, if not cell death (Parone et al., 2008; Wang et al., 2009; Chen et al., 2005).

Mitochondrial dynamics is a tightly regulated cellular process, with dedicated molecular machinery involving GTPases. Fission is regulated by at least two proteins: a large GTPase, dynamin-like protein 1, and a small molecule, Fis1, and fusion involves three large mitochondrial transmembrane proteins localized to the outer membrane: mitofusin 1, mitofusin 2, and optic atrophy protein 1 (Chan, 2006; Knott et al., 2008).

Mitochondria structurally abnormal have been reported in Alzheimer´s disease brains, for instance significant alterations in mitochondrial cristae (Hirai et al., 2001), the accumulation of osmiophylic material and significant decreases in mitochondrial size are found predominantly in neurons (Baloyannis, 2006). In addition, mitochondria are redistributed away of axons in the pyramidal (Wang et al., 2009). Electron-microscopic studies have showed an increase in mitochondrial fragmentation in human AD brains (Balayonnis, 2006; Wang et al., 2009). In cell-based experiments, β-amyloidproduction resulted in the appearance of fragmented and abnormally distributed mitochondria (Barsoum et al., 2006; Wang et al., 2008). The dynamic balance of fission and fusion in AD is greatly shifted toward fission, and, as a result, affected neurons contain abnormal mitochondria that are unable to meet the metabolic demands of the cell. Moreover, mitochondrial distribution in AD cells is perinuclear, with few metabolic organelles in the distal processes, where they are normally distributed in healthy cells and are needed for exocytosis, ion channel pumps, synaptic function and other activities.

### 2.3 Energetic impairment in AD brains

Normal synapse function requires concerted activity of a multitude of metabolic pathways, including the generation of gene products involved in membrane complex formation and maintenance; mitochondrial RNA, protein, and neurotransmitter synthesis and delivery; and most importantly, the maintenance of ion gradients across the plasma membranes, as they are critical for the generation of action potentials. These actions can only be performed efficiently when sufficient energetic substrates are supplied. Glucose metabolism in the brain provides about 95% of the energy required under normal circumstances, with fatty acids only making a minor contribution. This intense demand for energy is continual, even brief periods of oxygen or glucose deprivation result in neuronal death. However, in spite of this high energy requirement, the brain is rather uncompromising in its ability to utilize substrates for energy production (Costantini et al., 2008).

Early evidence for altered glucose metabolism in AD brain comes from *in vivo* fluorodeoxyglucose positron emission tomography measurements of the cerebral metabolic rate for glucose (de Leon et al., 1983). This change in glucose utilization is linked to cognitive performance (Constantini et al., 2008). Reductions up to 45% in cerebral glucose utilization in AD patients have been reported (Ishii K et al., 1997). Other studies have reported low brain's glucose consumption rate in hippocampal and entorhinal cortical regions (Swerdlow, 2007). The posterior cingulate cortex and the neighboring precuneus are metabolically affected in the earliest clinical and preclinical stages of AD and the primary visual cortex is relatively spared (Minoshima et al., 1997; Reiman et al., 1996). That reduction in glucose metabolism is the result of both decreased glucose transport (because of a decrease in the number of synapses) and a decrease in the number of neurons. Therefore, the decreased cerebral metabolism is a true loss of neurons and synapses rather than simply the decreased glucose metabolism expected from a smaller volume of tissue seen in patients with atrophy [Bokde, 2001; Ibanez et al., 1998)]. In addition, in alzheimer´s disease there is a generalized shift from glycolytic energy production toward use of an alternative fuel, ketone bodies. Patients with incipient alzheimer´s disease exhibit a utilization ratio of 2:1 glucose to ketone bodies, whereas comparably aged controls exhibit a ratio of 29:1, whereas young controls exclusively use glucose with a ratio of 100:0 (Hoyer, 1991). On the other hand, *in vitro* analyses of AD autopsy brain show reductions in glycolysis (Swerdlow & Kish, 2002). These findings have been consistently reproduced by a multitude of studies and this pattern of hypometabolism is therefore now widely accepted as a reliable *in vivo* hallmark of Alzheimer's disease, and accurately distinguishes AD from normal aging.

The defects in glucose utilization suggest possible abnormalities in mitochondrial function. In support of this view, a range of reports have shown altered mitochondrial properties in Alzheimer's disease, in particular, the energy extracting mechanisms of the mitochondria. For instance, the temporal and parietal cortical zones consistently exhibits abnormally high oxygen utilization in comparison to the amounts of glucose utilized, and reduced phosphocreatine levels, indicating impairment of the oxidative phosphorylation process in the mitochondria (Benson et al., 1981; Phelps et al., 1982; Friedland et al., 1983 Pettegrew et al, 1994). In addition, AD brain biopsies demonstrated mitochondrial uncoupling, a non-specific abnormality indicative of an impairment in conversion of ADP to ATP (Sims et al., 1987). Interestingly the abnormalities in cerebral metabolism precede the onset of neurological dysfunction as well as gross neuropathology of AD.

In vitro analyses of AD autopsy brain studies have shown that the most consistent defect in mitochondria in AD are the reductions in maximal activities of several key enzymes responsible for oxidative metabolism, including α-ketoglutarate dehydrogenase complex, isocitrate dehydrogenase, and pyruvate dehydrogenase complex, two enzymes involved in the rate-limiting step of tricarboxylic acid cycle (Parker et al., 1994; Gibson et al., 1998; Nagy et al., 1999; Swerdlow & Kish, 2002). In addition, studies have shown reduced cytochrome oxidase activity, the terminal enzyme in the electron transfer chain that is responsible for reducing molecular oxygen (Parker et al., 1994; Gibson et al., 1998; Maurer et al., 2000; Bosetti et al., 2002; Swerdlow & Kish, 2002).

Reductions in maximal activity of cytochrome c oxidase have been reported in several areas of the brain. For instance, it has been found that AD cases had lower cytochrome c oxidase activity than controls in the posterior cingulate cortex. That reduction was significantly greater than that in primary motor cortex (Valla et al., 2001). However, it is unclear to what extent maximal activity reduction reflects reduced COX enzyme expression or a structural change in the enzyme. Numerous studies have linked abnormal mitochondrial protein function to the altered neuronal expression of nuclear and mitochondrial genes encoding subunits of the mitochondrial electron transfer chain. Liang and collaborators (2008) showed that compared to controls, AD cases had the largest proportion (70 percent) of underexpressed genes comprising the nuclear genes encoding for subunits of the mitochondrial electron transfer chain complexes and translocases of the inner and outer mitochondrial membranes in the posterior cingulated cortex, a brain region which positron emission tomography studies found to be metabolically affected in the earliest stages of AD. The visual cortex, on the other hand, a brain region relatively spared in AD, contained significantly less underexpressed genes than the posterior cingulate cortices.

Interestingly, Reddy and Beal (2008) found mitochondrial genes in the NADH ubiquinone oxidoreductase of oxidative phosphorylation system to be downregulated in both early and definite AD brains, whereas complexes ubiquinone-cytochrome c reductase and cytochrome c oxidase showed increased mitochondrial RNA expressions. Several other studies have also reported this phenomenon (Hirai et al., 2001; Strazielle et al., 2003; Manczak et al., 2004; Reddy et al., 2004), which could be interpreted as a compensatory mechanism for the decreased cytochrome c oxidase function and the consequent increase in demand on energy production. As spectral analysis of the enzyme has indicated that cytochrome c oxidase is kinetically altered in AD and lacks one of its two substrate binding sites (Parker & Parks, 1995), altogether the data would imply that cytochrome c oxidase activity is reduced not because the quantity is decreased as a result of down-regulated gene expression, but because in AD, the enzyme is structurally different from that in controls. However, other studies have shown that cytochrome oxidase activity is reduced as a result of decreased mitochondrial RNA expression. Several studies demonstrated decreased mitochondrial RNA expression in NADH ubiquinone oxidoreductase and cytochrome c oxidase (Chandrasekaran et al., 1994, 1996, 1997) and decreased mRNA expression of nuclear-encoded mitochondrial genes in complexes cytochrome c oxidase and ATP synthase in brains of AD patients (Chandrasekaran et al., 1994, 1997; Simonian & Hyman, 1994). Clearly, at this point, it cannot be said whether reduced mitochondrial RNA expression, altered enzyme kinetics or both, contribute to reduced cytochrome c oxidase function in AD. Some studies suggest that mitochondrial DNA and mitochondrial number increase in AD, which would indicate altered cytochrome c oxidase kinetics, while others suggest that mitochondrial DNA and mitochondrial number decline, proposing reduced cytochrome c oxidase expression (De la Monte et al., 2000; Hirai et al., 2001; Baloyannis, 2006). Other studies have reported lowered biosynthesis of beta subunit of the ATP synthase, in the hippocampus and the ubiquinone-cytochrome c reductase core protein 1, respectively (Kim et al., 2000). How these changes in mitochondrial enzymes would translate into loss of specific neuronal populations, including cholinergic neurons in the forebrain, hippocampus, and neocortex is unclear. One possibility is that as yet unknown factors cause an imbalance that favours the generation of reactive oxygen species.

### 2.4 Mitochondria and oxidative stress

Oxidative stress is a relative increase in the ratio of free radicals to antioxidants. This may originate from an overproduction of reactive oxygen species or from a reduction in antioxidant capacity. Indeed, the activities of the antioxidant enzymes superoxide dismutase and catalase are significantly decreased in the frontal and temporal cortex of AD patients (Marcus et al., 1998). Not only that, antioxidant enzyme activity was shown to be spatially correlated with markers of lipid peroxidation (i.e. oxidative damage) and the brain areas particularly affected by neuronal loss in AD (Takeda et al., 2000). However, increased antioxidant activity in AD brains in response to increased free radical generation has also been reported (Lovell et al., 1995; Lu et al., 2004; Moreira et al., 2009). Thus, one explanation for the studies showing a lack of correlation between impaired mitochondrial function and oxidative stress is that in some AD cases, antioxidant defenses are able to counteract oxidative stress damage, whilst in others they cannot. However, this would automatically mean that in the AD cases with no oxidative stress, other impaired mechanisms must be causing AD.

Some studies show that brain tissue is especially vulnerable to oxidative attack due to its relatively low antioxidant capacity, high consumption of oxygen, high content of polyunsaturated fatty acids, and high content of redox-active transition metals such as iron (Butterfield et al., 2007). Iron can contribute to free radical damage by catalyzing the formation of the hydroxyl radical, inducing secondary initiation of lipid peroxidation and by promoting the oxidation of proteins. The increase in brain iron associated with several neurodegenerative diseases may lead to an increased production of free radicals via the Fenton reaction. Depending on the substrate attacked by the reactive oxygen species, oxidative damage will manifest as protein oxidation, DNA oxidation, or lipid peroxidation products.

Mitochondria are the primary source of cellular oxidants, taking into account that about 2–5% of molecular oxygen is not completely reduced to water at the electron transport chain and, therefore, a prime target of cumulative oxidative damage. Damage to mitochondrial proteins and mitocondrial DNA would be expected to decrease mitochondrial bioenergetics and efficiency (The underlying mechanism of abnormal mitochondrial reactive oxygen species production is the altered redox potential of mitochondrial respiratory chain carriers (due to hyperpolarization of mitochondrial membrane) and an increase in ubisemiquinone anion half-life time, resulting in slower electron transport, producing intermediates that stay reduced longer, thus increasing the chance that the electrons can escape to molecular oxygen, originating the reactive oxygen species (Sullivan & Brown 2005). Ultimately, ATP depletion will lead to necrotic cell death. Other forms of mitochondrial injury may lead to the release of pro-apoptotic factors, particularly of mitochondrial cytochrome c and the initiation of the cascade to apoptotic cell death.

### 2.5 Studies on platelets

The hypothesis that Alzheimer disease pathology is not brain-limited has led researchers to look for peripheral cells that may harbour changes related to this disease. On one such cell, the platelet, have the following similarities with neurons: 1) contain the amyloid precursor protein and secrete β-amyloid peptide (Di Luca et al., 2000; Sanchez-Gonzalez et al., 2006) 2) express neurotransmitters and some neuron-related proteins, such as NMDA receptors (Dreux & Launay, 1985). Interestingly, several of the enzymatic defects observed in AD brain are also found in noncerebral tissues. In addition, biochemical markers are likely to be important in the study of Alzheimer disease for several reasons. A clinical diagnosis of Alzheimer disease is inaccurate even among experienced investigators in about 10% to 15% of cases, and biomarkers might improve the accuracy of diagnosis. Importantly for the development of putative disease-modifying drugs for Alzheimer disease, biomarkers might also serve as indirect measures of disease severity. Usually biomarkers are assessed in different compartments including cerebrospinal fluid, skin fibroblasts, lymphocytes, blood and urine.

In our group of work we are analyzed platelets from Alzheimer disease patients and healthy subjects. Diagnosis of AD was made by using the: 1) mini mental state evaluation 2) Diagnostic and Statistical Manual of Mental Disorders-IV criteria for dementia and 3) National Institute of Neurological and Communicative Disorders and Stroke and the Alzheimer's Disease and Related Disorders Association criteria for diagnosis of probable dementia of Alzheimer type. Healthy control subjects were free of AD or any other disorder.

#### 2.5.1 ATP synthase and cytochrome c oxidase

To obtain direct evidence that mitochondrial functioning is altered in AD patients; we made measurements of the rate of the hydrolytic activity of ATP synthase and pH gradient driven by ATP hydrolysis, using platelet submitochondrial particles. The hydrolytic activity of ATP synthase in patients with probable AD was 41.7 ± 4.3 nmol $min^{-1}$ (mg protein)$^{-1}$, n =29, whereas in the control subjects was 29.1 ± 1.9 nmol nmol $min^{-1}$ (mg protein)$^{-1}$, n = 29. It is important to note that, in the male population with probable AD, we found that hydrolytic activity of ATP synthase increased as cerebral deterioration progressed. That increase in the hydrolytic activity of ATP synthase was statistically significant. Therefore, we made measurements of the pH gradient driven by ATP hydrolysis determined from the quenching of ACMA fluorescence induced upon 2 mM ATP addition. pH gradient was used as an indication of the enzyme proton channel function and of coupling between transport and catalysis. Data obtained showed a lower pH gradient in the submitochondrial particles of patients with probable AD (0.28 ± 0.08 pH units, n = 25) as compared to the controls (0.5 ± 0.1 pH units, n = 20). This suggests a functional alteration of the ATP synthase. In addition, proton gradient was completely abolished when 1 μM oligomycin was added to the submitochondrial particles. This indicates that the pH gradient was in fact due to the ATP-driven proton translocation through the membrane and that the proton transport activity of the enzyme from AD patients is as sensitive to the inhibitor as the control group (Martínez-Cano et al., 2004).

Functional impairment of mitochondrial ATP synthase can be explained by the following phenomena: If F0 and F1 sectors of the enzyme are separated by physical or kinetic decoupling; for an altered assembly of the regulatory subunits of the enzyme, in particular of the inhibitor protein IF1. Therefore, we made semi quantitative determinations of the inhibitor protein, IF1 in submitochondrial particles of platelets. Densitometric analyses of Western blot experiments indicated a 2-fold decrease of the relative content of the mitochondrial inhibitor protein (IF1) of the ATP synthase in platelets from AD samples compared to control subjects (Figure 1).

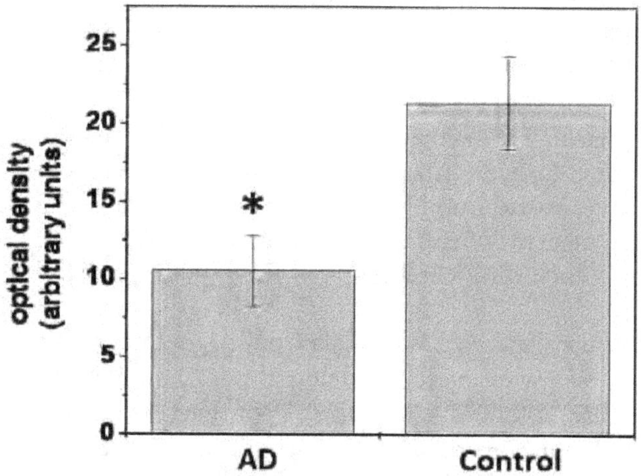


Fig. 1. Densitometric analyses of inhibitor protein IF1 in Alzheimer disease patients and control subjects. Statistical significance was assessed by Dunnett's test. *$P<0.05$ vs control group.

In order to assay the functional association of inhibitor protein IF1 with the ATP synthase in submitochondrial particles from Alzheimer and control group's samples, ATPase activity assays were carried out. Submitochondrial particles were incubated in conditions that induce a progressive release of IF1 to the media, i.e., pH 8.0, KCl 100 mM, and 40 °C. Additional experiments were conducted under conditions that favour the binding of the protein inhibitor of ATP synthase (sucrose medium). Figure 2 shows that the hydrolytic activity of ATP synthase of Alzheimer samples was unaffected by the medium of determination. In contrast, the activity of control samples was increased in a medium with KCl, i.e., in conditions that favours the disotiation of inhibitor protein IF1. Also note that the hydrolytic activity of the ATP synthase of the control samples, in a medium with KCl, did not reach the values of activity of samples from patients with AD, in the same medium. Taken together, these results suggest that that increased hydrolytic activity in patients with AD is partly due to a lower content of the inhibitor protein, IF1.

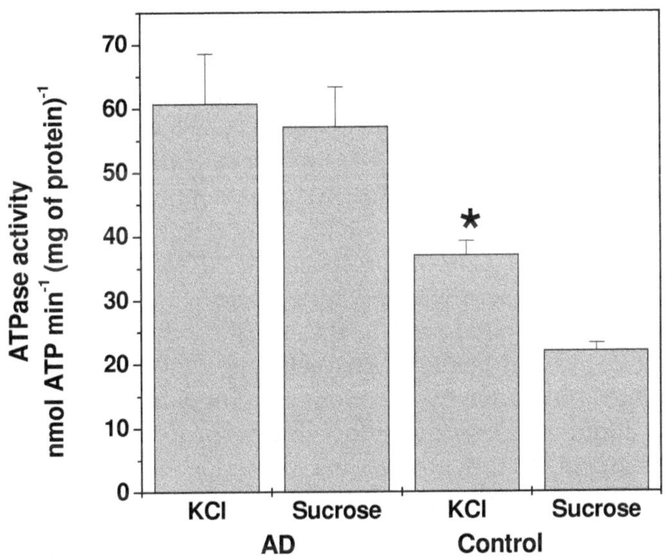


Fig. 2. Hydrolytic activity of ATP synthase in Alzheimer disease and control samples. Enzymatic activity was done at 40 °C, using a potassium chloride or sucrose medium of reaction. Data were subjected to an analysis of variance, and significant differences were assessed by Dunnett's test with $P < 0.05$ for comparison with the sucrose medium.

To our knowledge the hydrolytic activity of ATP synthase in patients with AD has been controversial since it has been reported that ATP hydrolysis activity in platelets was similar in patients with AD and controls (Boseti et al., 2002). Other authors reported a slightly increased in the frontal and occipital brain of AD. These data do not correlate with a 50-60% decrease in the level of mRNA encoding the β subunit of ATP synthase in the temporal cortex of AD patients (Chandrasekaran et al., 1996) or with the reduced amount of ATP synthase in the hippocampus of AD patients (Schagger & Ohm, 1995). Although it is unknown whether the deficiency of mitochondrial enzymes is a cause or an effect of Alzheimer disease, it has been speculated that can be a normal physiological response to a reduction in energy demand in the brains of patients (Jung et al, 2000; Chandrasekaran et al., 1996). So, the functional alterations in key enzymes of mitochondrial metabolism such as ATP synthase, can lead to a decrease in energy generation and can contribute to the neurodegenerative process. Thus, a reduction in cellular ATP concentration can activate specific protein kinases that phosphorylate tau protein, leading to the formation of neurofibrillary tangles (Stanley et al., 1996), and may cause increased susceptibility of neurons to excitatory amino acids, leading to neuronal degeneration by an excitotoxic process (Roder et al., 1993). On the other hand, mitochondrial dysfunction characterized by a combined deficiency of ATP synthase and cytochrome c oxidase can lead to the generation of free radicals that can damage proteins, nucleic acids and membranes and contribute to aggregation and plaque deposition of β-amyloid and neurofibrillary tangles formation (Beal, 1992; Troncoso et al., 1993).

By restriction analysis we identified the pathogenic mutation of the mitochondrial DNA in the gene encoding the subunit 6 of the ATP synthase. That mutations is T8993G converting the highly conserved leucine to arginine in a transmembrane helix. The mutation causes a severe impairment in the vectorial proton flow through F0 (García et al., 2000) and instability of the monomeric and dimeric forms of the ATP synthase without altering assembly or dimerization of the enzyme (Cortés-Hernández et al., 2007).

On the other hand several mutations in cytochrome c oxidase II gene have been previously described. Sequence chromatogram of mitochondrial cytochrome c oxidase II gene obtained from blood samples of our population revealed that four patients with probable Alzheimer´s disease had a point mutation A8027G (3 of them were identified as early onset, with familial history of the disease). Other four patients with early onset have the following mutations: A8003C, T8082C, C8201T and G7933A, respectively. To our knowledge none of these mutations were found in other neurodegenerative diseases.

It could argue that the mutations found in this work modified the protein conformation, since the different physichochemical characteristics of replaced aminoacids. That conformational change could alter the electrons binding site or the electrons transfer and this contributes to a diminution in enzymatic activity. The diminished cytochrome c activity could cause a decrease in ATP synthesis and diversion of electrons from their normal pathway resulting in increasing in superoxid radical production. Thus, cytochrome oxidase alterations can lead to increased reactive oxygen species generation, oxidative damage to mitochondrial membranes, and increased vulnerability to excitotoxins, and may be important in the pathogenesis of Alzheimer´s disease.

### 2.5.2 Membrane fluidity

It has been reported that cells of Alzheimer´s disease brains have altered phospholipid metabolism (Blusztajn et al., 1990; Ellison et al., 1987; Klunk et al., 1998; Nitsch et al., 1992) and a diminished unesterified cholesterol:phospholipid mole ratio (Mason et al., 1992), leading to altered membrane fluidity (Mecocci et al., 1996). On the other hand, submitochondrial particles are mainly constituted of inner mitochondrial membrane and are the site of oxidative phosphorylation and other enzymatic systems involved in the transport and utilization of metabolites. Therefore we assessed the membrane fluidity in platelet submitochondrial particles and erythrocyte membranes from Mexican patients with Alzheimer disease. That estimate was achieved from the excimer to monomer fluorescence intensity ratio (Ie/Im) of the fluorescent probe 1,3 dipyrenylpropane incorporated in membranes. That probe at submicromolar concentrations forms intramolecular excimers and its formation in membranes depends mainly of the medium microviscosity and temperature of determination. This method is very simple and does not require higher concentrations of other fluorescent lipophilic probes such as 1,6-diphenyl-1,3,5-hexatriene and its cationic derivative trimethylamino-,6-diphenyl-1,3,5-hexatriene. Thus, the risk of perturbation of the phospholipid phase inherent in the use of all probe molecules is minimized. Intramolecular excimer formation of this probe is related with the membrane fluidity, such the excimer formation depicts mainly the lateral motion of the probe within the membrane (Jurado et al., 1991). The higher the values of the excimer to monomer ratio, the more fluid the membrane, while the lower the ratio, the more rigid the membrane.

Therefore that ratio is directly proportional to membrane fluidity, which is reciprocal to membrane viscosity.

Similarly to the data reported from mitochondria in AD brains fluidity (Mecocci et al., 1996), a reduced fluidity in the platelet inner mitochondrial membrane was found. It can partially be due to increased levels of lipid peroxidation. Reduced membrane fluidity can diminish the activities of the enzymes of oxidative phosphorylation and other transport and receptor proteins, inasmuch as these enzymes are regulated by the physicochemical state of the lipid environment of the membrane. It may diminish significantly the ATP generation from the mitochondria. Interestingly, dysfunctional mitochondria and oxidative damage has been involved in Alzheimer's disease (Bonilla et al., 1999). In agreement with previous reports, membrane fluidity from erythrocyte was not altered in AD (Hajimohammadreza et al., 1990), regardless of increased lipid oxidation in erythrocyte AD patients. This suggests that, in AD, mitochondrial membranes are more sensitive to oxidative stress than erythrocytes.

In contrast to platelet inner mitochondrial membrane, it has been reported an increase in fluidity in whole membranes from platelets of AD patients (Zubenko et al., 1999). This increase results from the elaboration of an internal membrane compartment resembling endoplasmic reticulum that is functionally abnormal (Zubenko et al., 1987). At this regard, it is worth noting that the contribution of mitochondrial membranes to the whole cell membranes in platelets could be minimized since platelets contain few mitochondria (Fukami & Salganicoff, 1973).

On the other hand, Morais Cardoso et al. (2004), using DPH and TMA-DPH as fluorescent probes, found similar fluidity in mitocondrial membranes in platelets from AD patients and controls. That discrepancy with our data may be due to intrinsic differences in the populations tested, the purity of the used mitochondrial fraction and the nature of the probes used. Additionally, it's clear that the lipophilic probes are sensitive to slightly different membrane properties. For instance, DPH and TMA-DPH are rotational probes (Ameloot et al., 1984) and dipyrenylpropane is a lateral diffusion sensitive probe (Zachariasse et al., 1982). In addition, DPH partitions into the interior of the bilayer and its average location has been shown to be about 8 Å from the center of the bilayer. TMA-DPH is oriented in the membrane bilayer with its positive charge localized at the lipid-water interface. Its DPH moiety is localized at about 11 Å from the center of the bilayer and reports the interfacial region of the membrane (Kaiser & London, 1998). Whereas dipyrenylpropane is a highly hydrophobic probe which partitions into the membrane lipid bilayer (Zachariasse et al., 1982). At the moment we do not know whether the diminished membrane fluidity in AD is etiologically significant or a minor result of neurodegeneration

### 2.5.3 Amyloid precursor protein

Amyloid precursor proteins are transmembrane proteins of about 100 to 130 KDa, located primarily on the cell surface as well as on the endoplasmic reticulum, Golgi apparatus, and endosomes. Amyloid precursor protein may play a role in neuronal trafficking, migration and development (Van Gassen et al., 2000). Although a clear function of amyloid precursor protein has yet to be identified, it is the biochemical pathway leading to $\beta$-amyloid generation that demonstrates its link to AD pathogenesis. Amyloid precursor protein is subject to cleavage by three proteases, α, β, and γ secretases through two primary pathways. The first pathway involves cleavage of amyloid precursor protein 12 residues N-terminal to the transmembrane sequence by a group of integral membrane enzymes. Termed α-secretase cleavage, this cut creates a large, ectodomain fragment that is released from the cell surface as well asand a smaller C-terminal fragment (83 residues) attached to the membrane. Subsequent cleavage of this membrane-retained fragment by a unique complex of proteins, referred to as γ-secretase, releases a 3-kDa peptide unable to form amyloid fibrils. The second pathway involves an alternative cleavage by β-secretase, located at the N-terminus of the to *β*-amyloid sequence. This releases a unique ectodomain fragment and a C-terminal (C99) membrane-retained fragment. Then, cleavage of C99 by γ-secretase results in formation of to *β*-amyloid. The length of the C-terminal end of to *β*-amyloid varies depending on the specificity of γ-secretase cleavage, resulting in production of Aβ1-40 or a longer, more fibrillogenic *β*-amyloid 1-42/43 (Selkoe, 1998). The longer to *β*-amyloid peptide has a major role in to *β*-amyloid deposition because plaque formation follows a distinct pattern with the 42-43 amino acid peptide detected first followed by the more common to *β*-amyloid 1-40 (Lemere et al., 1996). The balance between α-secretase and β-secretase cleavage of amyloid precursor protein is important for to *β*-amyloid production and AD pathogenesis.

Western blotting experiments of amyloid precursor protein in platelets showed two main bands with molecular weights of 106 to 110 KDa and 130 KDa, respectively. The upper, 130 KDa, band corresponded to the full-length, mature of amyloid precursor protein. The lower, 106–110 KDa, band corresponded to the of amyloid precursor protein immature isoforms. The ratio of amyloid precursor protein isoforms between the 130 Kda amyloid precursor protein and 106–110 KDa amyloid precursor protein and odds ratios were obtained to determine risk factor of this component. Amyloid precursor protein ratio on AD subjects was lower than that of control subjects: $0.36 \pm 0.18$ vs. $0.67 \pm 0.10$, respectively. A low amyloid precursor protein ratio ($< 0.6$) showed an odds ratio of 4.63. When onset of disease was taken into account, an amyloid precursor protein ratio on early onset Alzheimer´s disease subjects of $0.39 \pm 0.19$ was found vs. $0.34 \pm 0.19$ on late onset Alzheimer´s disease subjects ($p > 0.05$). This suggests an increased degradation of amyloid precursor protein in AD platelets.

On the other hand we performed *ApoE* genotyping in AD platelets and controls. Data obtained showed that there was no association between amyloid precursor protein ratios and any specific ApoE allele (Sanchez-Gonzalez et al., 2006).

In concordance to previous studies, we observed a significant decreased amyloid precursor protein ratio on AD subjects as compared to that of control subjects (Utermann, 1987; Borroni et al., 2003). This means that an increased degradation of this precursor protein is being performed in peripheral tissues. Whether or not this phenomenon reflects a similar process occurring in the brain of AD subjects is still a matter of controversy. However, the existence of this phenomenon cannot be minimized, for processing and secretion of this precursor protein has been already demonstrated and its importance as a predictor for conversion to dementia of Alzheimer type in subjects with mild cognitive impairment has recently been proved (Borroni et al., 2003).

The precise mechanism of amelioration of amyloid precursor protein concentration is not deciphered yet. Modifications in the splicing mechanism, in the stability of messenger RNA encoding for amyloid precursor protein 751/770 or in the regulation of translation processes are some hypothesis (Di Luca et al., 1996). Our study is consistent with the results of Strittmatter et al., (1993) concerning an increased ApoE ε4 allele frequency in AD patients (Strittmatter & Saunders, 1993). A 4.5-times risk of presenting AD as related to the ApoE ε3/ε4 genotype and a 9.4-times risk related to the ε4 allele was also found. This is in accordance to studies published before showing an increased risk of presenting AD as

related to either ε4 heterozygocity or homozygocity (Amouyel et al., 1993; Anwar et al., 1993; Ben-Shlomo et al., 1993; Czech et al., 1993; Lucotte et al., 1993).
The coexistence of β-amyloid with the ApoE ε4 allele in the pathogenesis of AD has long been thought (Saunders et al., 1993) Increased risk of presenting AD in ApoE ε4 allele porters as well as augmented amyloid precursor protein degradation in platelets led us to consider the probability of relating both factors to determine a combined model for risk factor evaluation. We observed a 5-times risk of presenting the disease when both ε3/ε4 genotype and a low amyloid precursor protein ratio (taken as a ratio below (0.6) were stratified, and a 4-times risk with both the ε4/ε4 genotype and a low amyloid precursor protein ratio. These data confirms the relevance of peripheral amyloid precursor protein altered isoforms as an assessment of risk factor of the disease (Rosenberg et al., 1997). The stratified analysis helped us to exclude the effect of ApoE genotypes on the low amyloid precursor protein ratio. We observed no significant OR amelioration or increase of the low amyloid precursor protein ratio, thus strengthening the importance of a low amyloid precursor protein ratio in peripheral blood as an indicator of the disease.

## 3. Conclusion

Up to now several hypotheses about the complex etiology of Alzheimer´s disease have been proposed. According to the amyloid hypothesis, abnormal processing, and accelerated deposition of oligomeric forms of beta-amyloid are central mechanisms underlying pathological processes in Alzheimer disease. Although the amyloid hypothesis remains the main pathogenetic model of Alzheimer's disease, its role in the majority of sporadic Alzheimer cases is unclear. Therefore, other innovative proposals have been made in recent years, particularly the association of mitochondrial functional impairment in the development of the Alzheimer's disease. Immunohistochemical, biochemical, neuroimaging, electronic microscopy and molecular studies have demonstrated the existence of signs of mitochondrial impairment in Alzheimer´s disease brain. Interestingly, these changes are evident very early in Alzheimer disease progression. Current evidence shows that oxidative stress, mitochondrial impairment and altered mitochondrial dynamics contribute to the precipitation of Alzheimer´s disease pathology and thus cognitive decline.
On the other hand, using platelets as a model of study we found the following data: 1) an increased degradation of amyloid precursor protein; 2) an increased lipid oxidation products in mitochondria; 3) a dysfunction of mitochondrial ATP syntase; 4) lower levels of inhibitor protein (IF1) of ATP synthase; 5) reduce membrane fluidity in inner mitochondrial membrane; 6) point mutations of the mitochondrially encoded ATP synthase 6 and citochrome oxidase II genes.

## 4. References

Almeida, L. M.; Vaz, W. L.; Zachariasse, K. A. & Madeira, V. M. (1982). Fluidity of sarcoplasmic reticulum membranes investigated with dipyrenylpropane, an intramolecular excimer probe. *Biochemistry*, Vol. 21, No. 23, (Nov 9 1982), pp. 5972-5977, ISSN 0006-2960

Ameloot, M.; Hendrickx, H.; Herreman, W.; Pottel, H.; Van Cauwelaert, F. & van der Meer, W. (1984). Effect of orientational order on the decay of the fluorescence anisotropy in membrane suspensions. Experimental verification on unilamellar vesicles and lipid/alpha-lactalbumin complexes. *Biophys J*, Vol. 46, No. 4, (Oct 1984), pp. 525-539, ISSN 0006-3495

Amouyel, P.; Brousseau, T.; Fruchart, J. C. & Dallongeville, J. (1993). Apolipoprotein E-epsilon 4 allele and Alzheimer's disease. *Lancet*, Vol. 342, No. 8882, (Nov 20 1993), pp. 1309, ISSN 0140-6736

Anandatheerthavarada, H. K.; Biswas, G.; Robin, M. A. & Avadhani, N. G. (2003). Mitochondrial targeting and a novel transmembrane arrest of Alzheimer's amyloid precursor protein impairs mitochondrial function in neuronal cells. *J Cell Biol*, Vol. 161, No. 1, (Apr 14 2003), pp. 41-54, ISSN 0021-9525

Anantharaman, M.; Tangpong, J.; Keller, J. N.; Murphy, M. P.; Markesbery, W. R.; Kiningham, K. K. & St Clair, D. K. (2006). Beta-amyloid mediated nitration of manganese superoxide dismutase: implication for oxidative stress in a APPNLH/NLH X PS-1P264L/P264L double knock-in mouse model of Alzheimer's disease. *Am J Pathol*, Vol. 168, No. 5, (May 2006), pp. 1608-1618, ISSN 0002-9440

Anwar, N.; Lovestone, S.; Cheetham, M. E.; Levy, R. & Powell, J. F. (1993). Apolipoprotein E-epsilon 4 allele and Alzheimer's disease. *Lancet*, Vol. 342, No. 8882, (Nov 20 1993), pp. 1308-1309, ISSN 0140-6736

Atamna, H. & Frey, W. H., 2nd (2007). Mechanisms of mitochondrial dysfunction and energy deficiency in Alzheimer's disease. *Mitochondrion*, Vol. 7, No. 5, (Sep 2007), pp. 297-310, ISSN 1567-7249

Baloyannis, S. J. (2006). Mitochondrial alterations in Alzheimer's disease. *J Alzheimers Dis*, Vol. 9, No. 2, (Jul 2006), pp. 119-126, ISSN 1387-2877

Barsoum, M.J; Yuan, H.; Gerencser, A. A.; Liot, G.; Kushnareva, Y.; Gräber, S.; Kovacs, I.; Lee, W. D.; Waggoner, J.; Cui, J.; White, A. D.; Bossy, B.; Martinou, J. C.; Youle, R. J.; Lipton, S. A.; Ellisman, M. H.; Perkins, G. A. & Bossy-Wetzel, E. (2006). Nitric oxide induced mitochondrial fission is regulated by dynamin-related GTPases in neurons. *EMBO J*, Vol. 25, No. 16, (Aug 23), pp.3900–3911, ISSN 0261-4189

Beal, M. F. (1992). Does impairment of energy metabolism result in excitotoxic neuronal death in neurodegenerative illnesses? *Ann Neurol*, Vol. 31, No. 2, (Feb 1992), pp. 119-130, ISSN 0364-5134

Benson, D. F.; Kuhl, D. E.; Phelps, M. E.; Cummings, J. L. & Tsai, S. Y. (1981). Positron emission computed tomography in the diagnosis of dementia. *Trans Am Neurol Assoc*, Vol. 106, No. 1981), pp. 68-71, ISSN 0065-9479

Blusztajn, J. K.; Lopez Gonzalez-Coviella, I.; Logue, M.; Growdon, J. H. & Wurtman, R. J. (1990). Levels of phospholipid catabolic intermediates, glycerophosphocholine and glycerophosphoethanolamine, are elevated in brains of Alzheimer's disease but not of Down's syndrome patients. *Brain Res*, Vol. 536, No. 1-2, (Dec 17 1990), pp. 240-244, ISSN 0006-8993

Bokde, A. L.; Pietrini, P.; Ibanez, V.; Furey, M. L.; Alexander, G. E.; Graff-Radford, N. R.; Rapoport, S. I.; Schapiro, M. B. & Horwitz, B. (2001). The effect of brain atrophy on cerebral hypometabolism in the visual variant of Alzheimer disease. *Arch Neurol*, Vol. 58, No. 3, (Mar 2001), pp. 480-486, ISSN 0003-9942

Bonilla, E.; Tanji, K.; Hirano, M.; Vu, T. H.; DiMauro, S. & Schon, E. A. (1999). Mitochondrial involvement in Alzheimer's disease. *Biochim Biophys Acta*, Vol. 1410, No. 2, (Feb 9 1999), pp. 171-182, ISSN 0006-3002

Borroni, B.; Colciaghi, F.; Caltagirone, C.; Rozzini, L.; Broglio, L.; Cattabeni, F.; Di Luca, M. & Padovani, A. (2003). Platelet amyloid precursor protein abnormalities in mild cognitive impairment predict conversion to dementia of Alzheimer type: a 2-year follow-up study. *Arch Neurol*, Vol. 60, No. 12, (Dec 2003), pp. 1740-1744, ISSN 0003-9942

Bosetti, F.; Brizzi, F.; Barogi, S.; Mancuso, M.; Siciliano, G.; Tendi, E. A.; Murri, L.; Rapoport, S. I. & Solaini, G. (2002). Cytochrome c oxidase and mitochondrial F1F0-ATPase (ATP synthase) activities in platelets and brain from patients with Alzheimer's disease. *Neurobiol Aging*, Vol. 23, No. 3, (May-Jun 2002), pp. 371-376, ISSN 0197-4580

Braak, H. & Braak, E. (1991). Neuropathological stageing of Alzheimer-related changes. *Acta Neuropathol*, Vol. 82, No. 4, 1991), pp. 239-259, ISSN 0001-6322

Butterfield, D. A.; Reed, T.; Newman, S. F. & Sultana, R. (2007). Roles of amyloid beta-peptide-associated oxidative stress and brain protein modifications in the pathogenesis of Alzheimer's disease and mild cognitive impairment. *Free Radic Biol Med*, Vol. 43, No. 5, (Sep 1 2007), pp. 658-677, ISSN 0891-5849

Campanella, M.; Casswell, E.; Chong, S.; Farah, Z.; Wieckowski, M. R.; Abramov, A. Y.; Tinker, A.; & Duchen, M. R. (2008). Regulation of mitochondrial structure and function by the F1Fo-ATPase inhibitor protein, IF1. *Cell Metab*, Vol. 8, No. 1 (Jul 2008), pp. 13-25, ISSN 1550-4131

Cardoso, S. M.; Proenca, M. T.; Santos, S.; Santana, I. & Oliveira, C. R. (2004). Cytochrome c oxidase is decreased in Alzheimer's disease platelets. *Neurobiol Aging*, Vol. 25, No. 1, (Jan 2004), pp. 105-110, ISSN 0197-4580

Chan, D. C. (2006). Mitochondria: dynamic organelles in disease, aging, and development. *Cell*, Vol. 125, No. 7, (Jun 30 2006), pp. 1241-1252, ISSN 0092-8674

Chandrasekaran, K.; Giordano, T.; Brady, D. R.; Stoll, J.; Martin, L. J. & Rapoport, S. I. (1994). Impairment in mitochondrial cytochrome oxidase gene expression in Alzheimer disease. *Brain Res Mol Brain Res*, Vol. 24, No. 1-4, (Jul 1994), pp. 336-340, ISSN 0169-328X

Chandrasekaran, K.; Hatanpaa, K.; Brady, D. R. & Rapoport, S. I. (1996). Evidence for physiological down-regulation of brain oxidative phosphorylation in Alzheimer's disease. *Exp Neurol*, Vol. 142, No. 1, (Nov 1996), pp. 80-88, ISSN 0014-4886

Chandrasekaran, K.; Hatanpaa, K.; Rapoport, S. I. & Brady, D. R. (1997). Decreased expression of nuclear and mitochondrial DNA-encoded genes of oxidative phosphorylation in association neocortex in Alzheimer disease. *Brain Res Mol Brain Res*, Vol. 44, No. 1, (Feb 1997), pp. 99-104, ISSN 0169-328X

Chen, H. & Chan, D. C. (2006). Critical dependence of neurons on mitochondrial dynamics. *Curr Opin Cell Biol*, Vol. 18, No. 4, (Aug 2006), pp. 453-459, ISSN 0955-0674

Chen, H.; Chomyn, A. & Chan, D. C. (2005). Disruption of fusion results in mitochondrial heterogeneity and dysfunction. *J Biol Chem*, Vol. 280, No. 28, (Jul 15 2005), pp. 26185-26192, ISSN 0021-9258

Cortés-Hernández, P.; Vázquez-Memije, M.E. & García, J.J. (2007). ATP6 homoplasmic mutations inhibit and destabilize the human F1F0-ATP synthase without preventing enzyme assembly and oligomerization. *J Biol Chem*, Vol. 282, no. 2, (Jan 12), pp. 1051-1058, ISSN 0021-9258

Coskun, P. E.; Beal, M. F. & Wallace, D. C. (2004). Alzheimer's brains harbor somatic mtDNA control-region mutations that suppress mitochondrial transcription and replication. *Proc Natl Acad Sci U S A*, Vol. 101, No. 29, (Jul 20 2004), pp. 10726-10731, ISSN 0027-8424

Costantini, L. C.; Barr, L. J.; Vogel, J. L. & Henderson, S. T. (2008). Hypometabolism as a therapeutic target in Alzheimer's disease. *BMC Neurosci*, Vol. 9 Suppl 2, No. 2008), pp. S16, ISSN 1471-2202

Czech, C.; Monning, V.; Tienari, P. J.; Hartmann, T.; Masters, C.; Beyreuther, K. & Forstl, H. (1993). Apolipoprotein E-epsilon 4 allele and Alzheimer's disease. *Lancet*, Vol. 342, No. 8882, (Nov 20 1993), pp. 1309, ISSN 0140-6736

de la Monte, S. M.; Luong, T.; Neely, T. R.; Robinson, D. & Wands, J. R. (2000). Mitochondrial DNA damage as a mechanism of cell loss in Alzheimer's disease. *Lab Invest*, Vol. 80, No. 8, (Aug 2000), pp. 1323-1335, ISSN 0023-6837

de Leon, M. J.; Ferris, S. H.; George, A. E.; Christman, D. R.; Fowler, J. S.; Gentes, C.; Reisberg, B.; Gee, B.; Emmerich, M.; Yonekura, Y.; Brodie, J.; Kricheff, II & Wolf, A. P. (1983). Positron emission tomographic studies of aging and Alzheimer disease. *AJNR Am J Neuroradiol*, Vol. 4, No. 3, (May-Jun 1983), pp. 568-571, ISSN 0195-6108

Di Luca, M.; Colciaghi, F.; Pastorino, L.; Borroni, B.; Padovani, A. & Cattabeni, F. (2000). Platelets as a peripheral district where to study pathogenetic mechanisms of alzheimer disease: the case of amyloid precursor protein. *Eur J Pharmacol*, Vol. 405, No. 1-3, (Sep 29 2000), pp. 277-283, ISSN 0014-2999

Dreux, C. & Launay, J. M. (1985). [Blood platelets: neuronal model in psychiatric disorders]. *Encephale*, Vol. 11, No. 2, (Mar-Apr 1985), pp. 57-64, ISSN 0013-7006

Dreyfus, G.; Gomez-Puyou, A. & Iuena de Gomez-Puyou, M. (1981). Electrochemical gradient induced displacement of the natural ATPase inhibitor protein from mitochondrial ATPase as directed by antibodies against the inhibitor protein. *Biochem Biophys Res Commun*, Vol. 100, No. 1, (May 15 1981), pp. 400-406, ISSN 0006-291X

Ellison, D. W.; Beal, M. F. & Martin, J. B. (1987). Phosphoethanolamine and ethanolamine are decreased in Alzheimer's disease and Huntington's disease. *Brain Res*, Vol. 417, No. 2, (Aug 11 1987), pp. 389-392, ISSN 0006-8993

Frederick, R. L. & Shaw, J. M. (2007). Moving mitochondria: establishing distribution of an essential organelle. *Traffic*, Vol. 8, No. 12, (Dec 2007), pp. 1668-1675, ISSN 1398-9219

Friedland, R. P.; Budinger, T. F.; Ganz, E.; Yano, Y.; Mathis, C. A.; Koss, B.; Ober, B. A.; Huesman, R. H. & Derenzo, S. E. (1983). Regional cerebral metabolic alterations in dementia of the Alzheimer type: positron emission tomography with [18F]fluorodeoxyglucose. *J Comput Assist Tomogr*, Vol. 7, No. 4, (Aug 1983), pp. 590-598, ISSN 0363-8715

Fukami, M. H. & Salganicoff, L. (1973). Isolation and properties of human platelet mitochondria. *Blood*, Vol. 42, No. 6, (Dec 1973), pp. 913-918, ISSN 0006-4971

García, J.J.; Ogilvie, I.; Robinson, B. & Capaldi, R. A. (2000). Structure, functioning, and assembly of the ATP synthase in cells from patients with the T8993G mitochondrial DNA mutation. Comparison with the enzyme in Rho0 cells completely lacking mtDNA. *J Biol Chem*, Vol. 275, No. 15, (April 14), pp. 11075-11081, ISSN 0021-9258

García, J.J.; Morales-Rios, E.; Cortés-Hernández, P. & Rodríguez-Zavala, J. S. (2006). The inhibitor protein (IF1) promotes dimerization of the mitochondrial F1F0-ATP synthase. *Biochemistry*, Vol. 45, No. 42, (Oct 24), pp. 12695-12703, ISSN 0006-2960

García-Trejo, J. J. & Morales-Ríos, E. (2008). Regulation of the F1F0-ATP synthase rotary nanomotor in its monomeric-bacterial and dimeric-mitochondrial forms. *J Biol Phys*, Vol. 34, No. 1-2, (Apr 2008), pp. 197-212, ISSN: 0092-0606

Hajimohammadreza, I.; Brammer, M. J.; Eagger, S.; Burns, A. & Levy, R. (1990). Platelet and erythrocyte membrane changes in Alzheimer's disease. *Biochim Biophys Acta*, Vol. 1025, No. 2, (Jun 27 1990), pp. 208-214, ISSN 0006-3002

Hatefi, Y. (1985). The mitochondrial electron transport and oxidative phosphorylation system. *Annu Rev Biochem*, Vol. 54, No. 1985), pp. 1015-1069, ISSN 0066-4154

Hirai, K.; Aliev, G.; Nunomura, A.; Fujioka, H.; Russell, R. L.; Atwood, C. S.; Johnson, A. B.; Kress, Y.; Vinters, H. V.; Tabaton, M.; Shimohama, S.; Cash, A. D.; Siedlak, S. L.; Harris, P. L.; Jones, P. K.; Petersen, R. B.; Perry, G. & Smith, M. A. (2001). Mitochondrial abnormalities in Alzheimer's disease. *J Neurosci*, Vol. 21, No. 9, (May 1 2001), pp. 3017-3023, ISSN 0270-6474

Hoyer, S. (1991). Abnormalities of glucose metabolism in Alzheimer's disease. *Ann N Y Acad Sci*, Vol. 640, No. 1991), pp. 53-58, ISSN 0077-8923

Ibanez, V.; Pietrini, P.; Alexander, G. E.; Furey, M. L.; Teichberg, D.; Rajapakse, J. C.; Rapoport, S. I.; Schapiro, M. B. & Horwitz, B. (1998). Regional glucose metabolic abnormalities are not the result of atrophy in Alzheimer's disease. *Neurology*, Vol. 50, No. 6, (Jun 1998), pp. 1585-1593, ISSN 0028-3878

Ishii, K.; Sasaki, M.; Kitagaki, H.; Yamaji, S.; Sakamoto, S.; Matsuda, K. & Mori, E. (1997). Reduction of cerebellar glucose metabolism in advanced Alzheimer's disease. *J Nucl Med*, Vol. 38, No. 6, (Jun 1997), pp. 925-928, ISSN 0161-5505

Jung, C.; Higgins, C. M. & Xu, Z. (2000). Measuring the quantity and activity of mitochondrial electron transport chain complexes in tissues of central nervous system using blue native polyacrylamide gel electrophoresis. *Anal Biochem*, Vol. 286, No. 2, (Nov 15 2000), pp. 214-223, ISSN 0003-2697

Jurado, A. S.; Almeida, L. M. & Madeira, V. M. (1991). Fluidity of bacterial membrane lipids monitored by intramolecular excimerization of 1.3-di(2-pyrenyl)propane. *Biochem Biophys Res Commun*, Vol. 176, No. 1, (Apr 15 1991), pp. 356-363, ISSN 0006-291X

Kaiser, R. D. & London, E. (1998). Location of diphenylhexatriene (DPH) and its derivatives within membranes: comparison of different fluorescence quenching analyses of membrane depth. *Biochemistry*, Vol. 37, No. 22, (Jun 2 1998), pp. 8180-8190, ISSN 0006-2960

Kim, S. H.; Vlkolinsky, R.; Cairns, N. & Lubec, G. (2000). Decreased levels of complex III core protein 1 and complex V beta chain in brains from patients with Alzheimer's disease and Down syndrome. *Cell Mol Life Sci*, Vol. 57, No. 12, (Nov 2000), pp. 1810-1816, ISSN 1420-682X

Klunk, W. E.; Panchalingam, K.; McClure, R. J.; Stanley, J. A. & Pettegrew, J. W. (1998). Metabolic alterations in postmortem Alzheimer's disease brain are exaggerated by Apo-E4. *Neurobiol Aging*, Vol. 19, No. 6, (Nov-Dec 1998), pp. 511-515, ISSN 0197-4580

Knott, A. B.; Perkins, G.; Schwarzenbacher, R. & Bossy-Wetzel, E. (2008). Mitochondrial fragmentation in neurodegeneration. *Nat Rev Neurosci*, Vol. 9, No. 7, (Jul 2008), pp. 505-518, 1471-003X

Lemere, C. A.; Blusztajn, J. K.; Yamaguchi, H.; Wisniewski, T.; Saido, T. C. & Selkoe, D. J. (1996). Sequence of deposition of heterogeneous amyloid beta-peptides and APO E in Down syndrome: implications for initial events in amyloid plaque formation. *Neurobiol Dis*, Vol. 3, No. 1, (Feb 1996), pp. 16-32, ISSN 0969-9961

Liang, W. S.; Reiman, E. M.; Valla, J.; Dunckley, T.; Beach, T. G.; Grover, A.; Niedzielko, T. L.; Schneider, L. E.; Mastroeni, D.; Caselli, R.; Kukull, W.; Morris, J. C.; Hulette, C. M.; Schmechel, D.; Rogers, J. & Stephan, D. A. (2008). Alzheimer's disease is associated with reduced expression of energy metabolism genes in posterior cingulate neurons. *Proc Natl Acad Sci U S A*, Vol. 105, No. 11, (Mar 18 2008), pp. 4441-4446, ISSN 0027-8424

Lovell, M. A.; Ehmann, W. D.; Butler, S. M. & Markesbery, W. R. (1995). Elevated thiobarbituric acid-reactive substances and antioxidant enzyme activity in the brain in Alzheimer's disease. *Neurology*, Vol. 45, No. 8, (Aug 1995), pp. 1594-1601, ISSN 0028-3878

Lu, T.; Pan, Y.; Kao, S. Y.; Li, C.; Kohane, I.; Chan, J. & Yankner, B. A. (2004). Gene regulation and DNA damage in the ageing human brain. *Nature*, Vol. 429, No. 6994, (Jun 24 2004), pp. 883-891, ISSN 0028-0836

Manczak, M.; Park, B. S.; Jung, Y. & Reddy, P. H. (2004). Differential expression of oxidative phosphorylation genes in patients with Alzheimer's disease: implications for early mitochondrial dysfunction and oxidative damage. *Neuromolecular Med*, Vol. 5, No. 2, 2004), pp. 147-162, ISSN 1535-1084

Martinez-Cano, E.; Ortiz-Genaro, G.; Pacheco-Moises, F.; Macias-Islas, M. A.; Sanchez-Nieto, S. & Rosales-Corral, S. A. (2005). [Functional disorders of FOF1-ATPase in submitochondrial particles obtained from platelets of patients with a diagnosis of probable Alzheimer's disease]. *Rev Neurol*, Vol. 40, No. 2, (Jan 16-31 2005), pp. 81-85, ISSN 0210-0010

Mason, R. P.; Shoemaker, W. J.; Shajenko, L.; Chambers, T. E. & Herbette, L. G. (1992). Evidence for changes in the Alzheimer's disease brain cortical membrane structure mediated by cholesterol. *Neurobiol Aging*, Vol. 13, No. 3, (May-Jun 1992), pp. 413-419, ISSN 0197-4580

Maurer, I.; Zierz, S. & Moller, H. J. (2000). A selective defect of cytochrome c oxidase is present in brain of Alzheimer disease patients. *Neurobiol Aging*, Vol. 21, No. 3, (May-Jun 2000), pp. 455-462, ISSN 0197-4580

Mecocci, P.; Cherubini, A.; Beal, M. F.; Cecchetti, R.; Chionne, F.; Polidori, M. C.; Romano, G. & Senin, U. (1996). Altered mitochondrial membrane fluidity in AD brain. *Neurosci Lett*, Vol. 207, No. 2, (Mar 29 1996), pp. 129-132, ISSN 0304-3940

Minauro-Sanmiguel, F.; Wilkens, S. & Garcia, J. J. (2005). Structure of dimeric mitochondrial ATP synthase: novel F0 bridging features and the structural basis of mitochondrial cristae biogenesis *Proc Natl Acad Sci U S A*, Vol. 102, No. 35, (Aug 30 2005), pp. 12356-12358, ISSN 0027-8424

Minoshima, S.; Giordani, B.; Berent, S.; Frey, K. A.; Foster, N. L. & Kuhl, D. E. (1997). Metabolic reduction in the posterior cingulate cortex in very early Alzheimer's disease. *Ann Neurol*, Vol. 42, No. 1, (Jul 1997), pp. 85-94, ISSN 0364-5134

Moreira, P. I.; Duarte, A. I.; Santos, M. S.; Rego, A. C. & Oliveira, C. R. (2009). An integrative view of the role of oxidative stress, mitochondria and insulin in Alzheimer's disease. *J Alzheimers Dis*, Vol. 16, No. 4, 2009), pp. 741-761, ISSN 1387-2877

Mosconi, L.; Brys, M.; Switalski, R.; Mistur, R.; Glodzik, L.; Pirraglia, E.; Tsui, W.; De Santi, S. & de Leon, M. J. (2007). Maternal family history of Alzheimer's disease predisposes to reduced brain glucose metabolism. *Proc Natl Acad Sci U S A*, Vol. 104, No. 48, (Nov 27 2007), pp. 19067-19072, ISSN 0027-8424

Nagy, Z.; Esiri, M. M.; LeGris, M. & Matthews, P. M. (1999). Mitochondrial enzyme expression in the hippocampus in relation to Alzheimer-type pathology. *Acta Neuropathol*, Vol. 97, No. 4, (Apr 1999), pp. 346-354, ISSN 0001-6322

Nitsch, R. M.; Blusztajn, J. K.; Pittas, A. G.; Slack, B. E.; Growdon, J. H. & Wurtman, R. J. (1992). Evidence for a membrane defect in Alzheimer disease brain. *Proc Natl Acad Sci U S A*, Vol. 89, No. 5, (Mar 1 1992), pp. 1671-1675, ISSN 0027-8424

Ortiz, G. G.; Pacheco-Moises, F.; El Hafidi, M.; Jimenez-Delgado, A.; Macias-Islas, M. A.; Rosales Corral, S. A.; de la Rosa, A. C.; Sanchez-Gonzalez, V. J.; Arias-Merino, E. D. & Velazquez-Brizuela, I. E. (2008). Detection of membrane fluidity in submitochondrial particles of platelets and erythrocyte membranes from Mexican patients with Alzheimer disease by intramolecular excimer formation of 1,3 dipyrenylpropane. *Dis Markers*, Vol. 24, No. 3, 2008), pp. 151-156, ISSN 0278-0240

Parker, W. D., Jr.; Parks, J.; Filley, C. M. & Kleinschmidt-DeMasters, B. K. (1994). Electron transport chain defects in Alzheimer's disease brain. *Neurology*, Vol. 44, No. 6, (Jun 1994), pp. 1090-1096, ISSN 0028-3878

Parker, W. D., Jr. & Parks, J. K. (1995). Cytochrome c oxidase in Alzheimer's disease brain: purification and characterization. *Neurology*, Vol. 45, No. 3 Pt 1, (Mar 1995), pp. 482-486, ISSN 0028-3878

Parone, P. A.; Da Cruz, S.; Tondera, D.; Mattenberger, Y.; James, D. I.; Maechler, P.; Barja, F. & Martinou, J. C. (2008). Preventing mitochondrial fission impairs mitochondrial function and leads to loss of mitochondrial DNA. *PLoS One*, Vol. 3, No. 9, 2008), pp. e3257, ISSN 1932-6203

Pettegrew, J. W.; Panchalingam, K.; Klunk, W. E.; McClure, R. J. & Muenz, L. R. (1994). Alterations of cerebral metabolism in probable Alzheimer's disease: a preliminary study. *Neurobiol Aging*, Vol. 15, No. 1, (Jan-Feb 1994), pp. 117-132, ISSN 0197-4580

Phelps, M. E.; Mazziotta, J. C. & Huang, S. C. (1982). Study of cerebral function with positron computed tomography. *J Cereb Blood Flow Metab*, Vol. 2, No. 2, 1982), pp. 113-162, ISSN 0271-678X

Poole, A. C.; Thomas, R. E.; Andrews, L. A.; McBride, H. M.; Whitworth, A. J. & Pallanck, L. J. (2008). The PINK1/Parkin pathway regulates mitochondrial morphology. *Proc Natl Acad Sci U S A*, Vol. 105, No. 5, (Feb 5 2008), pp. 1638-1643, ISSN 0027-8424

Power, J.; Cross, R. L. & Harris, D. A. (1983). Interaction of F1-ATPase, from ox heart mitochondria with its naturally occurring inhibitor protein. Studies using radio-iodinated inhibitor protein. *Biochim Biophys Acta*, Vol. 724, No. 1, (Jul 29 1983), pp. 128-141, ISSN 0006-3002

Pullman, M. E. & Monroy, G. C. (1963). A Naturally Occurring Inhibitor of Mitochondrial Adenosine Triphosphatase. *J Biol Chem*, Vol. 238, No. (Nov 1963), pp. 3762-3769, ISSN 0021-9258

Qiu, X.; Chen, Y. & Zhou, M. (2001). Two point mutations in mitochondrial DNA of cytochrome c oxidase coexist with normal mtDNA in a patient with Alzheimer's disease. *Brain Res*, Vol. 893, No. 1-2, (Mar 2 2001), pp. 261-263, ISSN 0006-8993

Rapoport, S. I.; Hatanpaa, K.; Brady, D. R. & Chandrasekaran, K. (1996). Brain energy metabolism, cognitive function and down-regulated oxidative phosphorylation in Alzheimer disease. *Neurodegeneration*, Vol. 5, No. 4, (Dec 1996), pp. 473-476, ISSN 1055-8330

Reddy, P. H. & Beal, M. F. (2008). Amyloid beta, mitochondrial dysfunction and synaptic damage: implications for cognitive decline in aging and Alzheimer's disease. *Trends Mol Med*, Vol. 14, No. 2, (Feb 2008), pp. 45-53, ISSN 1471-4914

Reddy, P. H.; McWeeney, S.; Park, B. S.; Manczak, M.; Gutala, R. V.; Partovi, D.; Jung, Y.; Yau, V.; Searles, R.; Mori, M. & Quinn, J. (2004). Gene expression profiles of transcripts in amyloid precursor protein transgenic mice: up-regulation of mitochondrial metabolism and apoptotic genes is an early cellular change in Alzheimer's disease. *Hum Mol Genet*, Vol. 13, No. 12, (Jun 15 2004), pp. 1225-1240, ISSN 0964-6906

Reiman, E. M.; Caselli, R. J.; Yun, L. S.; Chen, K.; Bandy, D.; Minoshima, S.; Thibodeau, S. N. & Osborne, D. (1996). Preclinical evidence of Alzheimer's disease in persons homozygous for the epsilon 4 allele for apolipoprotein E. *N Engl J Med*, Vol. 334, No. 12, (Mar 21 1996), pp. 752-758, ISSN 0028-4793

Roder, H. M.; Eden, P. A. & Ingram, V. M. (1993). Brain protein kinase PK40erk converts TAU into a PHF-like form as found in Alzheimer's disease. *Biochem Biophys Res Commun*, Vol. 193, No. 2, (Jun 15 1993), pp. 639-647, ISSN 0006-291X

Roder, H. M. & Ingram, V. M. (1991). Two novel kinases phosphorylate tau and the KSP site of heavy neurofilament subunits in high stoichiometric ratios. *J Neurosci*, Vol. 11, No. 11, (Nov 1991), pp. 3325-3343, ISSN 0270-6474

Rosenberg, R. N.; Baskin, F.; Fosmire, J. A.; Risser, R.; Adams, P.; Svetlik, D.; Honig, L. S.; Cullum, C. M. & Weiner, M. F. (1997). Altered amyloid protein processing in platelets of patients with Alzheimer disease. *Arch Neurol*, Vol. 54, No. 2, (Feb 1997), pp. 139-144, ISSN 0003-9942

Roses, A. D.; Strittmatter, W. J.; Pericak-Vance, M. A.; Corder, E. H.; Saunders, A. M. & Schmechel, D. E. (1994). Clinical application of apolipoprotein E genotyping to Alzheimer's disease. *Lancet*, Vol. 343, No. 8912, (Jun 18 1994), pp. 1564-1565, ISSN 0140-6736

Sanchez-Bustamante, V. J.; Darszon, A. & Gomez-Puyou, A. (1982). On the function of the natural ATPase inhibitor protein in intact mitochondria. *Eur J Biochem*, Vol. 126, No. 3, (Sep 1 1982), pp. 611-616, ISSN 0014-2956

Sanchez-Gonzalez, V. J.; Ortiz, G. G.; Gallegos-Arreola, P.; Macias-Islas, M. A.; Arias-Merino, E. D.; Loera-Castaneda, V.; Martinez-Cano, E.; Velazquez-Brizuela, I. E.; Rosales-Corral, S. A.; Curiel-Ortega, C. R.; Pacheco-Moises, F. & Garcia, J. J. (2006). Altered beta-amyloid precursor protein isoforms in Mexican Alzheimer's Disease patients. *Dis Markers*, Vol. 22, No. 3, 2006), pp. 119-125, ISSN 0278-0240

Saunders, A. M.; Strittmatter, W. J.; Schmechel, D.; George-Hyslop, P. H.; Pericak-Vance, M. A.; Joo, S. H.; Rosi, B. L.; Gusella, J. F.; Crapper-MacLachlan, D. R. & Alberts, M. J. (1993). Association of apolipoprotein E allele epsilon 4 with late-onset familial and sporadic Alzheimer's disease. *Neurology*, Vol. 43, No. 8, (Aug 1993), pp. 1467-1472, ISSN 0028-3878

Schagger, H. & Ohm, T. G. (1995). Human diseases with defects in oxidative phosphorylation. 2. F1F0 ATP-synthase defects in Alzheimer disease revealed by blue native polyacrylamide gel electrophoresis. *Eur J Biochem*, Vol. 227, No. 3, (Feb 1 1995), pp. 916-921, ISSN 0014-2956

Schwerzmann, K. & Pedersen, P. L. (1981). Proton--adenosinetriphosphatase complex of rat liver mitochondria: effect of energy state on its interaction with the adenosinetriphosphatase inhibitory peptide. *Biochemistry*, Vol. 20, No. 22, (Oct 27 1981), pp. 6305-6311, ISSN 0006-2960

Selkoe, D. J. (2004). Cell biology of protein misfolding: the examples of Alzheimer's and Parkinson's diseases. *Nat Cell Biol*, Vol. 6, No. 11, (Nov 2004), pp. 1054-1061, ISSN 1465-7392

Simonian, N. A. & Hyman, B. T. (1994). Functional alterations in Alzheimer's disease: selective loss of mitochondrial-encoded cytochrome oxidase mRNA in the hippocampal formation. *J Neuropathol Exp Neurol*, Vol. 53, No. 5, (Sep 1994), pp. 508-512, ISSN 0022-3069

Sims, N. R.; Finegan, J. M.; Blass, J. P.; Bowen, D. M. & Neary, D. (1987). Mitochondrial function in brain tissue in primary degenerative dementia. *Brain Res*, Vol. 436, No. 1, (Dec 8 1987), pp. 30-38, ISSN 0006-8993

Strittmatter, W. J.; Saunders, A. M.; Schmechel, D.; Pericak-Vance, M.; Enghild, J.; Salvesen, G. S. & Roses, A. D. (1993). Apolipoprotein E: high-avidity binding to beta-amyloid and increased frequency of type 4 allele in late-onset familial Alzheimer disease. *Proc Natl Acad Sci U S A*, Vol. 90, No. 5, (Mar 1 1993), pp. 1977-1981, ISSN 0027-8424

Su, B.; Wang, X.; Nunomura, A.; Moreira, P. I.; Lee, H. G.; Perry, G.; Smith, M. A. & Zhu, X. (2008). Oxidative stress signaling in Alzheimer's disease. *Curr Alzheimer Res*, Vol. 5, No. 6, (Dec 2008), pp. 525-532, ISSN 1567-2050

Sullivan, P. G. & Brown, M. R. (2005). Mitochondrial aging and dysfunction in Alzheimer's disease. *Prog Neuropsychopharmacol Biol Psychiatry*, Vol. 29, No. 3, (Mar 2005), pp. 407-410, ISSN 0278-5846

Swerdlow, R. H. (2007). PET sheds light on Alzheimer's disease genetic risk. *Proc Natl Acad Sci U S A*, Vol. 104, No. 48, (Nov 27 2007), pp. 18881-18882, ISSN 0027-8424

Swerdlow, R. H. & Kish, S. J. (2002). Mitochondria in Alzheimer's disease. *Int Rev Neurobiol*, Vol. 53, No. 2002), pp. 341-385, ISSN 0074-7742

Takeda, A.; Smith, M. A.; Avila, J.; Nunomura, A.; Siedlak, S. L.; Zhu, X.; Perry, G. & Sayre, L. M. (2000). In Alzheimer's disease, heme oxygenase is coincident with Alz50, an epitope of tau induced by 4-hydroxy-2-nonenal modification. *J Neurochem*, Vol. 75, No. 3, (Sep 2000), pp. 1234-1241, ISSN 0022-3042

Troncoso, J. C.; Costello, A.; Watson, A. L., Jr. & Johnson, G. V. (1993). In vitro polymerization of oxidized tau into filaments. *Brain Res*, Vol. 613, No. 2, (Jun 11 1993), pp. 313-316, ISSN 0006-8993

Utermann, G. (1987). Apolipoprotein E polymorphism in health and disease. *Am Heart J*, Vol. 113, No. 2 Pt 2, (Feb 1987), pp. 433-440, ISSN 0002-8703

Valla, J.; Berndt, J. D. & Gonzalez-Lima, F. (2001). Energy hypometabolism in posterior cingulate cortex of Alzheimer's patients: superficial laminar cytochrome oxidase associated with disease duration. *J Neurosci*, Vol. 21, No. 13, (Jul 1 2001), pp. 4923-4930, ISSN 0270-6474

Van Gassen, G.; Annaert, W. & Van Broeckhoven, C. (2000). Binding partners of Alzheimer's disease proteins: are they physiologically relevant? *Neurobiol Dis*, Vol. 7, No. 3, (Jun 2000), pp. 135-151, ISSN 0969-9961

Wang, X.; Su, B.; Lee, H. G.; Li, X.; Perry, G.; Smith, M. A. & Zhu, X. (2009). Impaired balance of mitochondrial fission and fusion in Alzheimer's disease. *J Neurosci*, Vol. 29, No. 28, (Jul 15 2009), pp. 9090-9103, ISSN 0270-6474

Wang, X.; Su, B.; Siedlak, S. L.; Moreira, P. I.; Fujioka, H.; Wang, Y.; Casadesus, G. & Zhu, X. (2008). Amyloid-beta overproduction causes abnormal mitochondrial dynamics via differential modulation of mitochondrial fission/fusion proteins. *Proc Natl Acad Sci U S A*, Vol. 105, No. 49, (Dec 9 2008), pp. 19318-19323, ISSN 0027-8424

Zachariasse, K. A.; Vaz, W. L.; Sotomayor, C. & Kuhnle, W. (1982). Investigation of human erythrocyte ghost membranes with intramolecular excimer probes. *Biochim Biophys Acta*, Vol. 688, No. 2, (Jun 14 1982), pp. 323-332, ISSN 0006-3002

Zubenko, G. S.; Kopp, U.; Seto, T. & Firestone, L. L. (1999). Platelet membrane fluidity individuals at risk for Alzheimer's disease: a comparison of results from fluorescence spectroscopy and electron spin resonance spectroscopy. *Psychopharmacology (Berl)*, Vol. 145, No. 2, (Jul 1999), pp. 175-180, ISSN 0033-3158

Zubenko, G. S.; Malinakova, I. & Chojnacki, B. (1987). Proliferation of internal membranes in platelets from patients with Alzheimer's disease. *J Neuropathol Exp Neurol*, Vol. 46, No. 4, (Jul 1987), pp. 407-418, ISSN 0022-3069

3

# The Role of Glycogen Synthase Kinase-3 (GSK-3) in Alzheimer's Disease

Miguel Medina[1] and Jesús Avila[2]
[1]*Noscira S.A., Tres Cantos*
[2]*Centro de Biología Molecular "Severo Ochoa" CSIC-UAM, Cantoblanco*
*Spain*

## 1. Introduction

Despite its initial discovery as one of five protein kinases activities found to phosphorylate glycogen synthase (GS) in fractioned extracts of rabbit skeletal muscle (Embi et al., 1980; Hemmings et al., 1981), Glycogen Synthase Kinase 3 (GSK-3) is by no means restricted to a role in glycogen metabolism. Indeed, the enzyme targets a wide variety of proteins involved in signalling, metabolism, structural proteins and a remarkable number of transcription factors and plays a far more pleiotropic role than first imagined (Woodgett, 2006). Genetic analyses and the use of selective inhibitors have shown that GSK-3 plays critical roles in development, metabolic homeostasis, neuronal growth and differentiation (Hur & Zhon, 2010), cell polarity, cell fate and apoptosis. Its unique position in modulating the function of a diverse series of proteins in combination with its association with a wide variety of human disorders, from neurodegenerative diseases, stroke, bipolar disorder to diabetes and cancer, has attracted significant attention to the protein both as a therapeutic target and as a means to understand the molecular basis of these disorders.

In particular, the involvement of GSK-3 in several key pathophyisiological pathways leading to Alzheimer's disease (AD) and neurodegenerative diseases has placed this enzyme in a central position in this disorder. Thus, GSK-3 has recently been proposed as a link between the two major pathological pathways in AD, amyloid and tau (Hernández et al., 2010; Muyllaert et al., 2008) and even a "GSK-3 hypothesis of AD", suggesting that GSK-3 might be a casual mediator of the disease, has been put forward (Hooper et al., 2008). This review will focus on describing the key role that GSK-3 plays in AD pathobiology and the use of GSK-3 inhibition as a potential therapeutic approach to treat this disease.

## 2. GSK-3 structure and regulation

GSK-3 is a highly conserved protein kinase belonging to the CMGC family of serine/threonine protein kinases, as genes encoding the enzyme have been identified in every eukaryotic genome that has been investigated, such as *Dictyostelium discoideum* (Kim et al., 1999), *Xenopus laevis* (Itoh et al., 1995), *Drosophila melanogaster* (Ruel et al., 1993) or parasites such like *Plasmodium falciparum*, *Trypanosoma brucei* or *Leishmania donovani* (Osolodkin et al., 2011). Mammalian GSK-3 is encoded by two genes, *gsk-3a* and *gsk-3β*

(Frame & Cohen, 2001; Grimes & Jope, 2001), that encode proteins of 51 and 47 kDa, respectively and which display 84% overall identity (98% within their catalytic domains), with the main difference being an extra Gly-rich stretch in the N-terminal domain of GSK-3α (Woodgett, 1990). Mammalian GSK-3α and β are each widely expressed although some tissues show preferential levels of some of the two proteins. Furthermore, an alternatively splicing event between exons 8 and 9 of GSK-3β gives rise in neurons to a splice variant (GSK-3β2) containing a 13 amino acids insertion within the kinase domain near to the substrate binding pocket (Mukai et al., 2002). How this insertion affects kinase activity or regulation remains unclear, although some differences between GSK-3β1 and GSK-3β2 isoforms have already been described (see below).

Crystallographic studies have revealed the three-dimensional structure of GSK-3β (Dajani et al., 2001; ter Haar et al., 2001), having the overall shape common to most kinases, with a small N-terminal lobe mostly consisting of β-sheets and a large C-terminal lobe essentially formed of α-helices (Noble et al., 2005). The ATP binding pocket is located between the two lobes and it is well conserved among kinases (Bain et al., 2007). Very recently, a comparison of the human and parasite GSK-3 ATP binding sites has opened the possibility of developing selective drugs specifically affecting parasite GSK-3 (Osolodkin et al., 2011).

Some GSK-3 substrates do not require a very specific sequence but rather a previous *(primed)* phosphorylation by a *priming* kinase on a Ser or Thr residue located four amino acids C-terminal to the Ser or Thr residue to be modified by GSK-3 (see below for regulation through primed phosphorylation). The crystal structure of human GSK-3β has also provided a model for the binding of pre-phosphorylated substrates to the kinase. According to it, primed Ser/Thr is recognized by a positively charged binding pocket formed by residues Arg96, Arg180 and Lys205 that facilitates the binding of the phosphate group of primed substrates. GSK-3β uses the phosphorylated serine or threonine at position +4 of the substrate to align the two domains for optimal catalytic activity (Dajani et al., 2001; ter Haar et al., 2001).

Furthermore, crystal structures of GSK-3β complexes with interacting proteins FRAT/GBP and axin have allowed defining the molecular basis for those interactions, which play critical roles in some signalling pathways (see below for regulation through protein complex formation). These studies confirm the partial overlap of the binding sites of axin and FRAT1/GBP predicted from genetic and biochemical studies (Ferkey & Kimelman, 2002; Fraser et al., 2002) but reveal significant differences in the detailed interactions, and identify key residues mediating the differential interaction with both proteins. This ability of GSK-3β to bind two different proteins with high specificity *via* the same binding site is mediated by the conformational plasticity of the 285-299 loop, while some residues in this versatile binding site are involved in interactions with both axin and FRAT, others are involved uniquely with one or the other (Dajani et al., 2003).

GSK-3 is ubiquitously expressed and, unlike most kinases, has a relatively high activity in resting, unstimulated cells while it is normally reduced in response to a variety of extracellular stimuli (Frame & Cohen, 2001). In mammals, GSK-3α and β are each expressed widely at both the RNA and protein levels, although some tissues show preferential levels of some of the two proteins as for instance, both isoforms are highly expressed in neural tissue. Neither gene appears to be acutely regulated at the transcriptional level whereas the proteins are controlled post-translationally, largely through protein-protein interactions or by post-translational regulation.

Given that chemical inhibitors of GSK-3 are unable to discriminate between the various GSK-3 isoforms, evaluation of isoform-specific functions it is not possible by using these compounds. However, evidence for isoform-specific roles has now emerged from mouse models (see below). For instance, some recent findings suggest that there are tissue- and isoform-specific roles in regulation of glucose metabolism (Patel et al., 2008; Mol Cell Biol), as GSK-3α seems to be the predominant regulator of GS and glycogen synthesis in liver whereas GSK-3β has a more prevalent role within skeletal muscle and pancreas. Also, although the effect of the inserted sequence on kinase activity, substrate specificity or requirement for priming of substrates remains unclear, the neuron-specific alternatively spliced GSK-3β2 isoform appears to phosphorylate unprimed residues on tau and MAP1B to a lesser extent than GSK-3β1 (Mukai et al. 2002, Wood-Kaczmar *et al.* 2009).

Three decades after its discovery as a protein kinase involved in glycogen metabolism, GSK-3 has revealed as a key enzyme in regulating many critical cellular processes, providing a link between many different substrates and various signalling pathways as well as gene expression. Modulation of its activity has also turned out to be much more complex than originally thought. As already mentioned above, one of the main characteristics of GSK-3 is that its activity is high in resting, unstimulated cells while regulated by extracellular signals that typically induce a rapid and reversible decrease in enzymatic activity. Control of GSK-3 activity occurs by complex mechanisms that are each dependent upon specific signalling pathways (for a recent review see Medina & Wandosell, 2011).

Early on, GSK-3 was proved to be a dual specificity kinase differentially regulated by tyrosine and serine/threonine phosphorylation (Wang et al., 1994). The first regulatory mechanism described of GSK-3 activity involved the phosphorylation of specific residues of GSK-3 by other kinases; and more recently through auto-phosphorylation (Frame & Cohen, 2001; Harwood, 2001). Thus, four different regions and residues have been described in the GSK-3 molecule. First, it has been clearly established that phosphorylation of serine residue at positions 21 in GSK-3α and 9 in GSK-3β, correlates with the inhibition of its kinase activity (Frame et al., 2001; Stambolic et al., 1994; Sutherland et al., 1993). Many protein kinases are capable of phosphorylating GSK-3 at this residue, such as Akt, ILK, PKA, p90Rsk (Delcommenne et al., 1998; Fang et al., 2000), and many physiological situations of inhibition of GSK-3 correlate with serine phosphorylation, such as Insulin/IGF1, NGF, or Estradiol treatments, not only in neurons but also in other cell types (Cardona-Gomez et al., 2004). In addition, phosphorylation at threonine 43, present only in the isoform GSK-3β, by ERK also correlates with GSK-3 inhibition (Ding et al., 2005), whereas residues serine 389 and threonine 390 present in GSK-3β have been shown to be phosphorylated by p38 MAPK (Thornton et al., 2008), increasing the capacity of Ser-9 to be phosphorylated rather than promoting a direct inhibition.

In contrast, tyrosine phosphorylation present in positions 279 in GSK-3α or 216 in GSK-3β, correlates with an increase of its kinase activity (Hughes et al., 1993). Different candidate kinases such as Pyk-2 and Fyn have been reported to be able to phosphorylate GSK-3 on this residue *in vitro*, as MEK1/2 has been shown to do it in mammalian fibroblasts (Hartigan et al., 2001; Lesort et al., 1999) or ZAK1 in *Dictyostelium discoideum* (Kim et al., 1999; 2002), although no homologue of this latter kinase has been found in mammals. More recently, it has been suggested that phosphotyrosine in GSK-3 in mammalian systems might arise from a chaperone-dependent intra-molecular autophosphorylation event perhaps regulated by Hsp90 (Cole et al., 2004 Biochem J; Lockhead et al., 2006; Wang et al., 1994). Molecular dynamics and crystallographic studies clearly suggest that pTyr216 renders the kinase active through interactions with Arg220 and Arg223, stabilizing the activation loop and allowing full substrate accessibility (Buch et al., 2010; Cohen & Goedert, 2004). Very recently, it has been also shown that the extent of phosphorylation at both Ser9 and Tyr216 residues is very similar in both GSK-3β splice variants, β1 and β2 (Soutar et al., 2010).

On the other hand, tyrosine phosphorylation of residue 216 or 279 increased in neuronal cells following exposure to LPA (Sayas et al., 1999) and also upon exposure of neurons to β-amyloid or PrP (Muñoz-Montaño et al., 1997; Perez et al., 2003; Takashima et al., 1998) in a clear correlation with an increase on GSK-3 activity. In addition, in many neuronal cells the pharmacological inhibition of tyrosine phosphatases with *ortho*-vanadate increases the basal level of GSK-3-pTyr (Simon et al., 2008). Thus, taken all together, in addition to the reported tyrosine 216/279 autophosphorylation mechanism proposed, some as-yet-unidentified tyrosine kinases and/or phosphatases may also regulate GSK-3 activity by phosphorylation of this particular residue.

Another mechanism of GSK-3 regulation through post-translational modification involves the removal by calpain of a fragment from the N-terminal region of GSK-3, including the regulatory serines 9/21. After removal of that fragment GSK-3 becomes activated (Goñi-Oliver et al., 2007). The same study showed that both isoforms α and β are cleaved by calpain, although with different susceptibility. Moreover, GSK-3 truncation has been observed in human and mouse post-mortem brain tissue (Goñi-Oliver et al., 2009a). It is noteworthy to consider that a similar mechanism has been described for β-catenin in hippocampal neurons, where after NMDA-receptor-dependent activation; calpain induces the cleavage of β-catenin at the N-terminus, generating stable and truncated forms which maintain its transcriptional capacity (Abe & Takeichi, 2007). Likewise, GSK-3 truncation is mediated by extracellular calcium and can be inhibited by memantine (Goñi-Oliver et al., 2009b), a NMDA antagonist used for the treatment of Alzheimer's disease. Interestingly, GSK-3β has also been recently shown to be cleaved at the N-terminus (and subsequently activated) by matrix metallo-proteinase 2 (MMP-2) in cardiomyoblasts (Kanadasamy & Schulz, 2009).

Besides post-translational modifications, GSK-3 activity can also be regulated by protein complex association, for instance through its interaction with structural (scaffold) proteins. It is well known that GSK-3 contributes to Wnt signalling by participating in a multiprotein complex formed by axin, β-catenin and adenomatous polyposis coli (APC), among others (for review see, i.e. Moon et al., 2004). Indeed, in the absence of the Wnt ligand, GSK-3 it is able to phosphorylate β-catenin and targeting it for proteasome degradation (Aberle et al., 1997) whereas in its presence GSK-3 is unable to do that, increasing β-catenin cytosolic levels and eventually mediating TCF/LEF-mediated transcription at the nucleus. Recent data suggest that this complex may be specific for the GSK-3β2 splice isoform (Castaño et al., 2010). Recent evidence also supports a neuroprotective role for *Wnt* signaling in neurodegenerative disorders such as AD (Inestrosa & Toledo, 2008).

Moreover, another GSK-3-binding protein (GBP or FRAT) has been reported to regulate GSK-3 enzymatic activity (Itoh et al., 1995; Li et al., 1999). From the three different FRATs that have been cloned and characterized, FRAT1 appears to act as an inhibitory system (Yost et al., 1998) whereas FRAT2 appears to preferentially increase GSK-3-mediated phosphorylation in some residues (Stoothoff et al., 2005). Surprisingly, the triple FRAT-knockout mouse lacks any major defect in brain development (van Amerongen et al., 2005), which underlines the need to better define the precise role of FRAT in GSK-3 regulation and brain physiology. Furthermore, using the binding site on GSK-3 for FRAT/GBP, a GSK-3-interacting protein (GSKIP) has been identified that can block phosphorylation of different substrates and functions as a negative regulator of GSK-3β (Chou et al., 2006). Other proteins have also been proposed to further contribute to GSK-3 regulation through physical interaction with it. Thus, DISC-1 (Disrupted In Schizophrenia-1) regulates neural progenitor proliferation via the β-catenin/GSK-3β pathway, whereby DISC-1 stabilizes β-catenin by inhibiting GSK-3β activity through a direct binding (Mao et al., 2009). Finally, the dimeric scaffold protein 14-3-3 has been shown to co-elute from brain microtubules together with tau and GSK-3β and this interaction has been proposed to facilitate the interaction of the kinase with some of its substrates (Agarwal-Mawal et al., 2003).

As already mentioned, an unusual property of GSK3 is that most of its substrates require prior phosphorylation (priming) at a residue 4 or 5 amino acids C-terminal to the target residue (Frame & Cohen 2001), thus providing another mechanism of regulation of the GSK-3 activity. Some priming kinases have been identified, such as cdk5 (Alonso et al., 2006; Noble et al., 2003; Sengupta et al., 1997), PAR-1 (Nishimura et al., 2004), casein kinase I (Amit et al. 2002), PKC (Liu et al., 2003) or PKA (Sengupta et al., 1997). That said, there are examples of unprimed substrates reported, although is not entirely clear as yet whether this second set of unprimed substrates may define a different group of functions (Twomey & McCArthy, 2006).

## 3. GSK-3 activity in AD brain

Compared to age-matched control samples, increased levels of GSK-3 have been found in post-mortem analysis of brains from AD patients (Pei et al., 1997) while a spatial and temporal pattern of increased active GSK-3β expression correlating with the progression of neurofibrillary tangles (NFT) and neurodegeneration has also been shown (Leroy et al., 2002). Thus, GSK-3 has been shown to localize to pre-tangle neurons, dystrophic neurites and NFTs in AD brain (Pei et al., 1997). Neurons actively undergoing granulovacuolar degeneration are also immunopositive for active GSK3β (Leroy et al., 2002). Taken all together, although direct evidence might be lacking, all these studies strongly suggest that GSK-3β activity is increased in the brains of patients suffering from AD.

GSK-3β is the major kinase to phosphorylate tau protein both *in vitro* and *in vivo*. Furthermore, GSK-3β has been proposed as the link between the two major histopathological hallmarks of AD, the extracellular amyloid plaques and the intracellular NFT (Hernández et al., 2010; Ittner and Götz, 2011; Muyllaert et al., 2008). Exposure of primary neuronal cultures to Aβ induces activation of GSK-3β, tau phosphorylation and cell death, whereas blockade of GSK-3 expression by antisense oligonucleotides or its activity by lithium inhibits Aβ-induced toxicity (Alvarez et al., 1999; Hoshi et al., 2003; Wei et al., 2000).

GSK-3β-deficient mice die during embryonic development (Hoeflich *et al.* 2000, Liu *et al.* 2007) whereas GSK-3β heterozygous (+/-) mice are viable, although they show some neurological abnormalities, including reduced aggression, increased anxiety, reduced exploratory activity, poor memory consolidation and reduced responsiveness to amphetamine (O'Brien *et al.* 2004, Kimura *et al.* 2008, Beaulieu *et al.* 2008). Conversely, transgenic mice over-expressing GSK-3β result in behavioural changes that appear to recapitulate hyperactivity observed in the manic phase of bipolar disorder (Prickaerts *et al.* 2006).

On the other hand, mice lacking GSK-3α are viable and develop normally (MacAulay *et al.* 2007), but display enhanced glucose tolerance and insulin sensitivity accompanied by reduced fat mass. Interestingly, GSK-3α knock-out mice show reduced exploratory activity and aggression, similar to the GSK-3β heterozygotes, but in addition have decreased locomotion, impaired co-ordination and a deficit in fear conditioning (Kaidanovich-Beilin *et al.* 2009). These different in phenotypes in mice lacking one isoform or the other suggest non-redundant functions of the GSK-3 genes in the brain, while the overlapping behavioural problems between GSK-3α knockout (KO) and GSK-3β heterozygous (+/-) mice suggest some common substrates.

Furthermore, loss of both GSK-3 isoforms specifically in the brain results in increased self-renewal of neuronal progenitor cells, but reduced neurogenesis (Kim *et al.* 2009), while double GSK3α/β knock-in mice in which endogenous isoforms are replaced by mutant proteins where Ser21/9 have been mutated to Ala21/9 respectively, thus preventing repression by growth factor signalling, exhibit impaired neuronal precursor cell proliferation (Eom & Jope 2009). These data underscore the critical role that proper regulation of expression and activity of GSK-3 play in the maturation of these cells during mammalian brain development.

However, we must be careful when interpreting data from transgenic or KO animals since some strain specificity has been recently observed, at least in the case of improved insulin sensitivity and hepatic glucose homeostasis phenotype observed upon global inactivation of GSK-3α (Patel et al., 2011).

All these observations and the ones described below strongly suggest a central role of GSK-3 in AD pathogenesis and have also led to several efforts trying to identify sequence variations in the *gsk-3* gene and its promoter. Despite early reports of a lack of genetic association between the *gsk-3* coding sequence or its promoter with AD (Russ et al., 2001), several groups have now reported this association. Thus, a polymorphism in the promoter region (-50) of the *gsk-3β* gene appears associated with a two-fold increased risk for sporadic AD when analysing 333 sporadic AD patients and 307 control subjects from Spain (Mateo et al., 2006). More recently, a case-control study has found a rare intronic polymorphism in *gsk-3β* that occurred twice more frequently in AD patients than in aged healthy controls (Schaffer et al., 2010), strongly supporting the notion of a genetic association of the *gsk-3β* gene with AD. Furthermore, two additional independent studies have reported synergistic effects (epistasis) between the *gsk-3β* and either the *MAPT* (tau) genes (Kwok et al., 2008) or the p35 subunit of cdk5 (Mateo et al., 2009) in late-onset AD, further supporting a genetic association between *gsk-3β* and AD. Interestingly, a genetic polymorphism that increases the ratio of GSK-3β1 to GSK-3β2 interacts with tau haplotypes and modifies risk in Parkinson's and Alzheimer's disease (Kwok et al. 2005, 2008).

## 4. The role of GSK-3 in tau phosphorylation

Tau protein is a microtubule-associated protein (MAP) that in normal physiological conditions binds to microtubules (MT), regulating their assembly, dynamic behaviour, and spatial organization (Drechsel et al., 1992; LoPresti et al., 1995). Later on, tau has also been shown to regulate the axonal transport of organelles, including mitochondria (Ebneth et al., 1998). Tau is primarily, though not exclusively, a neuronal protein encoded by a single gene but with six major isoforms derived by alternative splicing (Goedert et al., 1989; Himmler et al., 1989). The interaction between tau and tubulin is mediated by four imperfect repeat domains (31-32 residues) encoded by exons 9-12 (Lee et al., 1989). Alternative splicing of exon 10 gives rise to isoforms with 3 or 4 binding domains (3R and 4R tau) (Goedert et al., 1989). Adult human brain shows a 1:1 ratio of 3R and 4R isoforms whereas foetal brain, however, only expresses 3R tau, demonstrating developmental regulation of exon 10 splicing. Different brain regions also differ in the relative levels of 3R and 4R isoforms with granule cells in the hippocampal formation reported to have only 3R tau (Goedert et al., 1989). Disturbances in this ratio are a common feature in most neurodegenerative tauopathies, including AD.

Within neurons, tau is predominantly found in axons as a highly soluble phosphoprotein. As mentioned in the case of alternative splicing, phosphorylation is also developmentally regulated, with a high tau phosphorylation level during embryogenesis and early development, when only the shortest of the isoforms is being expressed. By contrast, adult brain expresses all six isoforms with relatively reduced phosphorylation levels compared with the foetal one (see [Hanger et al., 2009] for a review).

Upon abnormal phosphorylation, the microtubule-associated protein tau reduces its affinity for and dissociates from microtubules. In AD brains tau accumulates in the neuronal perikarya and processes as paired helical filaments (PHF). It has been suggested that at the single-cell level the defects start with a modification of tau by phosphorylation, resulting in a destabilization of microtubules giving rise to a "pre-tangle" stage. After this stage, the destabilization of microtubules leads to loss of dendritic microtubules and synapses, plasma membrane degeneration, and eventually cell death (Iqbal et al., 2009).

The knowledge accumulated in the last years strongly suggest that tau-induced neurodegeneration is most likely a consequence of a combination of loss of (tau) function as well as gain of (toxic) function. On one hand, tau detachment from microtubules after hyperphosphorylation (or mutations) causes impaired microtubule function and axonal transport and eventually synaptic dysfunction and neurodegeneration (Jaworski et al., 2010). On the other hand, hyperphosphorylated tau molecules tend to self-assemble into filaments such as PHF or straight filaments (SF) that form the NFT. But hyperphosphorylated tau seems to also have the capacity of sequestering normal tau molecules (and perhaps other microtubule-associated proteins) into the aggregates, which will also have a negative impact on the normal microtubule function. At some point after detaching from microtubules and getting into the aggregation process, tau molecules also suffer other post-translational modifications such as truncation (Delobel et al., 2008; Gamblin et al., 2003; Nvak et al., 1993), glycosylation (Wang et al., 1996), O-GlcNAcylation (Arnold et al., 1996; Hart et al., 1996), and ubiquitination (Bancher et al., 1991; Mori et al., 1987), which could also contribute to the pathology. For a recent review on the molecular mechanisms by which tau induces neurodegeneration please refer to (Brunden et al., 2009; Iqbal et al., 2009).

Interestingly, recent data strongly indicates that some soluble, oligomeric (pre-filament, immature filaments) tau species, rather than the tangles, are indeed the pathogenic ones (Bretteville & Planel, 2008, Congdon & Duff, 2008), reminiscent of what has happened in recent years in the amyloid field regarding plaques and intermediate Aβ oligomers (Haass & Selkoe, 2007; Walsh & Selkoe, 2007). For a very long time, tangles or fibrils have been considered to be the pathological species, but it has become clear now that, much like amyloid plaques, NFT are the final stages of a pathological process, but the real damage might actually be done by some intermediate hyperphosphorylated, most likely soluble tau species (Brunden et al., 2009; Iqbal et al., 2009; Jaworski et al., 2010). In fact, there is some evidence suggesting that NFT might be protective indeed, as tangle-bearing neurons seem to survive for long periods of time (Andorfer et al., 2005; de Calignon et al., 2009; Morsch et al., 1999). More recently, some novel mechanisms of propagation of tau protein misfolding from the extracellular to the intracellular space, both *in vitro* (Frost et al., 2009) and *in vivo* (Clavaguera et al., 2010) have been described. The demonstration of a link between tau oligomers and brain pathology in animal models has lately sparked the interest of tau immunotherapies (Boutajangout et al., 2010; Kayed & Jackson, 2009; Medina, 2011; Sigurdsson, 2008).

GSK-3 induces tau phosporylation in several primed and unprimed PHF phosphoepitopes, both *in vitro* and in cell cultures. Activation of the insulin or Wnt signalling pathways increase tau phosphorylation mediated by GSK-3 (Caricasole et al., 2004; Lesort et al., 1999). Furthermore, some genetic studies show an association of Wnt signalling with AD through the low-density lipoprotein receptor-related protein 6 (LRP6), a co-receptor for Wnt signalling, which has been identified as a genetic risk for a subpopulation of late onset AD (De Ferrari et al., 2007). In addition, epidemiological and genetic studies also associate diabetes and insulin resistance with AD (Biessels & Kappelle, 2005; Hamilton et al., 2007; Reiman et al., 2007).

Persistent tau phosphorylation might results in neuritic dystrophy. Lipophosphatidic acid treated neurons result in GSK-3-dependent persistent tau phosphorylation followed by neurite retraction and growth cone collapse (Sayas et al., 2002). Several animal models, which exhibit persistent tau phosphorylation, also display neuritic dystrophy. For instance mice lacking either Reelin, mammalian disabled (mDab1), or VLDLR2 and ApoER2 exhibit persistent tau phosphorylation and have neuritic dystrophy and cytoskeletal abnormalities associated with them (Hiesberger et al., 1999; Sheldon et al., 1997). It is conceivable that persistent phosphorylation by GSK-3 results in neuritic dystrophy and subsequent cytoskeletal breakdown. In *Drosophila,* tau overexpression in combination with phosphorylation by the *Drosophila* GSK-3 homolog *Shaggy,* exacerbated neurodegeneration induced by tau overexpression alone, leading to neurofibrillary pathology (Jackson et al., 2002).

Recent evidence points out to GSK-3 linking tau and neuronal polarity through a protein called CRMP-2 (collapsing response mediator protein-2) which is essential for regulating axon growth and promotes assembly of microtubules (Cole et al., 2004). GSK-3 not only phosphorylates tau but also several CRMPs (Cole et al., 2006), including CRMP-2 (Yoshimura et al., 2005) at Thr514, a residue crucial for controlling its activity. Low levels of phosphorylated CRMP-2 at that residue are present in the growth cone and are associated with axon growth, which is consistent with previous data demonstrating that inhibition of GSK-3 results in enhanced neurite outgrowth (Muñoz-Montaño et al., 1999). These data were substantially backed up by a different group (Jiang et al., 2005) that also found that GSK-3 is spatially regulated, with the ratio of inactive (phosphorylated at S9) versus active (unphosphorylated) being highest in the axon tips, consistent with the fact that higher levels of unphosphorylated CRMP-2 drive axon development, and hence, neural polarity.

## 5. The role of GSK-3 in Aβ formation and neurotoxicity

While not universally accepted, the so-called amyloid hypothesis of AD has provided the main conceptual framework for studying the causes of the diseases and developing new therapeutic interventions during the last quarter of century. According to it, the gradual cerebral accumulation of soluble and insoluble assemblies of the amyloid Aβ peptide triggers a cascade of biochemical and cellular alterations that produce the clinical phenotype of AD (Hardy & Higgins, 1992; Hardy & Selkoe, 2002; Selkoe, 1991). The reasons for elevated Aβ levels in most patients with sporadic, late-onset AD are unknown, but recent evidence suggest that these could turn out to include increased neuronal release of Aβ during some kind of synaptic activity (Selkoe, 2002; 2008).

GSK-3 inhibition *per se* decreases Aβ production in cells and in an animal model of amyloidosis, as shown using non-isoform selective pharmacological inhibitors such as lithium, kenpaullone as well as small interfering RNA against the α isoform of GSK-3 (Phiel et al., 2003; Su et al., 2004; Sun et al., 2002). The exact mechanism by which this occurs remains unclear and in fact the isoform specificity of the effect on Aβ production is still highly controversial. However, the observation that amyloid precursor protein (APP) C-terminal fragments accumulate in the presence of these inhibitors suggests that GSK-3 may influence γ-secretase activity. γ-secretase activity is a multiprotein complex that is necessary for the terminal cleavage of APP to generate the Aβ fragment. Interestingly, inhibition of GSK-3 failed to demonstrate accumulation of C-terminal fragments of the Notch protein, which is also a substrate for γ-secretase (Phiel et al., 2003). Actually, GSK-3 has been shown to bind and phosphorylate presenilin 1 (PS1), the catalytic component of the γ-secretase complex, acting perhaps as a docking protein and regulating phosphorylation of some GSK-3 substrates such as tau and β-catenin (Palacino et al., 2001; Su et al., 2004; Takashima et al., 1998; Tesco & Tanzi, 2002; Twomey & McCarthy, 2006). PS1 has been shown to inactivate GSK-3 through PI3K/Akt signalling, preventing tau phosphorylation and apoptosis. Interestingly, PS1 FAD mutations inhibit PS1-dependent PI3K/Akt signalling, facilitating GSK-3 and thus tau phosphorylation (Baki et al., 2004). Furthermore, APP has also been shown to be a substrate for GSK-3 *in vitro* (Aplin et al., 1996) and *in vivo* (Rockenstein et al., 2007), suggesting a role of GSK-3 in APP transport and maturation (da Cruz e Silva & da Cruz e Silva, 2003; Lee et al., 2003) from the early secretory pathway through the axon terminals, perhaps controlling APP processing. Finally, modulation of the GSK-3 signalling pathway by chronic lithium treatment of transgenic animals has been shown to have neuroprotective effects by regulating APP maturation and processing (Rockenstein et al., 2007).

A substantial body of evidence has established the toxic properties of extracellular Aβ peptides on neuronal cells (Selkoe, 2008). Non-neuronal cells however are generally resistant to Aβ treatment, with some exceptions such as endothelial cells and smooth muscle cells (Suhara et al., 2003). On the other hand, oligomers of the Aβ peptide have been reported to act as antagonists for insulin (Towsend et al. 2007) or Wnt (Magdesian et al. 2008) receptors, resulting in an increase in GSK-3 activity. Also, a PS1 lack of function by mutations such as those present in some familial AD patients has been suggested to result in an increase of GSK-3 activity (Baki et al., 2004).

As mentioned, the aggregation of Aβ peptide into soluble oligomers is considered an early event in Alzheimer's disease and the presence of these aggregates seems to lead to neurodegeneration in the context of this disease. However, the mechanisms underlying Aβ-induced neurotoxicity are not completely understood. Although previous studies in mice have suggested that GSK-3 alters Aβ levels via modulation of APP processing (Phiel et al., 2003; Rockenstein et al., 2007), the direct effects of the enzyme on Aβ toxicity, and in the adult nervous system, have not been examined in depth. A recent study has tackled this particular issue of the specific role of GSK-3 in regulating Aβ42 toxicity in adult neurons *in vivo*, by modulating its activity in an adult-onset *Drosophila* model of Alzheimer's disease (Sofola et al., 2010). This study shows that GSK-3 inhibition ameliorates Aβ42 toxicity in adult flies, and also highlights a novel mechanism of protection by which GSK-3 directly regulates Aβ42 levels in the absence of any effects on APP processing.

## 6. The role of GSK-3 in synaptic plasticity, learning and memory

GSK-3 has also been shown to phosphorylate and inhibit kinesin-mediated motility. Fast axonal transport misregulation has been hypothesized to play a role in Alzheimer's disease pathogenesis (Morfini et al., 2002). Fibrillar Aβ binds to and induces the clustering of the integrin receptors, leading to the activation of paxillin and focal adhesion kinases. Interestingly, active GSK-3 associates with focal adhesion proteins suggesting the possibility that GSK-3 might mediate neuritic dystrophy via these interactions (Grace & Busciglio, 2003). Abnormal increase in GSK-3 activity has been shown to cause neurodegeneration and interfere with synaptic plasticity (for review see Bhat & Budd, 2002; Bhat & Froelich-Fabre, 2004).

Another important aspect of GSK-3 function is its role in the assembly and disassembly of synapses determining synaptic plasticity. Regarding memory, some states of synaptic plasticity may be considered as a balance between long-term potentiation (LTP) and long-term depression (LTD), with the former strengthening synaptic connections and the latter weakening them. Interestingly, GSK-3 appears to be a key factor in swaying that balance (Hooper et al., 2007; Peineau et al., 2007) since after LTP induction, GSK-3 becomes temporarily inactivated, support for LTD is lost and LTP comes out on top. This is relevant from the drug discovery point of view, since it implies that inhibition of GSK-3 might boost LTP and depress LTD, in principle a good thing for learning and memory. The precise molecular mechanism by which GSK-3 influences these processes remains to be elucidated, although some preliminary data seems to suggest that installation or maintenance of AMPA receptors might play a role (Peinau et al., 2007). Several GSK-3 downstream substrates such as CRMP-2 or the cAMP responsive element-binding protein (CREB) are also involved in synaptic remodelling, a key process required for memory formation. All this evidence has led to propose that GSK-3 acts as a gate through which LTP and memory are established (Hooper et al., 2008) and that memory failure in AD may be due to the inhibition of LTP by GSK-3 overactivity, with neuronal loss ensuing during disease progression.

It is well established that Aβ oligomers inhibit LTP and enhance LTD (Shieh et al., 2003; Walsh et al., 2002; Selkoe, 2008), although the precise mechanisms by which Aβ interferes with long-term plasticity have remained largely unknown. Very recently, GSK-3 has revealed as a key enzyme in mediating Aβ-induced LTP inhibition (Jo et al., 2011). In this study, treatment of rat hippocampal slices with Aβ oligomers induced caspase 3-mediated cleavage of Akt-1, resulting in GSK-3 activation. Consistent with it, treatment with a GSK-3 inhibitor completely prevented Aβ oligomers from inhibiting LTP.

## 7. Lithium as a GSK-3 inhibitor

The finding that the mood stabilizing drug lithium directly inhibited GSK-3 initially sparked the interest for this enzyme as a potential target for mood disorders. Lithium and valproic acid are mood stabilizers widely used in the chronic treatment of bipolar disorders. Lithium ions directly inhibit GSK-3 (Klein & Melton, 1996), most likely by competing with magnesium, while valproic acid inhibits GSK-3 activity in relevant therapeutic concentrations in human neuroblastoma cells (Chen et al., 1999), most likely through an indirect mechanism (Rosenberg, 2007).

The mechanism of action by which lithium exerts its therapeutic effects is not known but it is conceivable that the acute effects on GSK-3 results in changes in gene regulation and cellular changes which could affect the neuronal plasticity over time (Gould & Manji, 2002; Jope, 1999; Lennox & Hahn, 2000). Lithium also inhibits at least four phosphomonoesterases (including inositol monophosphatase) (York et al., 1995), and phosphoglucomutase (Ray & Szymanki, 1978; Stambolic & Woodgett, 1994), apart from GSK-3 (Klein & Melton, 1996; Li-Smerin et al., 2001). That said, GSK-3 is significantly inhibited at therapeutic lithium concentrations (Gould & Manji, 2002; Phiel et al., 2003; Shaldubina et al., 2001). Thus, if a significant proportion of lithium's therapeutic actions in bipolar disorder results from the inhibition of GSK-3, then this enzyme would be an important target for bipolar disorder (Li et al., 2002; Rowe et al., 2007).

In spite of these attributes, lithium has a narrow therapeutic window (blood serum levels 0.6 to 1.2 mM) above which side effects are intolerable. Overdose can lead to severe neurological dysfunction and in some cases death. Non-CNS side effects of lithium (not uncommonly within therapeutic levels) include tremor, polyuria, polydipsia, nausea, and weight gain. Lithium can have adverse reactions with other drug classes including diuretics, NSAIDS, and other drugs that alter kidney function (see Gould & Manji, 2006 for a review).

There are only a few observational studies that have attempted to address the clinical effect of lithium in patients with AD. A retrospective study with a large sample of patients with dementia resulted in an increased risk of AD in patients who had been treated with lithium within 4 years prior to diagnosis (Ayuso-Mateo et al., 2001), although it is possible that this is partially accounted for by the increased occurrence of depression associated with AD. Moreover, a single case study reported in dementia patient showed that lithium treatment alleviated symptoms of aggression and agitation, while cognition persisted after 1.5 years of treatment (Havens et al., 1982). Furthermore, a significantly increased global cognitive ability as measured by MMSE in non-demented patients appears associated with lithium intake (Terao et al., 2006). The study design and low sample size precludes however to draw any causative conclusion from those studies.

Some pilot studies have been carried out to directly address the effect of lithium treatment in AD patients. An open label feasibility and tolerability study on a small cohort of 22 subjects patients receiving a low dose of lithium was carried out in UK, reported a high discontinuation rate despite few, relatively mild and reversible side effects (MacDonald et al., 2008). A second randomized, single-blind, placebo-controlled, parallel group, multicentre 10-week study was carried out in Germany as a proof-of-principle (Hampel et al., 2009). A total of 71 patients with mild AD (MMSE scores between 21 and 26) were treated with lithium or placebo for 10 weeks after which neuropsychological and neuropsychiatric assessment was performed together with some biomarkers determinations in plasma (Aβ1-42), lymphocytes (GSK-3 activity) and CSF (total tau, phospho-tau, and Aβ1-42). In spite of the fact that lithium plasma levels were within the therapeutic range, no treatment effect was observed in any the cognition assessment scales used or the selected biomarkers. Given the short time of treatment of this study, the possibility that lithium has long-term effects on cognition or any other biomarker in AD remains to be tested.

## 8. Development of GSK-3 inhibitors and their therapeutic potential

The unique position of GSK-3 as a pivotal and central player in the pathogenesis of both sporadic and familial forms of AD has attracted significant attention to this enzyme as a therapeutic target and also as a means to understand the molecular basis underlying AD and related disorders. This has led to the synthesis of a high number of GSK-3 inhibitors, some of which are currently being tested in phase II proof-of-concept clinical trials (Mangialasche et al., 2010; Medina & Avila, 2010). Inhibition of GSK-3 with small molecules would be expected to slow down progression of neurodegeneration in AD and perhaps other tauopathies as well.

A number of novel potent and fairly selective small-molecule inhibitors of GSK-3 activity from different chemical families have recently been described, including hymenialdisine, indirubins, paullones, maleimides, amino pyrazoles, thiazoles, and 2,4-disubstituted thiadiazolidinones (TDZD) (reviewed in Medina & Castro, 2008). Most of them are ATP-competitive inhibitors, although more recently new small molecule derivatives that exhibit substrate competitive inhibition activity toward GSK-3 have been reported. Since the different GSK-3 isoforms display a high degree of homology within the ATP binding site, inhibitors are unable to exhibit isoform selectivity, as they all show similar potencies towards purified GSK-3α and GSK-3β.

Although the ATP-competitive inhibitors occupy the general area of the highly conserved ATP-binding site, they do explore other available space nearby depending upon their structure and it is possible to obtain selective inhibitors by taking advantage of the small differences that exist between the different kinases. Crystal structures of GSK-3β complexed with a variety of ligands, together with molecular modelling approaches, provide the necessary clues for enhancing selectivity towards GSK-3 (Patel et al., 2007; ter Haar et al., 2001). All ATP-binding site inhibitors make hydrogen bonds with backbone atoms of the kinase domain hinge (residues Asp 133 to Thr 138). The hydrogen bonds are the same as observed with ATP although different inhibitors make different combinations of hydrogen bonds. For instance, the two indirubin complexes (PDB 1UV5 and 1Q41) have four hydrogen bonds. In contrast, the Alsterpaullone complex (PDB 1Q3W) only has three hydrogen bonds (with the two backbone atoms of Val 135).

Some GSK-3 inhibitors also target other areas of the ATP pocket. For instance the nitro-group of the Alsterpaullone (PDB 1Q3W) and the chlorine of I-5 (3-anilino-4-arylmaleimide) interact with the conserved catalytic lysine, Lys 85. The bromine atom of 6-bromoindirubin (PDB 1UV5) is buried in the hydrophobic pocket of GSK-3β between residues Leu 132, Leu 130 and Met 101. This is a pocket that is often targeted to increase the selectivity of the inhibitor since it is one of the most diverse areas in the ATP-binding site of kinases and has been successfully used for instance to increase the selectivity in favour of p38α over ERK2. The GSK-3β ATP-binding site inhibitors do not cover the γ-phosphate transfer area. Targeting this part of the ATP-binding site does not appear to improve the selectivity of the inhibitor, although it may improve the potency as additional contacts between the inhibitor and the protein are established (ter Haar et al., 2006).

Some physiological peptides act as GSK-3 inhibitors, including GBP, a maternal *Xenopus* GSK-3 binding protein homologous to a mammalian T cell proto-oncogene (Yost et al., 1998) and p24, a heat resistant GSK-3 binding protein (Martín et al., 2002). That finding led to a synthetic strategy to develop new inhibitors, such as L803-mts, a peptidic inhibitor that binds to the substrate site (Plotkin et al., 2003). L803-mts has been more recently used to examine the impact of long-term *in vivo* inhibition of GSK-3 and its effects in specific tissues (Kaidanocih-Beilin & Eldar-Finkelman, 2006).

One classical approach for identifying GSK-3 inhibitors has exploited screening programs specifically aimed at finding new hits among compounds that exhibit other pharmacological profiles. However, the availability of X-ray crystallographic data of GSK-3β and several of its complexes with different inhibitors (ter Haar, 2006) in recent years has enabled the application of rational drug optimisation programs to discover new lead compounds. Molecular docking studies on the inhibitors of GSK-3 kinase in the enzyme binding sites of the X-ray complexes studies provide valuable insights into computational strategies useful for the identification of potential GSK-3 inhibitors (Gadakar et al., 2007). As a result of the great amount of information concerning current GSK-3 inhibitors, there are a huge number of reported empirical structure-activity relationships (SAR) that may guide a rational design of more potent and selective inhibitors. However, only a few studies based on Quantitative Structure-Activity Relationships (QSAR) are available for predicting the inhibitor potency against this specific kinase, and they involve mainly molecular modelling and 3D-QSAR (Medina & Castro, 2008).

The last few years have seen the synthesis of quite a number of fairly selective, potent GSK-3 inhibitors which have started to show *in vivo* efficacy in a diverse array of animal models of human diseases, including Alzheimer's disease. Despite the challenges faced by this approach with respect to safety and specificity, a number of efforts are underway to develop kinase inhibitors and in fact, Noscira's tideglusib (NP12), is already in phase II clinical trials for the treatment of both Alzheimer's disease and progressive supranuclear palsy (PSP), a tauopathy (Medina & Castro, 2008; Medina & Avila, 2010).

## 9. Conclusion

Three decades after its discovery as a protein kinase involved in glycogen metabolism, GSK-3 has revealed as a cellular nexus, integrating several signalling systems, including several second messengers and a wide selection of cellular stimulants. Modulation of its activity has also turned out to be much more complex than originally thought as control of GSK-3 activity occurs by complex mechanisms that are each dependent upon specific signalling pathways, including post-translational modifications, protein complex formation and subcellular localization. Although there seems to be a good degree of functional overlapping between the different isoforms, some tissue- and isoform-specific functions and substrates are starting to emerge and more will most likely be discovered within the next few years and will open the possibility to design better, more specific inhibitors.

Deregulation or abnormal GSK-3 activity appears to be associated with various relevant pathologies, including Alzheimer's disease, as the enzyme is uniquely positioned as a key, central player in AD pathogenesis, having a critical role in key events such as tau phosphorylation, Aβ formation and neurotoxicity, microtubule dynamics, synaptic plasticity, neuritic dystrophy, cognition, neuronal survival, and neurodegeneration. Furthermore, recent reports point out to a genetic association of the *gsk-3* gene with the risk of AD either by itself or synergistically with tau or cdk5 genes.

Drug discovery and development efforts for AD in the last two decades have primarily focused on targets defined by the amyloid cascade hypothesis, so far with disappointing results, underscoring the need of novel therapeutic approaches and targets. A significant effort has being made in the last few years to synthesize a high number of fairly selective, potent GSK-3 inhibitors, while some of them have shown *in vivo* efficacy in various animal models of AD. Some of the known drug discovery and development challenges will be faced: lack of good predictive animal models, lack of good validated biomarkers of disease progression, clinical trial design, early diagnosis and treatment, definition of target population, difficulties in demonstrating disease modifying effects, etc. Despite the challenges faced by this approach with respect to safety and specificity, a number of efforts are underway to develop GSK-3 inhibitors as useful drugs for the treatment of AD as some compounds have already reached phase II clinical trials and some proof-of-concept studies are currently ongoing or planned.

## 10. Acknowledgments

MM acknowledges grant support from EU-FP7 (Neuro.GSK3, project # 223276) and from CDTI's CENIT program (DENDRIA, project # CEN-20101023).

## 11. References

Abe K, and Takeichi M (2007) NMDA-receptor activation induces calpain-mediated beta-catenin cleavages for triggering gene expression. *Neuron* 53: 387-97.

Aberle H, Bauer A, Stappert J, Kispert A, Kemler R (1997) Beta-catenin is a target for the ubiquitin-proteasome pathway. *EMBO J* 16(13): 3797-804.

Agarwal-Mawal A, Qureshi HY, Cafferty PW, Yuan Z, Han D, Lin R, and Paudel HK (2003) 14-3-3 connects glycogen synthase kinase-3 beta to tau within a brain microtubule-associated tau phosphorylation complex. *J Biol Chem* 278 (15): 12722-8.

Alonso A del C, Li B, Grundke-Iqbal I, and Iqbal K (2006) Polymerization of hyperphosphorylated tau into filaments eliminates its inhibitory activity. *Proc Natl Acad Sci U S A* 103: 8864-9

Alvarez G, Muñoz-Montaño JR, Satrústegui J, Avila J, Bogónez E, Díaz-Nido J. (1999) Lithium protects cultured neurons against beta-amyloid-induced neurodegeneration. *FEBS Lett* 453(3): 260-4.

Amit S, Hatzubai A, Birman Y, Andersen JS, Ben-Shushan E, Mann M, Ben-Neriah Y, and Alkalay I (2002) Axin-mediated CKI phosphorylation of beta-catenin at Ser 45: a molecular switch for the Wnt pathway. *Genes Dev* 16: 1066-76

Andorfer C, Acker CM, Kress Y, Hof PR, Duff K, Davies P (2005) Cell-cycle reentry and cell death in transgenic mice expressing nonmutant human tau isoforms. *J Neurosci* 25(22): 5446-54.

Aplin AE, Gibb GM, Jacobsen JS, Gallo JM, Anderton BH. (1996) In vitro phosphorylation of the cytoplasmic domain of the amyloid precursor protein by glycogen synthase kinase-3b. *J. Neurochem.* 67(2):699-707

Arnold CS, Johnson GV, Cole RN, Dong DL, Lee M, Hart GW (1996) The microtubule-associated protein tau is extensively modified with O-linked N- acetylglucosamine. *J Biol Chem* 271(46): 28741-4.

Ayuso-Mateos JL, Vázquez-Barquero JL, Dowrick C, Lehtinen V, Dalgard OS, Casey P, Wilkinson C, Lasa L, Page H, Dunn G, Wilkinson G; ODIN Group (2001) Depressive disorders in Europe: prevalence figures from the ODIN study. *Br J Psychiatry* 179: 308-16.

Bain J, Plater L, Elliott M, Shpiro N, Hastie CJ, McLauchlan H, Klevernic I, Arthur JS, Alessi DR, and Cohen P (2007) The selectivity of protein kinase inhibitors: a further update. *Biochem J* 408: 297-315.

Baki L, Shioi J, Wen P, Shao Z, Schwarzman A, Gama-Sosa M, Neve R and Robakis NK (2004) PS1 activates PI3K thus inhibiting GSK-3 activity and tau overphosphorylation: effects of FAD mutations. *EMBO J* 23: 2586-96.

Baki, L., Shioi, J., Wen, P., Shao, Z., Schwarzman, A., Gama-Sosa, M., Neve, R. and Robakis, N.K. (2004) PS1 activates PI3K thus inhibiting GSK-3 activity and tau overphosphorylation: effects of FAD mutations. EMBO J. 23, 2586-96.

Bancher C, Grundke-Iqbal I, Iqbal K, Fried VA, Smith HT, Wisniewski HM (1991) Abnormal phosphorylation of tau precedes ubiquitination in neurofibrillary pathology of Alzheimer disease. *Brain Res* 539(1): 11-8.

Beaulieu JM, Zhang X, Rodriguez RM, Sotnikova TD, Cools MJ, Wetsel WC, Gainetdinov RR and Caron MG (2008) Role of GSK3 beta in behavioralabnormalities induced by serotonin deficiency. *Proc Natl Acad Sci USA* 105: 1333-1338.

Bhat R.V. and Froelich-Fabre S. (2004) Mechanisms of Tauopathies. *Drug Disc. Today Drug Disc.: Dis. Mech.*, 1, 391-8.

Bhat R.V., and Budd S. (2002) GSK3□ signaling: casting a wide net in Alzheimer´s Disease. *Neurosignals*, 11, 251-61.

Biessels GJ and Kappelle LJ (2005) Increased risk of Alzheime's disease in Type II diabetes: insulin resistance of the brain or insulin-induced amyloid pathology? *Biochem. Soc. Trans.* 33, 1041-4.

Boutajangout A, Quartermain D, Sigurdsson EM. (2010) Immunotherapy targeting pathological tau prevents cognitive decline in a new tangle mouse model. *J Neurosci* 30(49): 16559-66.

Bretteville A, Planel E (2008) Tau aggregates: toxic, inert, or protective species? *J Alzheimers Dis* 14(4): 431-6

Brunden KR, Trojanowski JQ, Lee VM (2009) Advances in tau-focused drug discovery for Alzheimer's disease and related tauopathies. *Nat Rev Drug Discov* 8(10): 783-93.

Buch I, Fishelovitch D, London N, Raveh B, Wolfson HJ, and Nussinov R (2010). Allosteric regulation of glycogen synthase kinase 3beta: a theoretical study. *Biochemistry* 49: 10890-901.

Cardona-Gomez P, Perez M, Avila J, Garcia-Segura LM, and Wandosell F (2004) Estradiol inhibits GSK3 and regulates interaction of estrogen receptors, GSK3, and beta-catenin in the hippocampus. *Mol Cell Neurosci* 25: 363-73.

Caricasole A, Copani A, Caraci F, Aronica E, Rozemuller AJ, Caruso A, Storto M, gaviraghi G, Terstappen GC and Nicoletti F (2004) Induction of Dikkopft-1, a negative modulator of the Wnt pathway, is associated with neuronal degeneration in Alzheimer's brain. *J. Neurosc*i. 24, 6021-27.

Castano Z, Gordon-Weeks PR and Kypta RM (2010) The neuron-specific isoform of glycogen synthase kinase-3beta is required for axon growth. *J Neurochem* 113: 117-130.

Chen G, Huang LD, Jiang YM, Manji HK (1999) The mood-stabilizing agent valproate inhibits the activity of glycogen synthase kinase-3. *J Neurochem* 72(3): 1327-30.

Chou HY, Howng SL, Cheng TS, Hsiao YL, Lieu AS, Loh JK, Hwang SL, Lin CC, Hsu CM, Wang C, Lee CI, Lu PJ, Chou CK, Huang CY, and Hong YR (2006) GSKIP is homologous to the Axin GSK3beta interaction domain and functions as a negative regulator of GSK3beta. *Biochemistry* 45: 11379-89.

Clavaguera F, Bolmont T, Crowther RA, Abramowski D, Frank S, Probst A, Fraser G, *et al.* (2010) Transmission and spreading of tauopathy in transgenic mouse brain. *Nat Cell Biol* 11(7): 909-13.

Cohen P, and Goedert M (2004) GSK3 inhibitors: development and therapeutic potential. *Nat Rev Drug Discov* 3: 479-87.

Cole A, Frame S, and Cohen P (2004) Further evidence that the tyrosine phosphorylation of glycogen synthase kinase-3 (GSK3) in mammalian cells is an autophosphorylation event. *Biochem J* 377: 249-55.

Cole AR, Causeret F, Yadirgi G, Hastie CJ, McLauchlan H, McManus EJ, Hernández F, Eickholt BJ, Nikolic M, and Sutherland C (2006) "Distinct priming kinases contribute to differential regulation of collapsin response mediator proteins by glycogen synthase kinase-3 in vivo" *J. Biol. Chem.* 281(24):16591-8.

Congdon EE, Duff KE (2008) Is tau aggregation toxic or protective? *J Alzheimers Dis* 14(4): 453-7.

da Cruz e Silva EF and da Cruz e Silva OA. (2003) Protein phosphorylation and APP metabolism. *Neurochem. Res.* 28(10): 1553-61.

Dajani R, Fraser E, Roe SM, Yeo M, Good VM, Thompson V, Dale TC, and Pearl LH (2003) Structural basis for recruitment of glycogen synthase kinase 3beta to the axin-APC scaffold complex. *EMBO J* 22: 494-501.

Dajani R, Fraser E, Roe SM, Young N, Good V, Dale TC, and Pearl LH (2001) Crystal structure of glycogen synthase kinase 3 beta: structural basis for phosphate-primed substrate specificity and autoinhibition. *Cell* 105: 721-32.

de Calignon A, Spires-Jones TL, Pitstick R, Carlson GA, Hyman BT (2009) Tangle-bearing neurons survive despite disruption of membrane integrity in a mouse model of tauopathy. *J Neuropathol Exp Neurol* 68(7): 757-61.

De Ferrari G.V., Papassotiropoulos A, Biechele T, Wavrant De-Vrieze F, Avila ME, Major MB, Myers A, Sáez K, Henríquez JP, Zhao A, Wollmer MA, Nitsch RM, Hock C, Morris CM, Hardy J, Moon RT. (2007) Common genetic variation within the low-density lipoprotein receptor-related protein 6 and late-onset Alzheimer's disease. *Proc. Natl. Acad. Sci.* 104, 9434-39.

Delcommenne M, Tan C, Gray V, Rue L, Woodgett J, and Dedhar S (1998) Phosphoinositide-3-OH kinase-dependent regulation of glycogen synthase kinase 3 and protein kinase B/AKT by the integrin-linked kinase. *Proc Natl Acad Sci U S A* 95: 11211-6.

Delobel P, Lavenir I, Fraser G, Ingram E, Holzer M, Ghetti B, Spillantini MG, Crowther RA, Goedert M. (2008) Analysis of tau phosphorylation and truncation in a mouse model of human tauopathy. *Am J Pathol* 172(1): 123-31.

Ding Q, Xia W, Liu JC, Yang JY, Lee DF, Xia J, Bartholomeusz G, Li Y, Pan Y, Li Z, Bargou RC, Qin J, Lai CC, Tsai FJ, Tsai CH, and Hung MC (2005) Erk associates with and primes GSK-3beta for its inactivation resulting in upregulation of beta-catenin. *Mol Cell* 19: 159-70.

Drechsel DN, Hyman AA, Cobb MH, Kirschner MW (1992) Modulation of the dynamic instability of tubulin assembly by the microtubule-associated protein tau. *Mol Biol Cell* 3(10): 1141-54.

Ebneth A, Godemann R, Stamer K, Illenberger S, Trinczek B, Mandelkow E (1998) Overexpression of tau protein inhibits kinesin-dependent trafficking of vesicles, mitochondria, and endoplasmic reticulum: Implications for Alzheimer's disease. *J Cell Biol* 143(3): 777-94.

Embi N, Rylatt DB, and Cohen P (1980) Glycogen synthase kinase-3 from rabbit skeletal muscle. Separation from cyclic-AMP-dependent protein kinase and phosphorylase kinase. *Eur. J. Biochem.* 107(2):519-27.

Eom TY and Jope RS (2009) Blocked inhibitory serine-phosphorylation of glycogen synthase kinase-3alpha/beta impairs in vivo neural precursor cell proliferation. *Biol Psychiatry* 66: 494-502.

Fang X, Yu SX, Lu Y, Bast RC Jr., Woodgett JR, and Mills GB (2000) Phosphorylation and inactivation of glycogen synthase kinase 3 by protein kinase A. *Proc Natl Acad Sci U S A* 97: 11960-5.

Ferkey DM & Kimelman D (2002) Glycogen synthase kinase-3 beta mutagenesis identifies a common binding domain for GBP and Axin. *J Biol Chem* 277: 16147-52.

Frame S and Cohen P (2001) GSK3 takes centre stage more than 20 years after its discovery. *Biochem J* 359: 1-16.

Frame S, Cohen P, and Biondi RM (2001) A common phosphate binding site explains the unique substrate specificity of GSK3 and its inactivation by phosphorylation. *Mol Cell* 7: 1321-7.

Fraser E, Young N, Dajani R, Franca-Koh J, Ryves J, Williams RS, Yeo M, Webster MT, Richardson C, Smalley CM, Pearl LH, Harwood A, and Dale TC (2002) Identification of the Axin and Frat binding region of glycogen synthase kinase-3. *J Biol Chem* 277: 2176-85.

Frost B, Jacks RL, Diamond MI. Propagation of tau misfolding from the outside to the inside of a cell (2009) *J Biol Chem* 284(19): 12845-52.

Gadakar PK, Phukan S, Dattatreya P, Balaji VN (2007) Pose prediction accuracy in docking studies and enrichment of actives in the active site of GSK-3beta. *J Chem Inf Model* 47(4):446-59.

Gamblin TC, Chen F, Zambrano A, Abraha A, Lagalwar S, Guillozet AL, Lu M, Fu Y, Garcia-Sierra F, LaPointe N, Miller R, Berry RW, Binder LI, Cryns VL (2993) Caspase cleavage of tau: linking amyloid and neurofibrillary tangles in Alzheimer's disease. *Proc Natl Acad Sci USA* 100(17): 10032-7

Goedert M, Spillantini MG, Potier MC, Ulrich J, Crowther RA (1989) Cloning and sequencing of the cDNA encoding an isoform of microtubule-associated protein tau containing four tandem repeats: differential expression of tau protein mRNAs in human brain. *EMBO J* 8(2): 393-9.

Goñi-Oliver P, Avila J, and Hernández F (2009a) Calpain-mediated truncation of GSK-3 in post-mortem brain samples. *J Neurosci Res* 87: 1156-61.

Goñi-Oliver P, Avila J, and Hernández F (2009b) Memantine inhibits calpain-mediated truncation of GSK-3 induced by NMDA: implications in Alzheimer's disease. *J Alzheimers Dis.* 18(4): 843-8.

Goñi-Oliver P, Lucas JJ, Avila J, and Hernández F (2007) N-terminal cleavage of GSK-3 by calpain: a new form of GSK-3 regulation. *J Biol Chem* 282: 22406-13.

Gould TD and Manji HK (2006) Glycogen synthase kinase 3: a target for novel mood disorder treatments. In: *Glycogen Synthase Kinase 3 (GSK-3) and Its Inhibitors-Drug discovery and Development.* Wang B (Ed), Ch 7, pp. 125-154. Wiley Series in Drug Discovery and Development. New Jersey, USA..

Gould TD, Manji HK (1995) The Wnt signaling pathway in bipolar disorder. *Neuroscientist* 8(5): 497-511.

Grace EA and Busciglio J (2003) Aberrant activation of focal adhesion proteins mediates fibrillar amyloid β-induced neuronal dystrophy. *J. Neurosci.* 23, 493-502.

Grimes CA, and Jope RS (2001) The multifaceted roles of glycogen synthase kinase 3beta in cellular signaling. *Prog Neurobiol* 65: 391-426.

Haass C, Selkoe DJ (2007) protein oligomers in neurodegeneration: Lessons from the Alzheimer's amyloid beta-peptide. *Nat Rev Mol Cell Biol* 8(2): 101-12.

Hamilton G, Proitsi P, Jehu L, Morgan A, Williams J, O'Donovan M, Owen MJ, Powell JF and Lovestone S (2007) Candidate gene association study of insulin signalling genes and Alzheimer's disease: evidence for SOS2, PCK1, and PPARgamma as susceptibility loci. *Am. J. Med. Genet. B Neuropsychiatr. Genet.* 144, 508-16.

Hampel H, Ewers M, Bürger K, Annas P, Mörtberg A, Bogstedt A, Frölich L, Schröder J, Schönknecht P, Riepe MW, Kraft I, Gasser T, Leyhe T, Möller HJ, Kurz A, Basun H (2009) Lithium trial in Alzheimer's disease: a randomized, single-blind, placebo-controlled, multicenter 10-week study. *J Clin Psychiatry* 70(6): 922-31.

Hanger DP, Anderton BH, Noble W (2009) Tau phosphorylation: The therapeutic challenge for neurodegenerative disease. *Trends Mol Med* 15(3): 112-9.

Hardy J, Selkoe DJ (2002) The amyloid hypothesis of Alzheimer's disease: progress and problems on the road to therapeutics. Science 297: 353–356.

Hardy JA, Higgins GA (1992) Alzheimer's disease: the amyloid cascade hypothesis. *Science* 256: 184–185.

Hart GW, Kreppel LK, Comer FI, Arnold CS, Snow DM, Ye Z, Cheng X, DellaManna D, Caine DS, Earles BJ, Akimoto Y, Cole RN, Hayes BK (1996) O-GlcNAcylation of key nuclear and cytoskeletal proteins: reciprocity with O-phosphorylation and putative roles in protein multimerization. *Glycobiology* 6(7): 711-6.

Hartigan JA, Xiong WC, and Johnson GV (2001) Glycogen synthase kinase 3beta is tyrosine phosphorylated by PYK2. *Biochem Biophys Res Commun* 284: 485-9.

Harwood AJ (2001) Regulation of GSK-3: a cellular multiprocessor. *Cell* 105: 821-4.

Havens WW 2nd, Cole J (1982) Successful treatment of dementia with lithium. *J Clin Psychopharmacol* 2(1): 71-2.

Hemmings BA, Yellowlees D, Kernohan JC, and Cohen P (1981) Purification of glycogen synthase kinase 3 from rabbit skeletal muscle. Copurification with the activating factor (FA) of the (Mg-ATP) dependent protein phosphatase. *Eur. J. Biochem.* 119(3):443-51.

Hernández F, Gómez de Barreda E, Fuster-Matanzo A, Lucas JJ, Avila J (2010) GSK3: a possible link between beta amyloid peptide and tau protein. *Exp Neurol.* 223(2): 322-5.

Hiesberger T., Trommsdorff M., Howell B. W., Goffinet A., Mumby M. C., Cooper J. A. and Herz J. (1999) Direct binding of Reelin to VLDL receptor and ApoE receptor 2 induces tyrosine phosphorylation of disabled-1 and modulates tau phosphorylation. *Neuron* 24, 481-9.

Himmler A, Drechsel D, Kirschner MW, Martin DW Jr (1989) Tau consists of a set of proteins with repeated C-terminal microtubule-binding domains and variable N-terminal domains. *Mol Cell Biol* 9(4): 1381-8.

Hoeflich KP, Luo J, Rubie EA, Tsao M-S, Jin O and Woodgett JR (2000) Requirement for GSK3beta in cell surival and NFkB activation. *Nature* 406: 86-90.

Hooper C, Killick R, and Lovestone S (2008) The GSK3 hypothesis of Alzheimer's disease. *J. Neurochem.* 104: 1433-9.

Hooper C, Markevich V, Plattner F, Killick R, Schofield E, Engel T, Hernandez F, Anderton B, Rosenblum K, Bliss T, Cooke SF, Avila J, Lucas JJ, Giese KP, Stephenson J, and Lovestone S (2007) Glycogen synthase kinase-3 inhibition is integral to long-term potentiation. Eur. J. Neurosci. 25(1): 81-6.

Hoshi M, Sato M, Matsumoto S, Noguchi A, Yasutake K, Yoshida N, Sato K (2003) Spherical aggregates of beta-amyloid (amylospheroid) show high neurotoxicity and activate tau protein kinase I/glycogen synthase kinase-3beta. *Proc Natl Acad Sci U S A* 100(11): 6370-6375.

Hsieh H, Boehm J, Sato C, Iwatsubo T, Tomita T, Sisodia S, Malinow R (2006) AMPAR removal underlies Abeta-induced synaptic depression and dendritic spine loss. Neuron 52(5): 831-43.

Hughes K, Nikolakaki E, Plyte SE, Totty NF, Woodgett JR (1993) Modulation of the glycogen synthase kinase-3 family by tyrosine phosphorylation. *EMBO J* 12(2): 803-8.

Hur EM and Zhon FP (2010) GSK3 signalling in neural development. *Nat Rev Neurosci* 11: 539-51.

Inestrosa NC, Toledo EM (2008) The role of Wnt signaling in neuronal dysfunction in Alzheimer's Disease. *Mol Neurodegener* 24: 3-9.

Iqbal K, Liu F, Gong CX, Alonso Adel C, Grundke-Iqbal I (2009) Mechanisms of tau-induced neurdegeneration. *Acta Neuropathol* 118(1): 53-69.

Itoh K, Tang TL, Neel BG, and Sokol SY (1995) Specific modulation of ectodermal cell fates in Xenopus embryos by glycogen synthase kinase. *Development* 121, 3979-88.

Ittner LM, Götz J (2011) Amyloid-β and tau--a toxic pas de deux in Alzheimer's disease. *Nat Rev Neurosci* 12(2): 65-72.

Jackson G. R., Wiedau-Pazos M., Sang T. K., Wagle N., Brown C. A., Massachi S. and Geschwind D. H. (2002) Human wild-type tau interacts with wingless pathway components and produces neurofibrillary pathology in Drosophila. *Neuron* 34, 509-19

Jaworski T, Kügler S, Van Leuven F (2010) Modeling of tau-mediated synaptic and neuronal degeneration in Alzheimer's disease. *Int J Alzheimers Dis.* pii: 573138.

Jiang H, Guo W, Liang X, Rao Y. (2005) Both the establishment and the maintenance of neuronal polarity require active mechanisms: critical roles of GSK-3β and its upstream regulators. Cell. 120:123-35.

Jo J, Whitcomb DJ, Olsen KM, Kerrigan TL, Lo SC, Bru-Mercier G, Dickinson B, Scullion S, Sheng M, Collingridge G, Cho K (2011) Aβ(1-42) inhibition of LTP is mediated by a signaling pathway involving caspase-3, Akt1 and GSK-3β. Nat Neurosci [Epub ahead of print]. PMID: 21441921.

Jope RS (1999) Anti-bipolar therapy: mechanism of action of lithium. *Mol Psychiatry* 4(2): 117-28.

Kaidanovich-Beilin O, Eldar-Finkelman H (2006) Long-term treatment with novel glycogen synthase kinase-3 inhibitor improves glucose homeostasis in ob/ob mice: molecular characterization in liver and muscle. *J Pharmacol Exp Ther* 316(1): 17-24.

Kaidanovich-Beilin O, Lipina TV, Takao K van Eede M, Hattori S, Laliberté C, Khan M, Okamoto K, Chambers JW, Fletcher PJ, MacAulay K, Doble BW, Henkelman M, Miyakawa T, Roder J, Woodgett JR. (2009) Abnormalities in brain structure and behavior in GSK-3alpha mutant mice. *Mol Brain* 2: 35.

Kandasamy AD, and Schulz R (2009) Glycogen synthase kinase-3beta is activated by matrix metalloproteinase-2 mediated proteolysis in cardiomyoblasts. *Cardiovasc Res* 83: 698-706.

Kayed R, Jackson GR. Prefilament tau species as potential targets for immunotherapy for Alzheimer disease and related disorders (2009) *Curr Opin Immunol* 21(3): 359-63.

Kim L, Harwood A, and Kimmel AR (2002) Receptor-dependent and tyrosine phosphatase-mediated inhibition of GSK3 regulates cell fate choice. *Dev Cell* 3: 23-32.

Kim L, Liu J, and Kimmel AR (1999).The novel tyrosine kinase ZAK1 activates GSK3 to direct cell fate specification. *Cell* 99: 399-408.

Kim WY, Wang X, Wu Y, Doble BW, Patel S, Woodgett JR and Snider WD (2009) GSK-3 is a master regulator of neural progenitor homeostasis. *Nat Neurosci* 12: 1390-1397.

Kimura T, Yamashita S, Nakao S, Park JM, Murayama M, Mizoroki T, Yoshiike Y, Sahara N and Takashima A (2008) GSK-3beta is required for memory reconsolidation in adult brain. *PLoS One,* 3(10): e3540.

Klein PS, Melton DA (1996) A molecular mechanism for the effect of lithium on development. *Proc Natl Acad Sci USA* 93(16): 8455-9.

Kwok JB, Hallupp M, Loy CT, Chan DK, Woo J, Mellick GD, Buchanan DD, Silburn PA, Halliday GM, Schofield PR (2005) GSK3B polymorphisms alter transcription and splicing in Parkinson's disease. *Ann Neurol* 58(6): 829-39.

Kwok JB, Loy CT, Hamilton G, Lau E, Hallupp M, Williams J, Owen MJ, Broe GA, Tang N, Lam L, Powell JF, Lovestone S, Schofield PR (2008) Glycogen synthase kinase-3beta and tau genes interact in Alzheimer's disease. *Ann Neurol* 64(4): 446-54.

Lee G, Neve RL, Kosik KS (1989) The microtubule binding domain of tau protein. *Neuron* 2(6): 1615-24.

Lee JH, Lau KF, Perkinton MS, Standen CL, Shemilt SJ, Mercken L, Cooper JD, McLoughlin DM, Miller CC. (2003) The neuronal adaptor protein X11a reduces Aβ levels in the brains of Alzheimer's APPswe Tg2576 transgenic mice. *J Biol Chem.* 278(47): 47025-9.

Lenox RH, Hahn CG (2000) Overview of the mechanism of action of lithium in the brain: fifty-year update. *J Clin Psychiatry* 61(Suppl 9): 5-15.

Leroy K, Boutajangout A, Authelet M, Woodgett JR, Anderton BH, and Brion JP (2002) The active form of glycogen synthase kinase-3b is associated with granulovacuolar degeneration in neurons in Alzheimer's disease. *Acta Neuropathol.* 103(2):91-9.

Lesort M, Jope RS, and Johnson GV (1999) Insulin transiently increases tau phosphorylation: involvement of glycogen synthase kinase-3beta and Fyn tyrosine kinase. *J Neurochem* 72: 576-84.

Li L, Yuan H, Weaver CD, Mao J, Farr GH 3rd, Sussman DJ, Jonkers J, Kimelman D, and Wu D (1999) Axin and Frat1 interact with dvl and GSK, bridging Dvl to GSK in Wnt-mediated regulation of LEF-1. *EMBO J* 18: 4233-40.

Li X, Bijur GN, Jope RS (2002) Glycogen synthase kinase-3beta, mood stabilizers, and neuroprotection. *Bipolar Disord* 4(2): 137-44.

Li-Smerin, Y, Levitan ES and Johnson JW (2001) Free intracellular Mg(2+) concentration and inhibition of NMDA responses in cultured rat neurons. *J Physiol* 533: 729-43.

Liu KJ, Arron JR, Stankunas K, Crabtree GR and Longaker MT (2007) Chemical rescue of cleft palate and midline defects in conditional GSK3b mice. *Nature* 446: 79-82.

Liu SJ, AH Zhang, Li HL, Wang Q, Deng HM, Netzer WJ, Xu H, and Wang JZ (2003) Overactivation of glycogen synthase kinase-3 by inhibition of phosphoinositol-3 kinase and protein kinase C leads to hyperphosphorylation of tau and impairment of spatial memory. *J Neurochem* 87: 1333-44.

Lochhead PA, Kinstrie R, Sibbet G, Rawjee T, Morrice N and Cleghon V (2006) A chaperone-dependent GSK3beta transitional intermediate mediates activation-loop autophosphorylation. *Mol Cell* 24: 627-633.

LoPresti P, Szuchet S, Papasozomenos SC, Zinkowski RP, Binder LI (1995) Functional implications for the microtubule-associated protein tau: Localization in oligodendrocytes. *Proc Natl Acad Sci USA* 92(22): 10369-73.

MacAulay K, Doble BW, Patel S, Hansotia T, Sinclair EM, Drucker DJ, Nagy A and Woodgett JR (2007) Glycogen synthase kinase 3alpha-specific regulation of murine hepatic glycogen metabolism. *Cell Metab* 6: 329-337.

Macdonald A, Briggs K, Poppe M, Higgins A, Velayudhan L, Lovestone S (2008) A feasibility and tolerability study of lithium in Alzheimer's disease. *Int J Geriatr Psychiatry* 23(7): 704-11.

Magdesian MH, Carvalho MM, Mendes FA, Saraiva LM, Juliano MA, Juliano L, Garcia-Abreu J, and Ferreira ST (2008) Amyloid-beta binds to the extracellular cysteine-rich domain of Frizzled and inhibits Wnt/beta-catenin signaling. *J Biol Chem.* 283(14): 9359-68

Mangialasche F, Solomon A, Winblad B, Mecocci P, Kivipelto M (2010) Alzheimer's disease: clinical trials and drug development. *Lancet Neurol* 9(7): 702-16.

Mao Y, Ge X, Frank CL, Madison JM, Koehler AN, Doud MK, Tassa C, Berry EM, Soda T, Singh KK, Biechele T, Petryshen TL, Moon RT, Haggarty SJ, and Tsai LH (2009) Disrupted in schizophrenia 1 regulates neuronal progenitor proliferation via modulation of GSK3beta/beta-catenin signaling. *Cell* 136 (6), 1017-31.

Martín CP, Vázquez J, Avila J, Moreno FJ (2002) P24, a glycogen synthase kinase 3 (GSK 3) inhibitor. Biochim Biophys Acta. 2002 Jan 2;1586(1):113-22.

Mateo I, Infante J, Llorca J, Rodríguez E, Berciano J, Combarros O (2006) Association between glycogen synthase kinase-3beta genetic polymorphism and late-onset Alzheimer's disease. *Dement Geriatr Cogn Disord* 21(4): 228-32.

Mateo I, Vázquez-Higuera JL, Sánchez-Juan P, Rodríguez-Rodríguez E, Infante J, García-Gorostiaga I, Berciano J, Combarros O (2009) Epistasis between tau phosphorylation regulating genes (CDK5R1 and GSK-3beta) and Alzheimer's disease risk. *Acta Neurol Scand* 120(2): 130-3.

Medina M & Wandosell F (2011) Deconstructing GSK-3: the fine regulation of its activity) *Int J Alz Dis* (in press).

Medina M (2011) Recent developments in tau-based therapeutics for neurodegenerative diseases. *Recent Pat CNS Drug Discov* 6(1): 20-30

Medina M, Avila J (2010) Glycogen synthase kinase-3 (GSK-3) inhibitors for the treatment of Alzheimer's disease. *Curr Pharm Des* 16(25): 2790-8.

Medina M, Castro A (2008) Glycogen synthase kinase-3 (GSK-3) inhibitors reach the clinic. *Curr Opin Drug Discov Devel* 11(4): 533-43.

Moon RT, Kohn AD, De Ferrari GV, and Kaykas A (2004) Wnt and beta-catenin signalling: diseases and therapies. *Nat Rev Genet* 5: 691-701.

Morfini G., Pigino G., Beffert U., Busciglio J. and Brady S. T. (2002) Fast axonal transport misregulation and Alzheimer's disease. *Neuromol. Med.* 2, 89-99.

Mori H, Kondo J, Ihara Y. (1987) Ubiquitin is a component of paired helical filaments in Alzheimer's disease. *Science* 235(4796): 1641-4.

Morsch R, Simon W, Coleman PD (1999) Neurons may live for decades with neurofibrillary tangles. *J Neuropathol Exp Neurol* 58(2): 188-97.

Mukai F, Ishiguro K, Sano Y, Fujita SC (2002) Alternative splicing isoform of tau protein kinase I/glycogen synthase kinase 3 beta. *J Neurochem.* 81(5):1073-83.

Muñoz-Montaño JR, Lim F, Moreno FJ, Avila J, and Díaz-Nido J. (1999) Glycogen Synthase Kinase-3 Modulates Neurite Outgrowth in Cultured Neurons: Possible Implications for Neurite Pathology in Alzheimer's Disease. *J. Alzheimers Dis.* 1(6):361-78.

Munoz-Montano JR, Moreno FJ, Avila J, and Diaz-Nido J (1997) Lithium inhibits Alzheimer's disease-like tau protein phosphorylation in neurons. *FEBS Lett* 411: 183-8.

Muyllaert D, Kremer A, Jaworski T, Borghgraef P, Devijver H, Croes S, Dewatcher I, and Van Leuven F. (2008) Glycogen synthase kinase-3beta, or a link between amyloid and tau pathology? *Genes Brain Behav.* 7 (suppl. 1): 57-66.

Nishimura I, Yang Y, and Lu B (2004) PAR-1 kinase plays an initiator role in a temporally ordered phosphorylation process that confers tau toxicity in Drosophila. *Cell* 116: 671-82.

Noble W, Olm V, Takata K, Casey E, Mary O, Meyerson J, Gaynor K, LaFrancois J, Wang L, Kondo T, Davies P, Burns M, Veeranna, Nixon R, Dickson D, Matsuoka Y, Ahlijanian M, Lau LF, and Duff K (2003) Cdk5 is a key factor in tau aggregation and tangle formation in vivo. *Neuron* 38: 555-65.

Noble W, Planel E, Zehr C, Olm V, Meyerson J, Suleman F, Gaynor K, Wang L, LaFrancois J, Feinstein B, Burns M, Krishnamurthy P, Wen Y, Bhat R, Lewis J, Dickson D, and Duff K (2005) Inhibition of glycogen synthase kinase-3 by lithium correlates with reduced tauopathy and degeneration in vivo. *Proc Natl Acad Sci U S A* 102: 6990-5.

O'Brien WT, Harper AD, Jove F, Woodgett JR, Maretto S, Piccolo S and Klein PS (2004) Glycogen synthase kinase-3beta haploinsufficiency mimics the behavioral and molecular effects of lithium. *J Neurosci* 24: 6791-6798.

Osolodkin DI, Zakharevich NV, Palyulin VA, Danilenko VN, and Zefirov NS (2011) Bioinformatic analysis of glycogen synthase kinase 3: human versus parasite kinases.*Parasitology* Feb 24: 1-11.

Palacino J.J., Murphy M.P., Murayama O., Iwasaki K., Fujiwara M., Takashima A., Golde T.E., and Wolozin B. (2001) Presenilin 1 regulates β-catenin-mediated transcription in a glycogen synthase kinase-3-independent fashion. *J. Biol. Chem.* 276(42):38563-9.

Patel DS, Dessalew N, Iqbal P, Bharatam PV (2007) Structure-based approaches in the design of GSK-3 selective inhibitors. *Curr Protein Pept Sci* 8(4):352-64.

Patel S, Doble BW, MacAulay K, Sinclair EM, Drucker DJ, Woodgett JR (2008) Tissue-specific role of glycogen synthase kinase 3beta in glucose homeostasis and insulin action. *Mol Cell Biol* 28(20): 6314-28.

Patel S, Macaulay K, Woodgett JR (2011) Tissue-specific analysis of glycogen synthase kinase-3α (GSK-3α) in glucose metabolism: effect of strain variation. *PLoS One* 6(1): e15845.

Pei JJ, Tanaka T, Tung YC, Braak E, Iqbal K, and Grundke-Iqbal I (1997) Distribution, levels, and activity of glycogen synthase kinase-3 in the Alzheimer disease brain. J *Neuropathol Exp Neurol*. 56(1):70-8.

Peineau S, Taghibiglou C, Bradley C, Wong TP, Liu L, Lu J, Lo E, Wu D, Saule E, Bouschet T, Matthews P, Isaac JT, Bortolotto ZA, Wang YT, and Collingridge GL (2007) LTP inhibits LTD in the hippocampus via regulation of GSK-3ba. *Neuron*. 53(5):703-17.

Perez M, Rojo AI, Wandosell F, Diaz-Nido J, and Avila J (2003) Prion peptide induces neuronal cell death through a pathway involving glycogen synthase kinase 3. *Biochem J* 372: 129-36.

Phiel CJ, Wilson CA, Lee VM, and Klein PS (2003) GSK-3alpha regulates production of Alzheimer's disease amyloid-b peptides *Nature*. 423(6938):435-9.

Plotkin B, Kaidanovich O, Talior I, Eldar-Finkelman H (2003) Insulin mimetic action of synthetic phosphorylated peptide inhibitors of glycogen synthase kinase-3. J Pharmacol Exp Ther 305(3): 974-80.

Prickaerts J, Moechars D, Cryns K, Lenaerts I, van Craenendonck H, Goris I, Daneels G, Bouwknecht JA and Steckler T (2006) Transgenic mice overexpressing glycogen synthase kinase 3beta: a putative model of hyperactivity and mania. *J Neurosci* 26: 9022-9029.

Ray WJ Jr, Szymanki ES, Ng L (1978) The binding of lithium and of anionic metabolites to phosphoglucomutase. *Biochim Biophys Acta* 522(2): 434-42.

Reiman EM, Webster JA, Myers AL, Hardy J, Dunckley T, Zismann VL, Joshipura KD, Pearson JV, Hu-Lince D, Huentelman MJ, Craig DW, Coon KD, Liang WS, Herbert RH, Beach T, Rohrer KC, Zhao AS, Leung D, Bryden L, Marlowe L, Kaleem M, Mastroeni D, Grover A, Heward CB, Ravid R, Rogers J, Hutton ML, Melquist S, Petersen RC, Alexander GE, Caselli RJ, Kukull W, Papassotiropoulos A, Stephan DA. (2007) GAB2 alleles modify Alzheimer's risk in ApoE4 carriers. *Neuron* 54, 713-20.

Rockenstein E, Torrance M, Adame A, Mante M, Bar-on P, Rose JB, Crews L, and Masliah E. (2007) Neuroprotective effects of regulators of the glycogen synthase kinase-3b signaling pathway in a transgenic model of Alzheimer's disease are associated with reduced amyloid precursor protein phosphorylation. *J. Neurosci.* 27(8):1981-91.

Rosenberg (2007) The mechanisms of action of valproate in neuropsychiatric disorders: can we see the forest for the trees? *Cell Mol Life Sci* 64(16): 2090-103.

Ruel L, Bourouis M, Heitzler P, Pantesco V, and Simpson P (1993) Drosophila shaggy kinase and rat glycogen synthase kinase-3 have conserved activities and act downstream of Notch. *Nature* 362 57-60.

Russ C, Lovestone S, Powell JF (2001) Identification of sequence variants and analysis of the role of the glycogen synthase kinase 3 beta gene and promoter in late onset Alzheimer's disease. *Mol Psychiatry* 6(3): 320-4

Sayas C. L., Avila J. and Wandosell F. (2002) Regulation of neuronal cytoskeleton by lysophosphatidic acid: role of GSK-3. *Biochim. Biophys. Acta* 1582, 144-53.

Sayas CL, Moreno-Flores MT, Avila J, Wandosell F (1999) The neurite retraction induced by lysophosphatidic acid increases Alzheimer's disease-like Tau phosphorylation. *J Biol Chem* 274(52): 37046-52.

Schaffer BA, Bertram L, Miller BL, Mullin K, Weintraub S, Johnson N, Bigio EH, Mesulam M, Wiedau-Pazos M, Jackson GR, Cummings JL, Cantor RM, Levey AI, Tanzi RE, Geschwind DH (2008) Association of GSK3B with Alzheimer disease and frontotemporal dementia. *Arch Neurol* 65(10): 1368-74.

Selkoe DJ (1991) The molecular pathology of Alzheimer's disease. *Neuron* 6: 487–498.

Selkoe DJ (2002) Alzheimer's disease is a synaptic failure. *Science* 298: 789–791.

Selkoe DJ (2008) Soluble oligomers of the amyloid β-protein impair synaptic plasticity and behaviour. *Behav Brain Res* 192(1): 106-13.

Sengupta A, Wu Q, Grundke-Iqbal I, Iqbal K, and Singh TJ (1997) Potentiation of GSK-3-catalyzed Alzheimer-like phosphorylation of human tau by cdk5. *Mol Cell Biochem* 167: 99-105.

Shaldubina A, Agam G, Belmaker RH (2001) The mechanism of lithium action: state of the art, ten years later. *Prog Neuropsychopharmacol Biol Psychiatry* 25(4): 855-66.

Sheldon M., Rice D. S., D'Arcangelo G., Yoneshima H., Nakajima K., Mikoshiba K., Howell B. W., Cooper J. A., Goldowitz D., and Curran T. (1997) Scrambler and yotari disrupt the disabled gene and produce a reeler-like phenotype in mice. *Nature* 389, 730-3.

Sigurdsson EM (2008). Immunotherapy targeting pathological tau protein in Alzheimer's disease and related tauopathies *J Alzheimers Dis* 15(2): 157-68.

Simon D, Benitez MJ, Gimenez-Cassina A, Garrido JJ, Bhat RV, Diaz-Nido J, and Wandosell F (2008) Pharmacological inhibition of GSK-3 is not strictly correlated with a decrease in tyrosine phosphorylation of residues 216/279. *J Neurosci Res* 86: 668-74.

Sofola O, Kerr F, Rogers I, Killick R, Augustin H, Gandy C, Allen MJ, Hardy J, Lovestone S, Partridge L (2010) Inhibition of GSK-3 ameliorates Abeta pathology in an adult-onset Drosophila model of Alzheimer's disease. *PLoS Genet* 6(9). pii: e1001087.

Soutar MP, Kim WY, Williamson R, Peggie M, Hastie CJ, McLauchlan H, Snider WD, Gordon-Weeks PR, and Sutherland C (2010) Evidence that glycogen synthase kinase-3 isoforms have distinct substrate preference in the brain. *J Neurochem* 115: 974-83.

Stambolic V, and Woodgett JR (1994) Mitogen inactivation of glycogen synthase kinase-3 beta in intact cells via serine 9 phosphorylation. *Biochem J* 303 (3): 701-4.

Stambolic V, Ruel L, Woodgett JR (1997) Lithium inhibits glycogen synthase kinase-3 activity and mimics wingless signalling in intact cells. *Curr Biol* 6(12): 1664-8.

Stoothoff WH, Cho JH, McDonald RP, and Johnson GV (2005) FRAT-2 preferentially increases glycogen synthase kinase 3 beta-mediated phosphorylation of primed sites, which results in enhanced tau phosphorylation. *J Biol Chem* 280: 270-6.

Su Y Ryder J., Li B., Wu X., Fox N., Solenberg, P., Brune K., Paul S., Zhou Y., Liu F., and Ni B. (2004) Lithium, a common drug for bipolar disorder treatment, regulates amyloid-β precursor protein processing. *Biochemistry* 43(22):6899-908.

Suhara T, Magrané J, Rosen K, Christensen R, Kim HS, Zheng B, McPhie DL, Walsh K, Querfurth H (2003) Abeta42 generation is toxic to endothelial cells and inhibits eNOS function through an Akt/GSK-3beta signaling-dependent mechanism. *Neurobiol Aging* 24(3): 437-51.

Sun X., Sato S., Murayama O., Murayama M., Park J.M., Yamaguchi H., and Takashima A. (2002) Lithium inhibits amyloid secretion in COS7 cells transfected with amyloid precursor protein C100. *Neurosci. Lett.* 321(1-2):61-4.

Sutherland C, Leighton IA, and Cohen P (1993) Inactivation of glycogen synthase kinase-3 beta by phosphorylation: new kinase connections in insulin and growth-factor signalling. *Biochem J* 296: 15-9.

Takashima A, Honda T, Yasutake K, Michel G, Murayama O, Murayama M, Ishiguro K, and Yamaguchi H (1998a) Activation of tau protein kinase I/glycogen synthase kinase-3beta by amyloid beta peptide (25-35) enhances phosphorylation of tau in hippocampal neurons. *Neurosci Res* 31: 317-23.

Takashima A., Murayama O., Kohno T., Honda T., Yasutake K., Nihonmatsu N., Mercken M., Yamaguchi H., Sugihara S., and Wolozin B. (1998b) Presenilin 1 associates with glycogen synthase kinase-3β and its substrate tau. *Proc. Natl. Acad. Sci. U S A.* 95(16):9637-41.

ter Haar E (2006) The crystal structure of glycogen synthase kinase 3. In: *Glycogen Synthase Kinase 3 (GSK-3) and Its Inhibitors-Drug discovery and Development.* Wang B (Ed), Ch 5, pp. 61-82. Wiley Series in Drug Discovery and Development. New Jersey, USA..

ter Haar E, Coll JT, Austen DA, Hsiao HM, Swenson L, and Jain J (2001) Structure of GSK3beta reveals a primed phosphorylation mechanism. *Nat Struct Biol* 8: 593-6.

Terao T, Nakano H, Inoue Y, Okamoto T, Nakamura J, Iwata N (2006) Lithium and dementia: a preliminary study. *Prog Neuropsychopharmacol Biol Psychiatry*30(6): 1125-8.

Tesco G. and Tanzi R.E. (2000) GSK-3β forms a tetrameric complex with endogenous PS1-CTF/NTF and β-catenin. Effects of the D257/D385A and FAD-linked mutations. *Ann. NY Acad. Sci.* 920:227-32.

Thornton TM, Pedraza-Alva G, Deng B, Wood CD, Aronshtam A, Clements JL, Sabio G, Davis RJ, Matthews DE, Doble B, and Rincon M (2008) Phosphorylation by p38 MAPK as an alternative pathway for GSK3beta inactivation. *Science* 320: 667-70.

Townsend M, Mehta T, and Selkoe DJ (2007) Soluble Abeta inhibits specific signal transduction cascades common to the insulin receptor pathway. *J Biol Chem* 282 (46): 33305-12.

Twomey C and McCarthy JV (2006) Presenilin-1 is an unprimed glycogen synthase kinase-3beta substrate. *FEBS Lett* 580: 4015-20.

van Amerongen R, Nawijn M, Franca-Koh J, Zevenhoven J, van der Gulden H, Jonkers J, and Berns A (2005) Frat is dispensable for canonical Wnt signaling in mammals. *Genes Dev* 19: 425-30.

Walsh DM, Klyubin I, Fadeeva JV, Cullen WK, Anwyl R, Wolfe MS, Rowan MJ, Selkoe DJ (2002) Naturally secreted oligomers of amyloid beta protein potently inhibit hippocampal long-term potentiation in vivo. Nature 416(6880): 535-9.

Walsh DM, Selkoe DJ (2007) A beta oligomers - a decade of discovery. *J Neurochem* 101(5): 1172-84

Wang JZ, Grundke-Iqbal I, Iqbal K (1996) Glycosylation of microtubule-associated protein tau: an abnormal posttranslational modification in Alzheimer's disease. *Nat Med* 2(8): 871-5.

Wang QM, Fiol CJ, DePaoli-Roach AA, and Roach PJ (1994) Glycogen synthase kinase-3 beta is a dual specificity kinase differentially regulated by tyrosine and serine/threonine phosphorylation. *J Biol Chem* 269: 14566-74.

Wei H, Leeds PR, Qian Y, Wei W, Chen R, Chuang D (2000) Beta-amyloid peptide-induced death of PC 12 cells and cerebellar granule cell neurons is inhibited by long-term lithium treatment. *Eur J Pharmacol* 392(3): 117-23.

Woodgett JR (2006) Glycogen synthase Kinase 3: an introductory synopsis. In: *Glycogen Synthase Kinase 3 (GSK-3) and Its Inhibitors-Drug discovery and Development.* Wang B (Ed), Ch 1, pp. 3-24. Wiley Series in Drug Discovery and Development. New Jersey, USA..

Woodgett JR: Molecular cloning and expression of glycogen synthase kinase-3/factor A. *EMBO J.* (1990) 9(8):2431-8.

Wood-Kaczmar A, Kraus M, Ishiguro K, Philpott KL and Gordon-Weeks PR (2009) An alternatively spliced form of glycogen synthase kinase-3beta is targeted to growing neurites and growth cones. *Mol Cell Neurosci* 42: 184-194.

York JD, Ponder JW, Majerus PW (1995) Definition of a metal-dependent/Li(+)-inhibited phosphomonoesterase protein family based upon a conserved three-dimensional core structure. *Proc Natl Acad Sci USA* 92(11): 5149-53.

Yoshimura T, Kawano Y, Arimura N, Kawabata S, Kikuchi A, Kaibuchi K. (2005) GSK-3β regulates phosphorylation of CRMP-2 and neuronal polarity. Cell 120:137-49.

Yost C, Farr GH 3rd, Pierce SB, Ferkey DM, Chen MM, and Kimelman D (1998)GBP, an inhibitor of GSK-3, is implicated in Xenopus development and oncogenesis. *Cell* 93: 1031-41.

# 4

# Pin1: A New Enzyme Pivotal for Protecting Against Alzheimer's Disease

Kazuhiro Nakamura, Suk Ling Ma and Kun Ping Lu
*Department of Medicine, Beth Israel Deaconess Medical Center*
*Harvard Medical School, Boston*
*USA*

## 1. Introduction

Alzheimer's disease (AD) affects more than 35 million people worldwide, and the prevalence of AD increases with age and doubles every 5 years after the age of 65 (Evans et al., 1989). AD is characterized by intracellular neurofibrillary tangles (NFTs) and extracellular amyloid fibrils composed of amyloid beta peptides (Aβ). Accordingly, both tau and amyloid have been the targets for development of treatment for AD.

Tau-mediated neurodegeneration may result from the combination of toxic gains-of-function acquired by the aggregates or their precursors and the detrimental effects that arise from the loss of the normal function(s) of tau in the disease state (Ballatore et al., 2007). The toxic gains-of-function includes sequestration of normal tau function by NFTs made of hyperphosphorylated tau. NFTs also become physical obstacles to the transport of vesicles and other cargos (Ballatore et al., 2007). The loss of the normal function of tau includes detachment of tau from microtubules that causes loss of microtubule-stabilizing function (Stoothoff & Johnson, 2005). Although dynamic tau phosphorylation occurs during embryonic development (Mawal-Dewan et al., 1994), aberrant tau phosphorylation in mature neurons is harmful to the neuron (Matsuo et al., 1994). Tau hyperphosphorylation is a key regulatory mechanism that leads to both such toxic gains-of-function and the loss of the normal function(s) of tau (Ballatore et al., 2007).

Upregulation of aberrant activation of tau kinases and downregulation of phosphatases are major mechanisms possibly involved in tau hyperphosphorylation (Ballatore et al., 2007). Consistently, tau phosphorylation on Ser/Thr-Pro by Pro-directed kinases (Illenberger et al., 1998; Pelech, 1995) or phosphatases such as phosphatase2A (PP2A) (Goedert et al., 2000; Sontag et al., 1996) play pivotal roles in tauopathy. Indeed, overexpression of glycogen synthase kinase-3β (GSK3β) or cyclin-dependent protein kinases (CDK5) and its activator p25 or inhibition of PP2A enhances or induces tau-related phenotypes in mice (Ahlijanian et al., 2000; Augustinack et al., 2002; Cruz et al., 2003; Kins et al., 2001; Noble et al., 2003). In addition, tau phosphorylation has been shown to promote tau degradation via chaperone-interacting protein/Hsp70 (Dickey et al., 2007; Kosik & Shimura, 2005; Petrucelli et al., 2004). These results indicate that kinases and phosphatases that increase and decrease phosphorylated tau, respectively, are crucial targets for treatment of AD. Design of inhibitors for these kinases is undertaken as potential drug targets (reviewed in (Mazanetz and Fischer, 2007).

Regarding amyloid, Aβ varies from 39 to 43 amino acids and arises from sequential β- and γ-secretases processing of the amyloid precursor protein (APP). Presenilin 1 (PS1) is a catalytic subunit of γ-secretase. Several active and passive immunotherapy approaches such as acceleration of clearance of Aβ from the brain of the AD patients using brain penetrant inhibitors of Aβ aggregation and anti-Aβ monoclonal antibodies are undertaken (Frisardi et al.). Inhibitors of proteases such as β- and γ-secretase regulating Aβ formation from APP and compounds that stimulate α-secretase, the enzyme responsible for the non-amyloidogenic metabolism of APP are also investigated (reviewed in Frisardi et al.).

In addition to inhibition of tau phosphorylation and clearance of Aβ, an approach that targets protein conformations of tau and APP has been proposed as a new therapeutic target treating AD. Phosphorylation of serine and threonine residues preceding proline (pSer/Thr–Pro) mediated by a large number of so-called Pro-directed protein kinases is a major signaling mechanism (Hunter, 1995; Lu, 2004; Lu et al., 2002). Specific pSer/Thr-Pro motifs in certain proteins such as tau can exist in 2 distinct *cis* and *trans* conformations, whose conversion can be greatly accelerated by Pin1 (protein interacting with NIMA 1), a unique prolyl *cis-trans* isomerase (Lu et al., 1996; Lu et al., 1999b; Yaffe et al., 1997; Zhou et al., 1999). Such Pin1-catalyzed conformational changes, which can now be visualized by nuclear magnetic resonance (NMR) (Pastorino et al., 2006), have a profound impact on phosphorylation signaling, achieved by regulating a spectrum of target activities (Lu, 2004; Lu & Zhou, 2007; Wulf et al., 2005). Pin1 is tightly regulated and its deregulation contributes to pathological conditions, notably AD and cancer (Butterfield et al., 2006; Lu, 2004; Lu & Zhou, 2007; Pastorino et al., 2006; Shen et al., 2005; Suizu et al., 2006; Wulf et al., 2005). Remarkably, deletion of Pin1 in mice causes progressive age-dependent tauopathy (Liou et al., 2003). The observation that deprivation of a single molecule causes tauopathy verifies the importance of Pin1 on tauopathy. Conversely, neuronal Pin1 overexpression decreases the stability of tau, and greatly inhibits the tauopathy phenotype in wild-type tau transgenic mice (Lim et al., 2008). In AD, Pin1 binds to and isomerizes the pThr231-Pro motif in tau to restore its ability to bind to microtubules and to promote their assembly (Lu et al., 1999a) by facilitating tau dephosphorylation by PP2A (Liou et al., 2003; Zhou et al., 2000). Moreover, Pin1 binds to the pThr668-Pro motif of APP in the *cis* and *trans* conformations, accelerates the isomerization rate (Pastorino et al., 2006) and promotes nonamyloidogenic APP processing, thereby producing neurotrophic αAPPs and reducing neurotoxic Aβ peptides (Pastorino et al., 2006).

Because such neurodegeneration-protecting effects by Pin1 are generally believed to be ascribable to *cis trans* conformational changes by Pin1, regulation of the conformations of tau and APP after phosphorylation likely serves as potential therapeutic target for AD.

In this chapter, we summarize the current understanding of the mechanisms on how Pin1 acts as a protecting molecule against neurodegeneration in AD mouse models, followed by evidences of the pivotal roles of Pin1 in human AD.

## 2. Contribution of *cis-trans* isomerization to neural functions

The unique stereochemistry of Pro means that it can adopt two completely different conformational states (*trans* and *cis*). The significance of this with respect to the fact that Pro is often found next to phosphorylated Ser/Thr residues was not appreciated for a long time (Lu, 2004; Wulf et al., 2005). A breakthrough in understanding the conformational importance of Pro-directed phosphorylation motifs was the discovery of a unique and conserved peptidyl-prolyl *cis/trans* isomerase (PPIase), Pin1 (Lu, 2004; Lu et al., 1996; Ranganathan et al., 1997; Yaffe et al., 1997). Although Pin1 belongs to the parvulin subfamily of PPIases, it is the only PPIase that specifically recognizes pSer/Thr-Pro peptide sequences (Lu, 2004; Lu et al., 1996; Ranganathan et al., 1997; Yaffe et al., 1997), which is especially important because Pro-directed kinases and phosphatases are conformation-specific and act only on the *trans* conformation (Brown et al., 1999; Weiwad et al., 2000; Zhou et al., 2000). The identification of Pin1 as a phosphorylation-specific PPIase led to a new concept that Pin1 catalytically regulates the conformation of substrates after their phosphorylation to further control protein function (Lu et al., 1999b; Ranganathan et al., 1997; Yaffe et al., 1997; Zhou et al., 1999).

Phosphorylation dramatically slows down the already slow rate of isomerization of Ser/Thr-Pro bonds and renders the phosphopeptide bond resistant to the catalytic action of conventional PPIases (Yaffe et al., 1997). Pro-directed phosphorylation also induces local structural changes that make it accessible to further modifications (Kipping et al., 2001). The striking substrate specificity of Pin1 towards certain pSer/Thr–Pro bonds results from its unique two domain structure consisting of an N-terminal WW domain and a C-terminal PPIase domain, which form a "double-check" mechanism (Ranganathan et al., 1997; Yaffe et al., 1997; Zhou et al., 2000). The WW domain of Pin1 binds only to specific pSer/Thr–Pro motifs, which are often critical regulatory phosphorylation sites in Pin1 substrates (Shen et al. 1998; Lu et al. 1999; Lu et al. 1999; Zhou et al. 2000; Ryo et al. 2001; Wulf et al. 2001; Lu et al. 2002). This WW domain binding targets the Pin1 catalytic domain close to its substrates, where the PPIase domain isomerizes specific pSer/Thr–Pro motifs and catalytically induces conformational changes in proteins (Lu et al., 1999b; Zhou et al., 2000). It remains to be solved why Pin1 binds only to specific pSer/Thr-Pro motifs in certain proteins but it may be due to combined primary (and other) structural determinants. Furthermore, the WW domain can increase or inhibit Pin1 isomerase activity depending on whether a peptide substrate is phosphorylated on a single site or on multiple sites *in vitro* (Smet et al., 2005), although the biological significance of these findings is unclear. The findings that many substrates contain a single phosphorylation target site for Pin1 suggest that when it is targeted to the substrate by the WW domain, the PPIase domain would have to act on the same pSer/Thr-Pro motif to accelerate its isomerization. Another possibility is that the WW domain and PPIase domain might act on different pSer/Thr-Pro motifs in the same protein or in different ones when a Pin1 substrate is multiphosphorylated or in a multiprotein complex. In contrast to most other constitutively active PPIases (Fischer & Aumuller, 2003), Pin1 function is tightly regulated at multiple levels under physiological conditions, as expected given the tight regulation of Pro-directed phosphorylation signalling. For example, in neurons, Pin1 expression is induced upon neuronal differentiation (Hamdane et al., 2006; Liou et al., 2003; Lu et al., 1999a). This observation raises the link between prolyl *cis-trans* isomerization and neural functions.

Indeed, prolyl *cis-trans* isomerization has been shown to control neural functions. The study that took an initiative in this field is *cis* and *trans* specific functions on the opening of a neurotransmitter-gated ion channel *in vitro* (Lummis et al., 2005). Serotonin (5-hydroxytryptamine type 3, 5-HT3) receptors are members of the cysteine-loop receptor superfamily (Lester et al., 2004). Neurotransmitter binding in these proteins triggers the opening of an ion channel by inducing *cis-trans* conformational change (Lummis et al., 2005).

5-HT3 receptors have a specific proline (P*8) located at the apex of the loop between the second and third transmembrane helices (M2 and M3). When P*8 is replaced with analogs that favor the *trans* conformation, closed channels are observed. Conversely, unnatural amino acids that have high *cis* preference resulted in irreversible open channels. These results suggest that neurotransmitter binding may trigger a conformational change that isomerizes P*8 from *trans* to *cis* (Lummis et al., 2005). Interestingly, proline is often found in the transmembrane regions of ion channels and transporters (Sansom & Weinstein, 2000), which suggests an important role for the conformational changes in regulating the gating of 5HT3 receptor channel. These results clearly show that prolyl *cis-trans* isomerization controls physiological neural functions *in vitro*. A finding that Pin1, a PPIase, enhances the ability of gephyrin to bind the β-subunit of glycine receptors, which is important for maintaining a high concentration of inhibitory glycine receptors juxtaposed to presynaptic releasing sites (Zita et al., 2007), further suggests an intriguing hypothesis that PPIases might be involved in neural functions, especially pathological neural functions.

Exploration of the contributions of Pin1, a PPIase, to pathological neural functions gave an answer for the hypothesis. Pin1 protects against spinal cord injury by preventing JNK3-induced MCL1 degradation, cytochrome *c* release and apoptosis *in vitro* and *in vivo* (Li et al., 2007), which are opposite to the *in vitro* findings that Pin1 acts on bimEL (also known as B-cell lymphoma protein-2 (bcl2)-like-11) to induce apoptosis (Becker & Bonni, 2006). Furthermore, evidences for Pin1's protection against neurodegeneration through tau and APP *in vitro* and *in vivo* as shown in the next section confirmed the pivotal role of the PPIase in pathological neural conditions.

## 3. Pin1 restores tauopathy phenotype in mice

### 3.1 Pin1 recognizes phosphorylated Thr231 in tau

Various isoforms of tau appear to be differentially expressed during development, however, the tau isoforms with 3 and 4 tubulin-binding repeats are expressed in a one-to-one ratio in most regions of the adult brain (Ballatore et al., 2007). The primary function of tau is to stabilize microtubules. Tau proteins promote tubulin polymerization and stabilize microtubule structure *in vivo* (Lindwall & Cole, 1984; Weingarten et al., 1975). Tau deletion also potentiates the phenotypes of axon tracts and neuronal layers in mice lacking MAP1B, another major MT-associated protein (Takei et al., 2000). In AD brains, neuronal cytoskeleton is progressively disrupted and replaced by NFTs (Alonso et al., 1996). NFTs in AD are composed of hyperphosphorylated tau in two forms (paired helical filaments (PHF) and straight filaments (SF)). Tau hyperphosphorylation appears to precede tangle formation and neurodegeneration in AD. Hyperphosphorylated tau shows defective microtubule binding, fails to promote microtubule assembly, and self-assembles into NFTs *in vitro* (Mandelkow, 1999). In contrast, dephosphorylation *in vitro* can restore the microtubule-binding function and abolish the aggregation of AD phospho-tau (ptau) (Alonso et al., 1996). Taken together, these results indicate that increased tau phosphorylation is a key and an early event in the pathogenesis of human tauopathies, and therefore, dephosphorylation of hyperphosphorylated tau could be an attractive way to restore physiological tau function.

Ser/Thr-Pro sites are major regulatory phosphorylation motif in cells (Blume-Jensen & Hunter, 2001; Lee & Tsai, 2003; Lu, 2004; Lu et al., 2003; Nigg, 2001). Enzymes that are responsible for such phosphorylation belong to a large superfamily of Pro-directed protein kinases, which include extracellular signal-regulated kinases (ERKs), stress-activated protein kinases/c-Jun-N-terminal kinases (SAPKs/JNKs), p38 kinases and Polo-like kinases (PLKs) in addition to CDKs and GSKs. These kinases have a crucial role in diverse cellular processes such as cell growth regulation, stress responses and neuronal survival, as well as in human diseases such as cancer and AD (Blume-Jensen & Hunter, 2001; Lee & Tsai, 2003; Lu, 2004; Lu et al., 2003; Nigg, 2001). Pin1 binds to tau in a phosphorylation-dependent manner and the binding site was mapped to pThr231 of tau *in vitro* (Lu et al., 1999a). This phospho-epitope has been proposed to be diagnostic for AD because its levels in the cerebrospinal fluid correlate with the progression of the disease (Hampel et al., 2001; Kohnken et al., 2000). In addition, the mobility shifted ptau was positively probed by both CP9, an antibody specific for pThr231, and TG3, an antibody detecting Alzheimer-specific conformation of pThr231. In AD brain sections, exogenous Pin1 specifically bound to NFTs and neurites, which were also reactive to Pin1 antibody and TG3, indicating endogenous Pin1 is also localized to the pThr231 site. Biochemically, Pin1 was co-purified with PHF. Thus, the Pin1 interaction with ptau has been established.

### 3.2 Pin1 restores normal tau function through dephosphorylation of pThr231 of tau in vitro

Tau phosphorylated by Cdc2 showed a marked decrease in microtubule binding compared to unphosphorylated tau in tau biochemical assay *in vitro* (Lu et al., 1999a). Pin1-directed restoration of tau's ability to bind to microtubule was revealed by several observations. The loss of ptau's affinity to microtubules could be dramatically rescued by the sole presence of Pin1. The functional consequence of application of Pin1 was derived when microtubule assembly from tubulin was measured based on turbidity changes detected by spectrophotometer. The ability of tau to promote tubulin polymerization was abolished after tau was phosphorylated by Cdc2. Wild-type Pin1, but not the binding of defective point mutant, restored the function.
The involvement of dephosphorylation in the restoration by Pin1 was led by the observations that many of phosphoproteins Pin1 binds to are also recognized by the mitosis- and phosphorylation-specific antibody (mAb) MPM-2, and induction of MPM-2 epitopes is a prominent common feature shared by AD, frontotemporal dementia and parkinsonism linked to chromosome 17 (FTDP-17), Down Syndrome, corticobasal degeneration, progressive supranuclear palsy and Pick's disease. Furthermore, various studies have shown that mitotic events, including Cdc2 kinase, are aberrantly activated in the AD brain (Vincent et al., 1997; Vincent et al., 1996) and the phosphorylation pattern of tau in mitotic cells is strikingly similar to that in the AD brain (Kondratick et al. 1996; Vincent et al. 1996; Vincent et al. 1997; Illenberger et al. 1998; Preuss et al. 1998; Vincent et al. 1998). Indeed, both mitotic and AD tau proteins are recognized by mitosis-specific or AD-specific mAbs that are phosphorylation-dependent. Pin1 binds to pSer/Thr–Pro sites of many MPM-2 antigens, including tau. The phosphorylation dependent *cis/trans*-isomerization of pSer/Thr–Pro of many MPM-2 antigens is important for cell cycle control (Ding et al., 2000; Lane & Nigg, 1996; Wells et al., 1999; Winkler et al., 2000). On the other hand, dephosphorylation of the MPM-2 epitopes by phosphatases, notably PP2A, also plays an essential role in the regulation of Cdc2 activation and mitosis (Evans & Stark, 1997; Kawabe et al., 1997; Kinoshita et al., 1990; Lee, 1995; Lin & Arndt, 1995; Sontag et al., 1995). Interestingly, using metabolically active rat brain slices as a model, Gong *et al.* (Gong et al., 2000) showed that down-regulation of PP2A by okadaic acid induced Alzheimer-like hyperphosphorylation of tau. In contrast, the inhibition of PP2B by cyclosporin A in the same system did not significantly affect tau phosphorylation.

The pure *cis* isomer of tau peptide can be obtained using *trans*-specific $\alpha$-chymotrypsin to eliminate the *trans* isomer (Zhou et al., 2000). In the absence of any PPIases, it took about 2.5 h to convert the pure *cis* peptide to equilibrium state, which is about 15% *cis*. Importantly, the pure *cis* peptides cannot be dephosphorylated by PP2A (Zhou et al., 2000). The pThr–Pro peptides were dephosphorylated by PP2A with a rate almost identical to that of *trans* isomer appearance. The *trans* isomer-dependent dephosphorylation was neither observed with alkaline phosphatase nor with a non-Pro-containing peptide. These experiments indicated that PP2A is a *trans* conformation-specific phosphatase. Indeed, the presence of Pin1 accelerated the dephosphorylation of tau by PP2A. However, the effect of Pin1 on PP2A dephosphorylation was not observed in tau Thr231Ala mutant. Taken together, Pin1 facilitates the dephosphorylation of pThr231-Pro site in tau through PP2A likely leads to the restoration of tau-mediated microtubule function.

### 3.3 Pin1 degrades hyperphosphorylated tau

Another effective way to treat tauopathy might be the elimination of hyperphosphorylated tau. It has been shown that tau phosphorylation regulates its degradation (Dickey et al., 2007; Kosik & Shimura, 2005; Petrucelli et al., 2004; Poppek et al., 2006) and that protein degradation is modulated by Pin1 (Lu & Zhou, 2007). These results suggest that Pin1 might act on the pThr231-Pro motif in tau to regulate the protein stability. Pin1 knockdown caused tau to become highly stable in neuron-like SH-SY5Y cells under cycloheximide experiment (Lim et al., 2008). Importantly, the effect of Pin1 knockdown on tau protein stability was completely abolished in the presence of the proteosome inhibitor MG132, demonstrating that the effect of Pin1 knockdown depends on functional proteosome, as shown for other Pin1 substrates (Lu & Zhou, 2007). The result was replicated in neurons isolated from mice. Transfected tau protein in primary cultured neurons and tau protein in brain slices from tau transgenic mouse were significantly more stable in Pin1-knockout background (Lu & Zhou, 2007). Further examination was carried out under Pin1 transgenic background in mice in which Pin1 transgene is expressed under Thy1.2 promoter that is active in neurons approximately 10 days after birth (Caroni, 1997). In the double transgenic mice having both tau transgene and Pin1 transgene, tau phosphorylation on Thr231 was reduced compared to tau transgene alone.

Tau phosphorylation has been shown to promote tau degradation via chaperone-interacting protein/Hsp70 (Dickey et al., 2007; Kosik & Shimura, 2005; Petrucelli et al., 2004) or inhibit tau degradation (Poppek et al., 2006). Interestingly, F-box proteins, which target phosphorylated proteins to ubiquitin-mediated proteolysis, bind to pSer/Thr-Pro motifs only in *trans*, but not *cis* (Orlicky et al., 2003). One model is that proteins targeting phosphorylated tau for degradation might bind to certain pSer/Thr-Pro motif(s) in tau only in *trans* conformation that would promote this interaction to promote degradation of tau. In this model, although tau is probably phosphorylated on certain Ser/Thr-Pro motifs such as the Thr231-Pro motif in *trans* due to the conformation specificity of kinases (Lu & Zhou, 2007), the pThr231-Pro motif in tau might have a tendency to be in the *cis* conformation due to local structural constraints after phosphorylation, as shown for APP (Ramelot & Nicholson, 2001). Therefore, in the nonequilibrium cellular environment, Pin1 overexpression might greatly accelerate the *cis* to *trans* isomerization to promote tau degradation, whereas Pin1 inhibition might allow a higher concentration of *cis* pThr231-Pro motif to be present for a longer time, which might inhibit tau degradation (Figure 1).

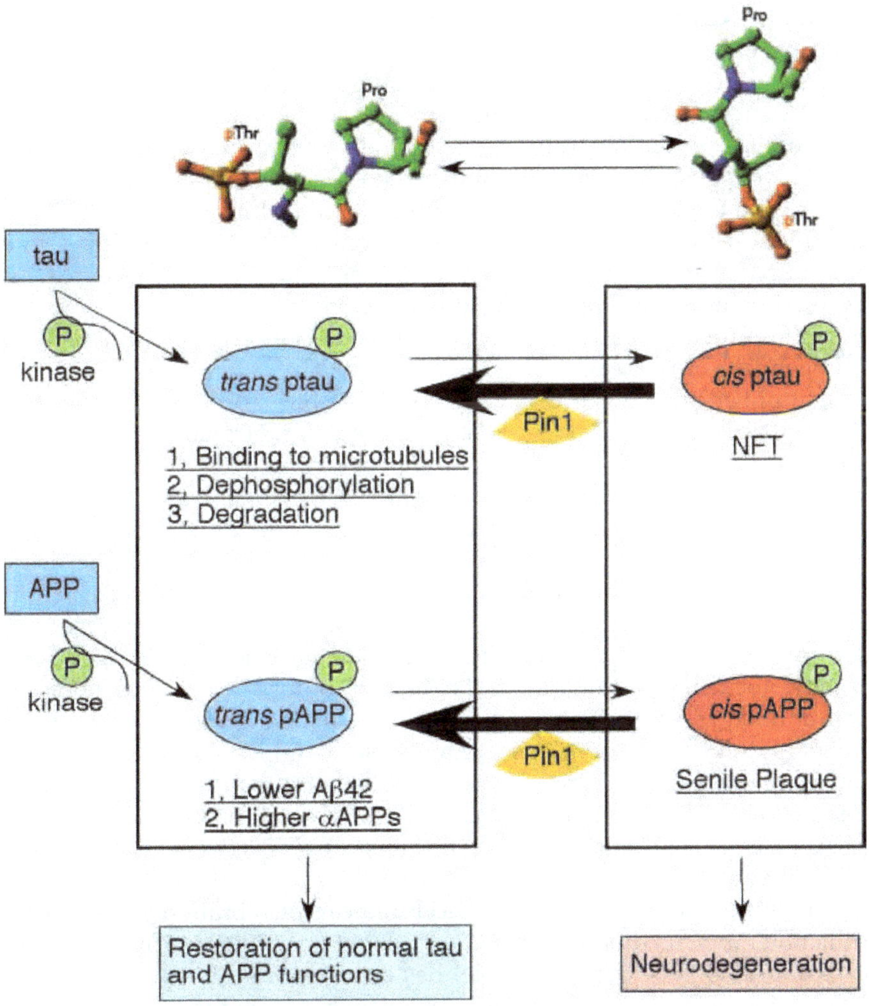


Tau and APP may be phosphorylated by protein kinases as part of their normal functions. *Cis*-ptau is resistant to binding to microtubules, protein phosphatases and degradation. By catalysing isomerization of the *cis* to *trans* conformation, Pin1 facilitates binding to microtubules and restores normal tau function. Pin1 also promotes tau dephosphorylation by phosphatases that contributes to the binding to microtubules. The *cis* to *trans* transition by Pin1 also facilitates degradation of phosphorylated tau. Regarding APP, *cis*-pAPP represents amyloidogenic APP processing. Pin1 catalyses isomerization of the *cis* to *trans* conformation, thereby, inducing decreased Aβ42 and increased αAPPs. The *trans*-conformations of ptau and pAPP may represent the physiological conformations that promote their normal functions.

Fig. 1. Restoration of tau and APP functions by Pin1.

Importantly, in 18-month-old tau transgenic mice, neuropathological changes, as demonstrated by the presence of some silver-positive neurons in the ventral horn of spinal cord and several degenerating or demyelinated axons within the sciatic nerves were found. However, neither silver-positive neurons in the spinal cord nor degenerated neurons within the sciatic nerve was observed in double transgenic mice having both Pin1 transgene and wild-type tau transgene (Lim et al., 2008). This result indicates that Pin1 overexpression effectively inhibits spinal and peripheral neuropathies induced by tau overexpression.

### 3.4 Deletion of Pin1 causes tauopathy in mice

Pin1 knockout mice (Liou et al., 2003) serves as a good tool to investigate the effect of Pin1 on endogenous tau *in vivo*. Pin1-deficient mice showed progressive age-dependent motor and behavioral deficits including abnormal limb-clasping reflexes, hunched postures and reduced mobility (Liou et al., 2003) similar to tau transgenic mice (Allen et al., 2002; Lewis et al., 2000). These phenotypes in Pin1 mutant mice are significant because the total level of NFTs correlates with the degree of cognitive impairment (Arriagada et al., 1992a; Arriagada et al., 1992b). Pioneering studies that used immunohistochemical techniques to determine the level of both NFTs and senile plaques in different brain regions of AD patients, as well as non-demented elderly individuals, demonstrated that the number of NFTs, but not the numbers of senile plaques, correlates with the degree of cognitive impairment (Arriagada et al., 1992a; Arriagada et al., 1992b).

Since neuron number in the parietal cortex of old, but not young mutant mice were significantly decreased, these phenotypes were caused by neuronal loss. A similar neuronal degeneration was found in spinal cords of the knockout mice (Liou et al., 2003). Tau hyperphosphorylation has been observed in aged mutant mice, with a dramatic mobility shift that is reversed by phosphatase treatment (Liou et al., 2003). The retarded forms of ptau in the mutant mice were also detected by various phospho-specific or Alzheimer-conformation-specific antibodies, such as AT180 and TG3. The phosphatase activity specific to pThr231 peptide motif was significantly reduced in the mutant mice, which is in agreement with Pin1's role in facilitating PP2A phosphatase activity. In aged Pin1-deficient mice, immunohistochemical staining of the hippocampus, cortex and spinal cord with specific ptau antibodies showed distinct somatodendritic signals, indicating pathological localization of tau. In Pin1-deficient mice, immunoelectronmicroscopic analysis showed that NFT-like tau filaments decorated by AT180 gold label were isolated from sarkosyl insoluble fractions (Liou et al., 2003). The tau filaments isolated resembled some of the human FTDP-17 mutants (Allen et al., 2002; Gotz et al., 2001; Lewis et al., 2000; Lim et al., 2001; Tanemura et al., 2002). Gallyas and thioflavin-staining, two established methods detecting NFTs in AD brains, were immense in entorhinal cortex and hippocampus, brain regions where impaired neuronal function appears initially in AD (Liou et al., 2003). These phenotypes are noteworthy because no gene deletion model has been reported to spontaneously cause tau pathology, thus no endogenous protective mechanism has been proposed.

## 4. Pin1 reduces Ab in mice

Tau and APP are two major molecules for AD. A growing body of evidence indicates some common features between the normal cell cycle and degenerated AD neurons, especially mitotic phosphorylation on certain Ser/Thr-Pro motifs (Lu et al., 2003; Yang & Herrup, 2007). Phosphorylation of APP on the Thr668-Pro motif, which occurs in mitotic cells (Suzuki et al., 1994), is also increased in AD brains and can elevate Aβ secretion *in vitro* (Lee et al., 2003).

Nuclear magnetic resonance (NMR) analysis of the action of Pin1 on APP has revealed the dynamic regulation of the intracellular domain of APP between the two completely distinct structures (Pastorino et al., 2006). APP possesses a Thr668-Pro motif that exists in *trans* before phosphorylation. The *cis* conformation appears only after phosphorylation due to local structural constraints, with ~10% of the phosphorylated motifs existing in the *cis* conformation (Ramelot & Nicholson, 2001). Pin1 binds to the pThr668-Pro motif in the *cis* and *trans* conformations and also accelerates the isomerization rate >1000-fold (in the millisecond timescale) compared with the typical uncatalysed reaction (which is in the minute timescale), with the catalysed *cis* to *trans* rate being 10-fold faster than the reverse rate (Pastorino et al., 2006), in contrast to a recent report that Pin1 does not act on full-length protein (Akiyama et al., 2005). Therefore, Pin1 would rapidly re-establish *cis/trans* equilibrium if either population was suddenly depleted in the cell.

APP processing is determined by APP subcellular localization and occurs through non-amyloidogenic processing at the plasma membrane by α-secretases or amyloidogenic processing at endosomes by β-secretase (De Strooper & Annaert, 2000; Esler & Wolfe, 2001; Hardy & Selkoe, 2002; Mattson, 2004; Selkoe et al., 1996). There is observation Pin1 co-localizes with APP at plasma membrane but not at endosomes, suggesting Pin1 affects APP intracellular localization and therefore affect APP processing and Aβ production (Pastorino et al., 2006). In addition, in Pin1 knockout mice, a significant increase in Aβ42 level in brain is observed (Pastorino et al., 2006).

Importantly, functional consequence of Pin1 deregulation revealed that the *cis* pThr668-Pro motif has a longer lifetime and its population relative to *trans* can be shifted far from its equilibrium depending on isomer-specific interactions, which might favor more amyloidogenic APP processing and Aβ production without proper Pin1 function (Figure 1). Therefore, in collaboration with other Alzheimer's disease factors, Pin1 deregulation might promote amyloidogenic APP processing and Aβ production and thus contribute to the pathology of AD (Pastorino et al., 2006).

## 5. Involvement of Pin1 in human AD

Positional cloning led to the identification of rare, disease-causing mutations in APP, PSEN1, and PSEN2 causing early-onset familial AD, followed by the discovery of ApoE as the only widely accepted and replicated risk factor for late-onset AD. In addition, recent genome-wide association approaches have delivered several additional AD susceptibility loci that are common in the general population (reviewed in Bertram & Tanzi, 2009).

Pin1 is mapped to 19p13.2, which has been identified as a novel locus for late onset AD that is independent of the effect of ApoE4 (Butler et al., 2009; Wijsman et al., 2004). Several common polymorphisms have been identified in the coding and promoter regions of Pin1. The relationship between Pin1 level and AD is of particular interest because Pin1 is downregulated and/or inhibited by oxidative modifications in AD (Liou et al., 2003; Sultana et al., 2006). Previous studies showed that Pin1 promoter single nucleotide polymorphism (SNP) (842G>C) is associated with reduced level of Pin1 in blood cells and increased risk for AD in an Italian cohort (Segat et al., 2007), although not in other cohorts (Lambert et al., 2009; Nowotny et al., 2007). Further studies have confirmed that this SNP abolishes Pin1 promoter activity and is associated with reduced risk for multiple cancers(Han et al., 2010). It is possible that the undetected population structure in studies with heterogeneous populations of subjects can lead to false positive results or failures in detecting the association with disease (Marchini et al., 2004) and this effect increased with samples size which might explain the conflicting results among the studies on Pin1 promoter polymorphisms. It has been shown that Chinese and Japanese subpopulations are more homogeneous and have a lower degree of population admixture (Marchini et al., 2004). Using Chinese subjects, we recently studied the onset of AD and Pin1 polymorphism. A functional polymorphism in the Pin1 promoter (rs2287839) was identified and this polymorphism was significantly associated with a 3-year delay in the onset of AD (Ma et al.). The base change of the SNP abolished the binding site of AP4 and increased the expression level of Pin1 in AD (Ma et al.). AP4 belongs to the basic helix-loop-helix leucine-zipper (bHLH-LZ) subgroup of bHLH proteins and recognizes the symmetrical DNA core sequence CAGCTG (Hu et al., 1990). Our result on AP4 RNAi and AP4 overexpression in H4 cells showed AP4 was able to repress the expression of Pin1 through the AP4 binding site in the promoter region of Pin1.

The above result is confirmed by biochemical and histochemical approaches using AD brain. Pin1 translocation from the soluble fractions to the insoluble fractions was reported in AD brains, while it was mainly present in the soluble fraction in age matched normal brain samples (Lu et al., 1999a). Further histological studies clarified Pin1's impact on AD. In the hippocampus and neocortex, the neurons in specific subregions are more prone to neurofibrillary degeneration than the neighboring subregions, indicating stereotypical patterns of neurodegeneration in AD. In the hippocampus, expression of Pin1 was relatively higher in CA4, CA3, CA2 and presubiculum, and lower in CA1 and subiculum. In the parietal cortex, expression of Pin1 was relatively higher in layer IIIb-c neurons, and lower in layer V neurons. The subregions with low expression of Pin1 coincide with the subregions that are more susceptible to neurofibrillary degeneration in AD, whereas those containing high Pin1 expression are not, showing an inverse correlation between Pin1 expression and predicted vulnerability (Liou et al., 2003). In AD brains, tangle-bearing neurons were enriched in CA1 and subiculum of the hippocampus and in layer V of the parietal cortex (Arriagada et al., 1992b; Davies et al., 1992; Hof & Morrison, 1991; Pearson et al., 1985). Overall, Pin1 level is generally low in these regions (Liou et al., 2003).

Because Pin1 is important in modulating APP processing in mice and has an inverse relationship with tau accumulation in human AD, increased Pin1 expression resulting from the base substitution of the SNP might delay the pathological process of AD, thus delaying the age of onset of AD (Figure 2). This result is significant because an intervention that could delay the average age of onset of AD by only 2 years has been predicted to reduce the expected prevalence by 23% by 2050 (Brookmeyer et al., 1998).

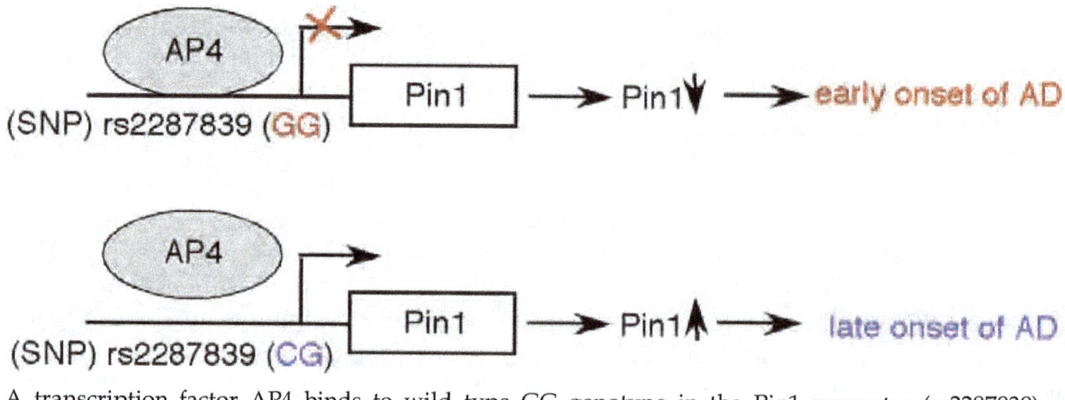


A transcription factor AP4 binds to wild type GG genotype in the Pin1 promoter (rs2287839) and represses its transcription. The polymorphism (CG) abolishes the binding site of AP4 and disinhibits the repression, thereby increases Pin1 expression level in AD. The polymorphism results in 3-year delay of the onset of AD.

Fig. 2. A Pin1 polymorphism associates with delayed onset of AD.

## 6. Conclusions

Tau and APP, two major causative molecules for AD, are reasonable and attractive therapeutic targets. The links between tau malfunctions and an overall imbalance in the activity levels or regulation of tau kinases and phosphatases have been established (Churcher, 2006; Mazanetz & Fischer, 2007). Although, attempts to identify AD-specific phosphorylation sites on tau have yet to yield conclusive results (Gordon-Krajcer et al., 2000; Schneider et al., 1999), the most probable candidates are Ser262 and the region around Thr231 and Ser235 (Hasegawa et al., 1992; Kohnken et al., 2000). Among these sites, Ser262 is identified as a Lys-Xaa-Gly-Ser motif recognized by Par1 kinase (microtubule associated regulating kinase) (Doerflinger et al., 2003; Drewes et al., 1995; Nishimura et al., 2004), whereas pSer/Thr–Pro sites of Thr231 and Ser235 are phosphorylated by CDKs, MAPKs, and/or GSKs (Ishiguro et al. 1993; Sperber et al. 1995; Zheng-Fischhofer et al. 1998; Ahlijanian et al. 2000; Reynolds et al. 2000; Takashima et al. 2001). These pro-directed kinases also target other pSer/Thr–Pro sites of tau. A hierarchy of phosphorylation regulation by different kinases has been implicated in the cascade of hyperphosphorylation and certain sites may play an initiative role (Jicha et al., 1999; Zheng-Fischhofer et al., 1998). GSK3β or CDK5 has been suggested to induce pre-tangle or NFT phenotypes, respectively (Lucas et al., 2001; Noble et al., 2003; Phiel et al., 2003). Thus, these tau kinases have received particular attention as targets for disease-modifying therapies using inhibitory compounds. Clearance of Aβ is also a logical therapeutic approach. If these inhibitor drugs can reach the brain efficiently from systemic circulation by crossing the blood–brain barrier, those might be attractive therapeutic approaches.

The discovery of the phosphorylation-specific PPIase Pin1 has established conformational regulation after phosphorylation as a new signaling mechanism. Pin1 could restore both tau and APP processing through their conformational changes. Thus, Pin1 might provide the opportunity for exploring more efficient therapy for AD than that targeting either tau or APP. A major challenge for the future will be to stably express Pin1 in the AD brain to normalize tau and APP processing.

## 7. References


Ahlijanian, M.K., Barrezueta, N.X., Williams, R.D., Jakowski, A., Kowsz, K.P., McCarthy, S., Coskran, T., Carlo, A., Seymour, P.A., Burkhardt, J.E., Nelson, R.B. & McNeish, J.D. (2000). Hyperphosphorylated tau and neurofilament and cytoskeletal disruptions in mice overexpressing human p25, an activator of cdk5. *Proceedings of the National Academy of Sciences USA*, Vol. 97, No. 6, pp. 2910-2915, ISSN 0027-8424

Akiyama, H., Shin, R.W., Uchida, C., Kitamoto, T. & Uchida, T. (2005). Pin1 promotes production of Alzheimer's amyloid beta from beta-cleaved amyloid precursor protein. *Biochemical and Biophysical Research Communications*, Vol. 336, No. 2, pp. 521-529, ISSN 0006-291X

Allen, B., Ingram, E., Takao, M., Smith, M.J., Jakes, R., Virdee, K., Yoshida, H., Holzer, M., Craxton, M., Emson, P.C., Atzori, C., Migheli, A., Crowther, R.A., Ghetti, B., Spillantini, M.G. & Goedert, M. (2002). Abundant tau filaments and nonapoptotic neurodegeneration in transgenic mice expressing human P301S tau protein. *Journal of Neuroscience*, Vol. 22, No. 21, pp. 9340-9351, ISSN 0270-6474

Alonso, A.C., Grundke-Iqbal, I. & Iqbal, K. (1996). Alzheimer's disease hyperphosphorylated tau sequesters normal tau into tangles of filaments and disassembles microtubules. *Nature Medicine*, Vol. 2, No. 7, pp. 783-787, ISSN 1078-8956

Arriagada, P.V., Growdon, J.H., Hedley-Whyte, E.T. & Hyman, B.T. (1992a). Neurofibrillary tangles but not senile plaques parallel duration and severity of Alzheimer's disease. *Neurology*, Vol. 42, No. 3 Pt 1, pp. 631-639, ISSN 0028-3878

Arriagada, P.V., Marzloff, K. & Hyman, B.T. (1992b). Distribution of Alzheimer-type pathologic changes in nondemented elderly individuals matches the pattern in Alzheimer's disease. *Neurology*, Vol. 42, No. 9, pp. 1681-1688, ISSN 0028-3878

Augustinack, J.C., Schneider, A., Mandelkow, E.M. & Hyman, B.T. (2002). Specific tau phosphorylation sites correlate with severity of neuronal cytopathology in Alzheimer's disease. *Acta Neuropathologica*, Vol. 103, No. 1, pp. 26-35, ISSN 0001-6322

Ballatore, C., Lee, V.M. & Trojanowski, J.Q. (2007). Tau-mediated neurodegeneration in Alzheimer's disease and related disorders. *Nature Reviews Neuroscience*, Vol. 8, No. 9, pp. 663-672, ISSN 1471-0048

Becker, E.B. & Bonni, A. (2006). Pin1 mediates neural-specific activation of the mitochondrial apoptotic machinery. *Neuron*, Vol. 49, No. 5, pp. 655-662, ISSN 0896-6273

Bertram, L. & Tanzi, R.E. (2009). Genome-wide association studies in Alzheimer's disease. *Human Molecular Genetics*, Vol. 18 (R2), pp. R137-145, ISSN 0964-6906

Blume-Jensen, P. & Hunter, T. (2001). Oncogenic kinase signalling. *Nature*, Vol. 411, No. 6835, pp. 355-365, ISSN 0028-0836

Brookmeyer, R., Gray, S. & Kawas, C. (1998). Projections of Alzheimer's disease in the United States and the public health impact of delaying disease onset. *American Journal of Public Health*, Vol. 88, No. 9, pp. 1337-1342, ISSN 0090-0036

Brown, N.R., Noble, M.E., Endicott, J.A. & Johnson, L.N. (1999). The structural basis for specificity of substrate and recruitment peptides for cyclin-dependent kinases. *Nature Cell Biology*, Vol. 1, No.7, pp. 438-443, ISSN 1097-6256

Butler, A.W., Ng, M.Y., Hamshere, M.L., Forabosco, P., Wroe, R., Al-Chalabi, A., Lewis, C.M. & Powell, J.F. (2009). Meta-analysis of linkage studies for Alzheimer's disease--a web resource. *Neurobiology of Aging*, Vol. 30, No. 7, pp. 1037-1047, ISSN 0197-4580

Butterfield, D.A., Abdul, H.M., Opii, W., Newman, S.F., Joshi, G., Ansari, M.A. & Sultana, R. (2006). Pin1 in Alzheimer's disease. *Journal of Neurochemistry*, Vol. 98, No. 6, pp. 1697-1706, ISSN 0022-3042

Caroni, P. (1997). Overexpression of growth-associated proteins in the neurons of adult transgenic mice. *Journal of Neuroscience Methods*, Vol. 71, No. 1, pp. 3-9, ISSN 0165-0270

Churcher, I. (2006). Tau therapeutic strategies for the treatment of Alzheimer's disease. *Current Topics in Medicinal Chemistry*, Vol. 6, No. 6, pp. 579-595, ISSN 1568-0266

Cruz, J.C., Tseng, H.C., Goldman, J.A., Shih, H. & Tsai, L.H. (2003). Aberrant Cdk5 activation by p25 triggers pathological events leading to neurodegeneration and neurofibrillary tangles. *Neuron*, Vol. 40, No. 3, pp. 471-483, ISSN 0896-6273

Davies, D.C., Horwood, N., Isaacs, S.L. & Mann, D.M. (1992). The effect of age and Alzheimer's disease on pyramidal neuron density in the individual fields of the hippocampal formation. *Acta Neuropathologica*, Vol. 83, No. 5, pp. 510-517, ISSN 0001-6322

De Strooper, B. & Annaert, W. (2000). Proteolytic processing and cell biological functions of the amyloid precursor protein. *Journal of Cell Science*, Vol. 113 (Pt 11), pp. 1857-1870, ISSN 0021-9533

Dickey, C.A., Kamal, A., Lundgren, K., Klosak, N., Bailey, R.M., Dunmore, J., Ash, P., Shoraka, S., Zlatkovic, J., Eckman, C.B., Patterson, C., Dickson, D.W., Nahman, N.S., Jr., Hutton, M., Burrows, F. & Petrucelli, L. (2007). The high-affinity HSP90-CHIP complex recognizes and selectively degrades phosphorylated tau client proteins. *Journal of Clinical Investigation*, Vol. 117, No. 3, pp. 648-658, ISSN 0021-9738

Ding, X.L., Husseman, J., Tomashevski, A., Nochlin, D., Jin, L.W. & Vincent, I. (2000). The cell cycle Cdc25A tyrosine phosphatase is activated in degenerating postmitotic neurons in Alzheimer's disease. *American Journal of Pathology*, Vol. 157, No. 6, pp. 1983-1990, ISSN 1525-2191

Doerflinger, H., Benton, R., Shulman, J.M. & St Johnston, D. (2003). The role of PAR-1 in regulating the polarised microtubule cytoskeleton in the Drosophila follicular epithelium. *Development*, Vol. 130, No. 17, pp. 3965-3975, ISSN 0950-1991

Drewes, G., Trinczek, B., Illenberger, S., Biernat, J., Schmitt-Ulms, G., Meyer, H.E., Mandelkow, E.M. & Mandelkow, E. (1995). Microtubule-associated protein/microtubule affinity-regulating kinase (p110mark). A novel protein kinase that regulates tau-microtubule interactions and dynamic instability by phosphorylation at the Alzheimer-specific site serine 262. *Journal of Biological Chemistry*, Vol. 270, No. 13, pp 7679-7688, ISSN 0021-9258

Esler, W.P. & Wolfe, M.S. (2001). A portrait of Alzheimer secretases--new features and familiar faces. *Science*, Vol. 293, No. 5534, pp 1449-1454, ISSN 0036-8075

Evans, D.A., Funkenstein, H.H., Albert, M.S., Scherr, P.A., Cook, N.R., Chown, M.J., Hebert, L.E., Hennekens, C.H. & Taylor, J.O. (1989). Prevalence of Alzheimer's disease in a community population of older persons. Higher than previously reported. *JAMA*, Vol. 262, No. 18, pp. 2551-2556, ISSN 0002-9955

Evans, D.R. & Stark, M.J. (1997). Mutations in the Saccharomyces cerevisiae type 2A protein phosphatase catalytic subunit reveal roles in cell wall integrity, actin cytoskeleton organization and mitosis. *Genetics*, Vol. 145, No. 2, pp. 227-241, ISSN 0016-6731

Fischer, G. & Aumuller, T. (2003). Regulation of peptide bond cis/trans isomerization by enzyme catalysis and its implication in physiological processes. *Reviews of Physiology, Biochemistry & Pharmacology*, Vol. 148, pp. 105-150, ISSN 0303-4240

Frisardi, V., Solfrizzi, V., Imbimbo, P.B., Capurso, C., D'Introno, A., Colacicco, A.M., Vendemiale, G., Seripa, D., Pilotto, A., Capurso, A. & Panza, F. (2010). Towards disease-modifying treatment of Alzheimer's disease: drugs targeting beta-amyloid. *Current Alzheimer Research*, Vol. 7, No. 1, pp. 40-55, ISSN 1567-2050

Goedert, M., Satumtira, S., Jakes, R., Smith, M.J., Kamibayashi, C., White, C.L., 3rd & Sontag, E. (2000). Reduced binding of protein phosphatase 2A to tau protein with frontotemporal dementia and parkinsonism linked to chromosome 17 mutations. *Journal of Neurochemistry*, Vol. 75, No. 5, pp. 2155-2162, ISSN 0022-3042

Gong, C.X., Lidsky, T., Wegiel, J., Zuck, L., Grundke-Iqbal, I. & Iqbal, K. (2000). Phosphorylation of microtubule-associated protein tau is regulated by protein phosphatase 2A in mammalian brain. Implications for neurofibrillary degeneration in Alzheimer's disease. *Journal of Biological Chemistry*, Vol. 275, No. 8, pp. 5535-5544, ISSN 0021-9258

Gordon-Krajcer, W., Yang, L. & Ksiezak-Reding, H. (2000). Conformation of paired helical filaments blocks dephosphorylation of epitopes shared with fetal tau except

Ser199/202 and Ser202/Thr205. *Brain Research*, Vol. 856, No. 1-2, pp. 163-175, ISSN 0006-8993

Gotz, J., Chen, F., Barmettler, R. & Nitsch, R.M. (2001). Tau filament formation in transgenic mice expressing P301L tau. *Journal of Biological Chemistry*, Vol. 276, No. 1, pp. 529-534, ISSN 0021-9258

Hamdane, M., Dourlen, P., Bretteville, A., Sambo, A.V., Ferreira, S., Ando, K., Kerdraon, O., Begard, S., Geay, L., Lippens, G., Sergeant, N., Delacourte, A., Maurage, C.A., Galas, M.C. & Buee, L. (2006). Pin1 allows for differential Tau dephosphorylation in neuronal cells. *Molecular and Cellular Neurosciences*, Vol. 32, No. 1-2, pp. 155-160, ISSN 1044-7431

Hampel, H., Buerger, K., Kohnken, R., Teipel, S.J., Zinkowski, R., Moeller, H.J., Rapoport, S.I. & Davies, P. (2001). Tracking of Alzheimer's disease progression with cerebrospinal fluid tau protein phosphorylated at threonine 231. *Annals of Neurology*, Vol. 49, No. 4, pp. 545-546, ISSN 0364-5134

Han, C.H., Lu, J., Wei, Q., Bondy, M.L., Brewster, A.M., Yu, T.K., Buchholz, T.A., Arun, B.K. & Wang, L.E. (2010). The functional promoter polymorphism (-842G>C) in the PIN1 gene is associated with decreased risk of breast cancer in non-Hispanic white women 55 years and younger. *Breast cancer research and treatment*, Vol. 122, No. 1, pp. 243-249, ISSN 0167-6806

Hardy, J. & Selkoe, D.J. (2002). The amyloid hypothesis of Alzheimer's disease: progress and problems on the road to therapeutics. *Science*, Vol. 297, No. 5580, pp. 353-356, ISSN 0036-8075

Hasegawa, M., Morishima-Kawashima, M., Takio, K., Suzuki, M., Titani, K. & Ihara, Y. (1992). Protein sequence and mass spectrometric analyses of tau in the Alzheimer's disease brain. *Journal of Biological Chemistry*, Vol. 267, No. 24, pp. 17047-17054, ISSN 0021-9258

Hof, P.R. & Morrison, J.H. (1991). Neocortical neuronal subpopulations labeled by a monoclonal antibody to calbindin exhibit differential vulnerability in Alzheimer's disease. *Experimantal Neurology*, Vol. 111, No. 3, pp. 293-301, ISSN 0014-4886

Hu, Y.F., Luscher, B., Admon, A., Mermod, N. & Tjian, R. (1990). Transcription factor AP-4 contains multiple dimerization domains that regulate dimer specificity. *Genes & Development*, Vol. 4, No. 10, pp. 1741-1752, ISSN 0890-9369

Hunter, T. (1995). Protein kinases and phosphatases: the yin and yang of protein phosphorylation and signaling. *Cell*, Vol. 80, No. 2, pp. 225-236, ISSN 0092-8674

Illenberger, S., Zheng-Fischhofer, Q., Preuss, U., Stamer, K., Baumann, K., Trinczek, B., Biernat, J., Godemann, R., Mandelkow, E.M. & Mandelkow, E. (1998). The endogenous and cell cycle-dependent phosphorylation of tau protein in living cells: implications for Alzheimer's disease. *Molecular Biology of the Cell*, Vol. 9, No. 6, pp. 1495-1512, ISSN 1059-1524

Jicha, G.A., O'Donnell, A., Weaver, C., Angeletti, R. & Davies, P. (1999). Hierarchical phosphorylation of recombinant tau by the paired-helical filament-associated protein kinase is dependent on cyclic AMP-dependent protein kinase. *Journal of Neurochemistry*, Vol. 72, No. 1, pp. 214-224, ISSN 0022-3042

Kawabe, T., Muslin, A.J. & Korsmeyer, S.J. (1997). HOX11 interacts with protein phosphatases PP2A and PP1 and disrupts a G2/M cell-cycle checkpoint. *Nature*, Vol. 385, No. 6615, pp. 454-458, ISSN 0028-0836

Kinoshita, N., Ohkura, H. & Yanagida, M. (1990). Distinct, essential roles of type 1 and 2A protein phosphatases in the control of the fission yeast cell division cycle. *Cell*, Vol. 63, No. 2, pp. 405-415, ISSN 0092-8674

Kins, S., Crameri, A., Evans, D.R., Hemmings, B.A., Nitsch, R.M. & Gotz, J. (2001). Reduced protein phosphatase 2A activity induces hyperphosphorylation and altered compartmentalization of tau in transgenic mice. *Journal of Biological Chemistry*, Vol. 276, No. 41, pp. 38193-38200, ISSN 0021-9258

Kipping, M., Zarnt, T., Kiessig, S., Reimer, U., Fischer, G. & Bayer, P. (2001). Increased backbone flexibility in threonine45-phosphorylated hirudin upon pH change. *Biochemistry*, Vol. 40, No. 27, pp. 7957-7963, ISSN 0006-2960

Kohnken, R., Buerger, K., Zinkowski, R., Miller, C., Kerkman, D., DeBernardis, J., Shen, J., Moller, H.J., Davies, P. & Hampel, H. (2000). Detection of tau phosphorylated at threonine 231 in cerebrospinal fluid of Alzheimer's disease patients. *Neuroscience Letters*, Vol. 287, No. 3, pp. 187-190, ISSN 0304-3940

Kosik, K.S. & Shimura, H. (2005). Phosphorylated tau and the neurodegenerative foldopathies. *Biochimica et Biophysica Acta*, Vol. 1739, No. 2-3, pp. 298-310, ISSN 0006-3002

Lambert, J.C., Heath, S., Even, G., Campion, D., Sleegers, K., Hiltunen, M., Combarros, O., Zelenika, D., Bullido, M.J., Tavernier, B., Letenneur, L., Bettens, K., Berr, C., Pasquier, F., Fievet, N., Barberger-Gateau, P., Engelborghs, S., De Deyn, P., Mateo, I., Franck, A., Helisalmi, S., Porcellini, E., Hanon, O., de Pancorbo, M.M., Lendon, C., Dufouil, C., Jaillard, C., Leveillard, T., Alvarez, V., Bosco, P., Mancuso, M., Panza, F., Nacmias, B., Bossu, P., Piccardi, P., Annoni, G., Seripa, D., Galimberti, D., Hannequin, D., Licastro, F., Soininen, H., Ritchie, K., Blanche, H., Dartigues, J.F., Tzourio, C., Gut, I., Van Broeckhoven, C., Alperovitch, A., Lathrop, M. & Amouyel, P. (2009). Genome-wide association study identifies variants at CLU and CR1 associated with Alzheimer's disease. *Nature Genetics*, Vol. 41, No. 10, pp. 1094-1099, ISSN 1061-4036

Lane, H.A. & Nigg, E.A. (1996). Antibody microinjection reveals an essential role for human polo-like kinase 1 (Plk1) in the functional maturation of mitotic centrosomes. *Journal of Cell Biology*, Vol. 135, No. 6 Pt 2, pp. 1701-1713, ISSN 0021-9525

Lee, M.S., Kao, S.C., Lemere, C.A., Xia, W., Tseng, H.C., Zhou, Y., Neve, R., Ahlijanian, M.K. & Tsai, L.H. (2003). APP processing is regulated by cytoplasmic phosphorylation. *Journal of Cell Biology*, Vol. 163, No. 1, pp. 83-95, ISSN 0021-9525

Lee, M.S. & Tsai, L.H. (2003). Cdk5: one of the links between senile plaques and neurofibrillary tangles? *Journal of Alzheimer's Disease*, Vol. 5, No. 2, pp. 127-137, ISSN 1387-2877

Lee, T.H. (1995). The role of protein phosphatase type-2A in the Xenopus cell cycle: initiation of the G2/M transition. *Seminars in Cancer Biology*, Vol. 6, No. 4, pp. 203-209, ISSN 1044-579X

Lester, H.A., Dibas, M.I., Dahan, D.S., Leite, J.F. & Dougherty, D.A. (2004). Cys-loop receptors: new twists and turns. *Trends in Neurosciences*, Vol. 27, No. 6, pp. 329-336, ISSN 0166-2236

Lewis, J., McGowan, E., Rockwood, J., Melrose, H., Nacharaju, P., Van Slegtenhorst, M., Gwinn-Hardy, K., Paul Murphy, M., Baker, M., Yu, X., Duff, K., Hardy, J., Corral, A., Lin, W.L., Yen, S.H., Dickson, D.W., Davies, P. & Hutton, M. (2000). Neurofibrillary tangles, amyotrophy and progressive motor disturbance in mice expressing mutant (P301L) tau protein. *Nature Genetics*, Vol. 25, No. 4, pp. 402-405, ISSN 1061-4036

Li, Q.M., Tep, C., Yune, T.Y., Zhou, X.Z., Uchida, T., Lu, K.P. & Yoon, S.O. (2007). Opposite regulation of oligodendrocyte apoptosis by JNK3 and Pin1 after spinal cord injury. *Journal of Neuroscience*, Vol. 27, No. 31, pp. 8395-8404, ISSN 0270-6474

Lim, F., Hernandez, F., Lucas, J.J., Gomez-Ramos, P., Moran, M.A. & Avila, J. (2001). FTDP-17 mutations in tau transgenic mice provoke lysosomal abnormalities and Tau filaments in forebrain. *Molecular and Cellular Neurosciences*, Vol. 18, No. 6, pp. 702-714, ISSN 1044-7431

Lim, J., Balastik, M., Lee, T.H., Nakamura, K., Liou, Y.C., Sun, A., Finn, G., Pastorino, L., Lee, V.M. & Lu, K.P. (2008). Pin1 has opposite effects on wild-type and P301L tau stability and tauopathy. *Journal of Clinical Investigation*, Vol. 118, No. 5, pp. 1877-1889, ISSN 0021-9738

Lin, F.C. & Arndt, K.T. (1995). The role of Saccharomyces cerevisiae type 2A phosphatase in the actin cytoskeleton and in entry into mitosis. *EMBO Journal*, Vol. 14, No. 12, pp. 2745-2759, ISSN 0261-4189

Lindwall, G. & Cole, R.D. (1984). Phosphorylation affects the ability of tau protein to promote microtubule assembly. *The Journal of Biological Chemistry*, Vol. 259, No. 8, pp. 5301-5305, ISSN 0021-9258

Liou, Y.C., Sun, A., Ryo, A., Zhou, X.Z., Yu, Z.X., Huang, H.K., Uchida, T., Bronson, R., Bing, G., Li, X., Hunter, T. & Lu, K.P. (2003). Role of the prolyl isomerase Pin1 in protecting against age-dependent neurodegeneration. *Nature*, Vol. 424, No. 6948, pp. 556-561, ISSN 0028-0836

Lu, K.P. (2004). Pinning down cell signaling, cancer and Alzheimer's disease. *Trends in Biochemical Sciences*, Vol. 29, No. 4, pp. 200-209, ISSN 0968-0004

Lu, K.P., Hanes, S.D. & Hunter, T. (1996). A human peptidyl-prolyl isomerase essential for regulation of mitosis. *Nature*, Vol. 380, No. 6574, pp. 544-547, ISSN 0028-0836

Lu, K.P., Liou, Y.C. & Vincent, I. (2003). Proline-directed phosphorylation and isomerization in mitotic regulation and in Alzheimer's Disease. *Bioessays*, Vol. 25, No. 2, pp. 174-181, ISSN 0265-9247

Lu, K.P., Liou, Y.C. & Zhou, X.Z. (2002). Pinning down proline-directed phosphorylation signaling. *Trends in Cell Biology*, Vol. 12, No. 4, pp. 164-172, ISSN 0962-8924

Lu, K.P. & Zhou, X.Z. (2007). The prolyl isomerase PIN1: a pivotal new twist in phosphorylation signalling and disease. *Nature Reviews Molecular Cell Biology*, Vol. 8, No. 11, pp. 904-916, ISSN 1471-0072

Lu, P.J., Wulf, G., Zhou, X.Z., Davies, P. & Lu, K.P. (1999a). The prolyl isomerase Pin1 restores the function of Alzheimer-associated phosphorylated tau protein. *Nature*, Vol. 399, No. 6738, pp. 784-788, ISSN 0028-0836

Lu, P.J., Zhou, X.Z., Shen, M. & Lu, K.P. (1999b). Function of WW domains as phosphoserine- or phosphothreonine-binding modules. *Science*, Vol. 283, No. 5406, pp. 1325-1328, ISSN 0036-8075

Lucas, J.J., Hernandez, F., Gomez-Ramos, P., Moran, M.A., Hen, R. & Avila, J. (2001). Decreased nuclear beta-catenin, tau hyperphosphorylation and neurodegeneration in GSK-3beta conditional transgenic mice. *EMBO Journal*, Vol. 20, No. 1-2, pp. 27-39, ISSN 0261-4189

Lummis, S.C., Beene, D.L., Lee, L.W., Lester, H.A., Broadhurst, R.W. & Dougherty, D.A. (2005). Cis-trans isomerization at a proline opens the pore of a neurotransmitter-gated ion channel. *Nature*, Vol. 438, No. 7065, pp. 248-252, ISSN 0028-0836

Ma, S.L., Tang, N.L., Tam, C.W., Cheong Lui, V.W., Lam, L.C., Chiu, H.F., Driver, J.A., Pastorino, L. & Lu, K.P. (2010) A PIN1 polymorphism that prevents its suppression by AP4 associates with delayed onset of Alzheimer's disease. *Neurobiology of Aging*, ISSN 0197-4580

Mandelkow, E. (1999). Alzheimer's disease. The tangled tale of tau. *Nature*, Vol. 402, No. 6762, pp. 588-589, ISSN 0028-0836

Marchini, J., Cardon, L.R., Phillips, M.S. & Donnelly, P. (2004). The effects of human population structure on large genetic association studies. *Nature Genetics*, Vol. 36, No. 5, pp. 512-517, ISSN 1061-4036

Matsuo, E.S., Shin, R.W., Billingsley, M.L., Van deVoorde, A., O'Connor, M., Trojanowski, J.Q. & Lee, V.M. (1994). Biopsy-derived adult human brain tau is phosphorylated at many of the same sites as Alzheimer's disease paired helical filament tau. *Neuron*, Vol. 13, No. 4, pp. 989-1002, ISSN 0896-6273

Mattson, M.P. (2004). Pathways towards and away from Alzheimer's disease. *Nature*, Vol. 430, No. 7000, pp. 631-639, ISSN 0028-0836

Mawal-Dewan, M., Henley, J., Van de Voorde, A., Trojanowski, J.Q. & Lee, V.M. (1994). The phosphorylation state of tau in the developing rat brain is regulated by phosphoprotein phosphatases. *The Journal of Biological Chemistry*, Vol. 269, No. 49, pp. 30981-30987, ISSN 0021-9258

Mazanetz, M.P. & Fischer, P.M. (2007). Untangling tau hyperphosphorylation in drug design for neurodegenerative diseases. *Nature Reviews Drug Discovery*, Vol. 6, No. 6, pp. 464-479, ISSN 1474-1776

Nigg, E.A. (2001). Mitotic kinases as regulators of cell division and its checkpoints. *Nature Reviews Molecular Cell Biology*, Vol. 2, No. 1, pp. 21-32, ISSN 1471-0072

Nishimura, I., Yang, Y. & Lu, B. (2004). PAR-1 kinase plays an initiator role in a temporally ordered phosphorylation process that confers tau toxicity in Drosophila. *Cell*, Vol. 116, No. 5, pp. 671-682, ISSN 0092-8674

Noble, W., Olm, V., Takata, K., Casey, E., Mary, O., Meyerson, J., Gaynor, K., LaFrancois, J., Wang, L., Kondo, T., Davies, P., Burns, M., Veeranna, Nixon, R., Dickson, D., Matsuoka, Y., Ahlijanian, M., Lau, L.F. & Duff, K. (2003). Cdk5 is a key factor in tau aggregation and tangle formation in vivo. *Neuron*, Vol. 38, No. 4, pp. 555-565, ISSN 0896-6273

Nowotny, P., Bertelsen, S., Hinrichs, A.L., Kauwe, J.S., Mayo, K., Jacquart, S., Morris, J.C. & Goate, A. (2007). Association studies between common variants in prolyl isomerase Pin1 and the risk for late-onset Alzheimer's disease. *Neuroscience Letters*, Vol. 419, No. 1, pp. 15-17, ISSN 0304-3940

Orlicky, S., Tang, X., Willems, A., Tyers, M. & Sicheri, F. (2003). Structural basis for phosphodependent substrate selection and orientation by the SCFCdc4 ubiquitin ligase. *Cell*, Vol. 112, No. 2, pp. 243-256, ISSN 0092-8674

Pastorino, L., Sun, A., Lu, P.J., Zhou, X.Z., Balastik, M., Finn, G., Wulf, G., Lim, J., Li, S.H., Li, X., Xia, W., Nicholson, L.K. & Lu, K.P. (2006). The prolyl isomerase Pin1 regulates amyloid precursor protein processing and amyloid-beta production. *Nature*, Vol. 440, No. 7083, pp. 528-534, ISSN 0028-0836

Pearson, R.C., Esiri, M.M., Hiorns, R.W., Wilcock, G.K. & Powell, T.P. (1985). Anatomical correlates of the distribution of the pathological changes in the neocortex in Alzheimer disease. *Proceedings of the National Academy of Sciences USA*, Vol. 82, No. 13, pp. 4531-4534, ISSN 0027-8424

Pelech, S.L. (1995). Networking with proline-directed protein kinases implicated in tau phosphorylation. *Neurobiology of Aging*, Vol. 16, No. 3, pp. 247-256; discussion pp. 257-261, ISSN 0197-4580

Petrucelli, L., Dickson, D., Kehoe, K., Taylor, J., Snyder, H., Grover, A., De Lucia, M., McGowan, E., Lewis, J., Prihar, G., Kim, J., Dillmann, W.H., Browne, S.E., Hall, A., Voellmy, R., Tsuboi, Y., Dawson, T.M., Wolozin, B., Hardy, J. & Hutton, M. (2004). CHIP and Hsp70 regulate tau ubiquitination, degradation and aggregation. *Human Molecular Genetics*, Vol. 13, No. 7, pp. 703-714, ISSN 0964-6906

Phiel, C.J., Wilson, C.A., Lee, V.M. & Klein, P.S. (2003). GSK-3alpha regulates production of Alzheimer's disease amyloid-beta peptides. *Nature*, Vol. 423, No. 6938, pp. 435-439, ISSN 0028-0836

Poppek, D., Keck, S., Ermak, G., Jung, T., Stolzing, A., Ullrich, O., Davies, K.J. & Grune, T. (2006). Phosphorylation inhibits turnover of the tau protein by the proteasome: influence of RCAN1 and oxidative stress. *Biochemical Journal*, Vol. 400, No. 3, pp. 511-520, ISSN 0264-6021

Ramelot, T.A. & Nicholson, L.K. (2001). Phosphorylation-induced structural changes in the amyloid precursor protein cytoplasmic tail detected by NMR. *Journal of Molecular Biology*, Vol. 307, No. 3, pp. 871-884, ISSN 0022-2836

Ranganathan, R., Lu, K.P., Hunter, T. & Noel, J.P. (1997). Structural and functional analysis of the mitotic rotamase Pin1 suggests substrate recognition is phosphorylation dependent. *Cell*, Vol. 89, No. 6, pp. 875-886, ISSN 0092-8674

Sansom, M.S. & Weinstein, H. (2000). Hinges, swivels and switches: the role of prolines in signalling via transmembrane alpha-helices. *Trends in Pharmacological Sciences*, Vol. 21, No. 11, pp. 445-451, ISSN 0165-6147

Schneider, A., Biernat, J., von Bergen, M., Mandelkow, E. & Mandelkow, E.M. (1999). Phosphorylation that detaches tau protein from microtubules (Ser262, Ser214) also protects it against aggregation into Alzheimer paired helical filaments. *Biochemistry*, Vol. 38, No. 12, pp. 3549-3558, ISSN 0006-2960

Segat, L., Pontillo, A., Annoni, G., Trabattoni, D., Vergani, C., Clerici, M., Arosio, B. & Crovella, S. (2007). PIN1 promoter polymorphisms are associated with Alzheimer's disease. *Neurobiology of Aging*, Vol. 28, No. 1, pp. 69-74, ISSN 0197-4580

Selkoe, D.J., Yamazaki, T., Citron, M., Podlisny, M.B., Koo, E.H., Teplow, D.B. & Haass, C. (1996). The role of APP processing and trafficking pathways in the formation of amyloid beta-protein. *Annals of the New York Academy of Sciences*, Vol. 777, pp. 57-64, ISSN 1749-6632

Shen, Z.J., Esnault, S. & Malter, J.S. (2005). The peptidyl-prolyl isomerase Pin1 regulates the stability of granulocyte-macrophage colony-stimulating factor mRNA in activated eosinophils. *Nature Immunology*, Vol. 6, No. 12, pp. 1280-1287, ISSN 1529-2908

Smet, C., Wieruszeski, J.M., Buee, L., Landrieu, I. & Lippens, G. (2005). Regulation of Pin1 peptidyl-prolyl cis/trans isomerase activity by its WW binding module on a multi-phosphorylated peptide of Tau protein. *FEBS Letters*, Vol. 579, No. 19, pp. 4159-4164, ISSN 0014-5793.

Sontag, E., Nunbhakdi-Craig, V., Bloom, G.S. & Mumby, M.C. (1995). A novel pool of protein phosphatase 2A is associated with microtubules and is regulated during the cell cycle. *Journal of Cell Biology*, Vol. 128, No. 6, pp. 1131-1144, ISSN 0021-9525

Sontag, E., Nunbhakdi-Craig, V., Lee, G., Bloom, G.S. & Mumby, M.C. (1996). Regulation of the phosphorylation state and microtubule-binding activity of Tau by protein phosphatase 2A. *Neuron*, Vol. 17, No. 6, pp. 1201-1207, ISSN 0896-6273

Stoothoff, W.H. & Johnson, G.V. (2005). Tau phosphorylation: physiological and pathological consequences. *Biochimica et Biophysica Acta*, Vol. 1739, No. 2-3, pp. 280-297, ISSN 0006-3002

Suizu, F., Ryo, A., Wulf, G., Lim, J. & Lu, K.P. (2006). Pin1 regulates centrosome duplication, and its overexpression induces centrosome amplification, chromosome instability, and oncogenesis. *Molecular and Cellular Biology*, Vol. 26, No. 4, pp. 1463-1479, ISSN 0270-7306

Sultana, R., Boyd-Kimball, D., Poon, H.F., Cai, J., Pierce, W.M., Klein, J.B., Markesbery, W.R., Zhou, X.Z., Lu, K.P. & Butterfield, D.A. (2006). Oxidative modification and down-regulation of Pin1 in Alzheimer's disease hippocampus: A redox proteomics analysis. *Neurobiology of Aging*, Vol. 27, No. 7, pp. 918-925, ISSN 0197- 4580

Suzuki, T., Oishi, M., Marshak, D.R., Czernik, A.J., Nairn, A.C. & Greengard, P. (1994). Cell cycle-dependent regulation of the phosphorylation and metabolism of the Alzheimer amyloid precursor protein. *EMBO Journal*, Vol. 13, No. 5, pp. 1114-1122, ISSN 0261-4189

Takei, Y., Teng, J., Harada, A. & Hirokawa, N. (2000). Defects in axonal elongation and neuronal migration in mice with disrupted tau and map1b genes. *Journal of Cell Biology*, Vol. 150, No. 5, pp. 989-1000, ISSN 0021-9525

Tanemura, K., Murayama, M., Akagi, T., Hashikawa, T., Tominaga, T., Ichikawa, M., Yamaguchi, H. & Takashima, A. (2002). Neurodegeneration with tau accumulation in a transgenic mouse expressing V337M human tau. *Journal of Neuroscience*, Vol. 22, No. 1, pp. 133-141, ISSN 0270-6474

Vincent, I., Jicha, G., Rosado, M. & Dickson, D.W. (1997). Aberrant expression of mitotic cdc2/cyclin B1 kinase in degenerating neurons of Alzheimer's disease brain. *Journal of Neuroscience*, Vol. 17, No. 10, pp. 3588-3598, ISSN 0270-6474

Vincent, I., Rosado, M. & Davies, P. (1996). Mitotic mechanisms in Alzheimer's disease? *Journal of Cell Biology*, Vol. 132, No. 3, pp. 413-425, ISSN 0021-9525

Weingarten, M.D., Lockwood, A.H., Hwo, S.Y. & Kirschner, M.W. (1975). A protein factor essential for microtubule assembly. *Proceedings of the National Academy of Sciences USA*, Vol. 72, No. 5, pp. 1858-1862, ISSN 0027-8424

Weiwad, M., Kullertz, G., Schutkowski, M. & Fischer, G. (2000). Evidence that the substrate backbone conformation is critical to phosphorylation by p42 MAP kinase. *FEBS Letters*, Vol. 478, No. 1-2, pp. 39-42, ISSN 0014-5793

Wells, N.J., Watanabe, N., Tokusumi, T., Jiang, W., Verdecia, M.A. & Hunter, T. (1999). The C-terminal domain of the Cdc2 inhibitory kinase Myt1 interacts with Cdc2 complexes and is required for inhibition of G(2)/M progression. *Journal of Cell Science*, Vol. 112 (Pt 19), pp. 3361-3371, ISSN 0021-9533

Wijsman, E.M., Daw, E.W., Yu, C.E., Payami, H., Steinbart, E.J., Nochlin, D., Conlon, E.M., Bird, T.D. & Schellenberg, G.D. (2004). Evidence for a novel late-onset Alzheimer disease locus on chromosome 19p13.2. *Amwrican Journal of Human Genetics*, Vol. 75, No. 3, pp. 398-409, ISSN 0002-9297

Winkler, K.E., Swenson, K.I., Kornbluth, S. & Means, A.R. (2000). Requirement of the prolyl isomerase Pin1 for the replication checkpoint. *Science*, Vol. 287, No. 5458, pp. 1644-1647, ISSN 0036-8075

Wulf, G., Finn, G., Suizu, F. & Lu, K.P. (2005). Phosphorylation-specific prolyl isomerization: is there an underlying theme? *Nature Cell Biology*, Vol. 7, No. 5, pp. 435-441, ISSN 1097-6256

Yaffe, M.B., Schutkowski, M., Shen, M., Zhou, X.Z., Stukenberg, P.T., Rahfeld, J.U., Xu, J., Kuang, J., Kirschner, M.W., Fischer, G., Cantley, L.C. & Lu, K.P. (1997). Sequence-specific and phosphorylation-dependent proline isomerization: a potential mitotic regulatory mechanism. *Science*, Vol. 278, No. 5345, pp. 1957-1960, ISSN 0036-8075

Yang, Y. & Herrup, K. (2007). Cell division in the CNS: protective response or lethal event in post-mitotic neurons? *Biochimica et Biophysica Acta*, Vol. 1772, No. 4, pp. 457-466, ISSN 0006-3002

Zheng-Fischhofer, Q., Biernat, J., Mandelkow, E.M., Illenberger, S., Godemann, R. & Mandelkow, E. (1998). Sequential phosphorylation of Tau by glycogen synthase kinase-3beta and protein kinase A at Thr212 and Ser214 generates the Alzheimer-specific epitope of antibody AT100 and requires a paired-helical-filament-like conformation. *European Journal of Biochemistry*, Vol. 252, No. 3, pp. 542-552, ISSN 0014-2956

Zhou, X.Z., Kops, O., Werner, A., Lu, P.J., Shen, M., Stoller, G., Kullertz, G., Stark, M., Fischer, G. & Lu, K.P. (2000). Pin1-dependent prolyl isomerization regulates dephosphorylation of Cdc25C and tau proteins. Molecular *Cell*, Vol. 6, No. 4, pp. 873-883, ISSN 1097-2765

Zhou, X.Z., Lu, P.J., Wulf, G. & Lu, K.P. (1999). Phosphorylation-dependent prolyl isomerization: a novel signaling regulatory mechanism. *Cellular and Molecular Life Sciences*, Vol. 56, No. 9-10, pp. 788-806, ISSN 1420-682X

Zita, M.M., Marchionni, I., Bottos, E., Righi, M., Del Sal, G., Cherubini, E. & Zacchi, P. (2007). Post-phosphorylation prolyl isomerisation of gephyrin represents a mechanism to modulate glycine receptors function. *EMBO Journal*, Vol. 26, No. 7, pp. 1761-1771, ISSN 0261-4189

# 5

# Key Enzymes and Proteins in Amyloid-Beta Production and Clearance

Cecília R A Santos[1], Isabel Cardoso[2,3] and Isabel Gonçalves[1]
[1]*University of Beira Interior- Health Sciences Research Centre, Covilhã*
[2]*Escola Superior de Tecnologia da Saúde do Porto, Instituto Politécnico do Porto, Vila Nova de Gaia,*
[3]*Molecular Neurobiology Unit, IBMC- Instituto de Biologia Molecular e Celular, Porto, Portugal*

## 1. Introduction

Last century, in 1907, Alois Alzheimer first described the disease that now bears his name, relating a 54-year-old female case with presenile dementia. Alzheimer's disease (AD), an irreversible progressive neurodegenerative disorder, is actually the most common form of dementia. AD affects more than 24 million people all over the world, and is predicted to double every 20 years, becoming one of the medical burdens of our days. More than 90% of AD cases are sporadic late-onset, and have a complex idiopathic aetiology. The small number of early onset AD cases, is related to hereditary monogenic defects, and has provided important clues for understanding the AD pathology (Bertram, et al. 2007). Although the available drugs are able to delay the symptoms and progression of the disease and to positively influence the quality of life of the patients, at present there is still no cure for AD.

AD is characterized clinically by progressive decline in cognitive function and neuropatologically by the presence of neuropil threads and neuron loss, in addition to the molecular hallmarks of neurofibrillar tangles and neuritic (or senile) plaques in the brain. Neuritic plaques are extracellular amyloid deposits found abundantly in the hippocampus, in the neocortex and in the amygdala of AD brains. These pathological brain changes may occur 20 to 30 years prior to the onset of the clinical symptoms and the symptomatic phase of AD can last from 5 to 12 years (DeKosky and Marek 2003). The extracellular neuritic plaque deposits of amyloid were first investigated by (Glenner and Wong 1984), when they purified microvascular amyloid deposits from AD brains, and provided a partial sequence of a 4kDa subunit protein, that they named amyloid-beta (Aβ) peptide. Around the same time, the hyperphosphorylated tau (p-tau), a microtubule assembly protein, was identified as the main constituent of the neurofibrillar tangles (NFTs) that accumulate inside many neurons in AD brains (Grundke-Iqbal, et al. 1986). Amyloid deposition and neurofibrillar tangles, occur with some frequency in brains of young adults with Down's syndrome (Schochet, et al. 1973). The discovery that amyloid deposits in the brain from Down syndrome were composed of Aβ peptide (Glenner and Wong 1984), as well as the cloning of the beta amyloid precursor protein (APP), with its localization to the chromosome 21

(Korenberg, et al. 1989), led the scientists to search AD-causing mutations in the APP gene. Since that, several mutations associated with familial early onset forms of AD have been described, either in the APP gene (Kowalska 2003) or in preselin 1 (PS1) or preselin 2 (PS2) genes (Bertram et al. 2007). Either PS1 or PS2 can be the catalytic subunit of γ-secretase, which is the final endoprotease in the pathways that generate the Aβ peptide (see section 2). All these findings led to the amyloid cascade hypothesis, articulated by John Hardy and others (Hardy and Higgins 1992), in which the accumulation of Aβ peptide, generated from the proteolytic cleavage of APP in the brain, could trigger a complex downstream cascade that results in the symptoms of AD. This hypothesis states that gradual accumulation and aggregation of the hydrophobic Aβ peptide initiates a cascade that leads to synaptic alterations, astrocytic and microglial activation, the modification of the soluble tau protein into insoluble paired helical filaments, and progressive neuronal loss associated with multiple neurotransmitter deficiencies and cognitive failure (Hardy and Selkoe 2002). The cascade hypothesis suggests that stopping or slowing formation of the Aβ plaques would delay the onset of the disease symptoms. Aβ is found in the extracellular fluids of the brain, including cerebrospinal fluid (CSF), and in the interstitial fluid surrounding neurons and glial cells in brain lobes (Seubert, et al. 1992; Vigo-Pelfrey, et al. 1993). Over the last years, several key proteins have been described as being implicated in Aβ production and clearance, but further elucidation of the mechanisms involved in the process will be important for identifying new potential therapies to reduce Aβ accumulation and combat AD. This book chapter reviews the production of Aβ from APP and the proteins involved in its degradation and clearance .

## 2. Generation of amyloid beta peptides

The β amyloid precursor protein, APP, takes a central position in AD pathogenesis, as it is processed by the sequential action of β- and γ-secretase, generating the Aβ peptide, which is deposited as amyloid plaques in brains of AD individuals. APP is an integral membrane protein, with a large N-terminal extracellular domain and a short C-terminal cytoplasmatic domain, which is expressed ubiquitously in neuronal and non-neuronal cells.

The human APP gene is located on chromosome 21 (Korenberg et al. 1989) and alternative splicing results in protein isoforms of various lengths: two isoforms predominant in non-neuronal tissues (751- and 770-), and the 695-amino acid form, that is the predominant isoform in neurons (Kang and Muller-Hill 1990). APP belongs to a protein family that includes APP-like protein 1 (APLP1) and 2 (APLP2) (Eggert, et al. 2004), a group of type-I transmembrane proteins that are processed in the same fashion. APP is hydrolyzed into different fragments (Figure 1) during its intracellular trafficking, and these metabolites mediate various functions (Haass 2004; Haass and Selkoe 1993). APP is first cleaved by either α- or β-secretase at the α- or β-sites, respectively, which lie in the extracellular domain of the APP. These proteases compete for APP, originating: soluble APPα (sAPPα, for α-secretase) or soluble APPβ (sAPPβ, for β-secretase), which are released to the extracellular space, and a membrane anchored C-terminal end (C83 for α-secretase or C99 for β-secretase). Subsequently, in the lipid bilayer, γ-secretase acts in the C-terminal end, C83 or C99. The γ-cleavage of C83 generates the APP intracellular domain (AICD), with 6kDa, and the N-terminal peptide with 3kDa (p3) into the extracellular space. γ-cleavage of C99, in a specific sequence (Aβ domain) generates Aβ peptide and the AICD. This pathway of APP processing by β-secretase followed by γ-secretase leading to Aβ peptide is called the amyloidogenic pathway. Aberrant and/or cumulative Aβ production, have been postulated to be the main etiological basis of AD. The alternative pathway of APP processing by α-secretase followed by γ-secretase, in which no Aβ is formed, is termed nonamyloidogenic pathway.

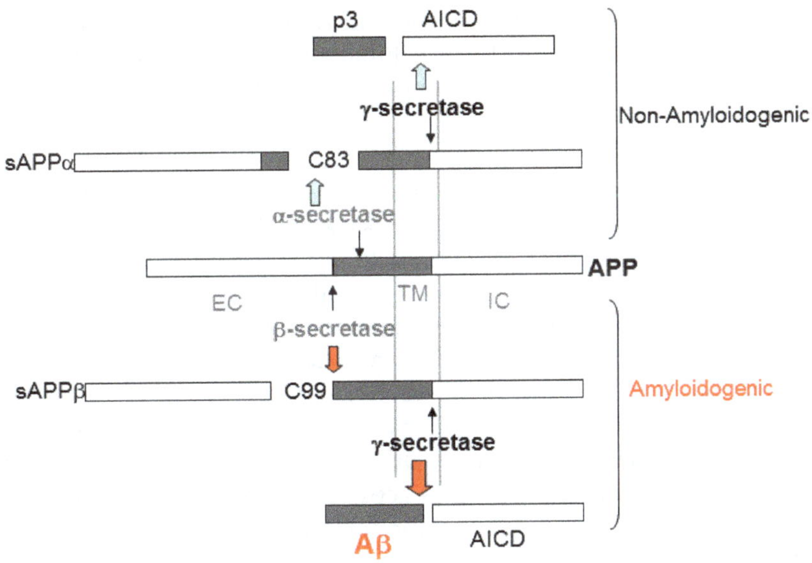


Fig. 1. Schematic diagram of APP processing (not drawn in scale). TM-transmembrane;EC-extracelular; IC- intracellular

Aβ is a ~4kDa peptide with 38 to 43 amino acids, depending on the site of γ-secretase cleavage. Aβ peptide is normally produced by cells and under physiological conditions there are two major species: Aβ40 and Aβ42. The major species produced is Aβ40 and corresponds to 90% of the total Aβ peptide. The minor species produced, Aβ42, is more prone to aggregation due to two additional hydrophobic amino acids, and therefore it is the predominant species accumulated in AD brain plaques.

A number of proteins influence the subcellular trafficking itinerary of APP and β-secretase between the cell surface, endosomes and the Trans-Golgi-Network (TGN). APP is synthesized in the endoplasmic reticulum (ER) and is transported through the Golgi apparatus to the TGN, where the highest concentration is found in steady state neurons (Greenfield, et al. 1999). From TGN, the APP can be transported, in TGN-derived vesicles, to cell surface where it is either cleaved by α-secretase to produce sAPPα, or internalized via the endosomal-lysosomal pathway (Caporaso, et al. 1994). The Aβ peptide is generated either in the ER and TGN (Greenfield et al. 1999), as in the endosomal/lysosomal system (Haass and Selkoe 1993). Available evidence suggests that co-residence of APP and β-secretase in the endosomal compartments promotes amyloidogenesis. Retrograde transport of APP, out of the endosome to the TGN, reduces Aβ production, while APP routed to, and kept at the cell surface, enhances its non-amyloidogenic processing (Tang 2009).

Very little is known about the physiological function of APP and its proteolytic products. APP knockout mice (KO) are viable and fertile, showing a slight abnormal phenotype

(Dawson, et al. 1999). APLP1 and APLP2 KO mice are also viable and fertile, but APP/APLP2 and APLP1/APLP2 double null mice and APP/APLP1/APLP2 triple null mice show early postnatal lethality (Heber, et al. 2000; von Koch, et al. 1997). APP/APLP1 double null mice are viable, suggesting redundant functions of amyloid precursor protein family members (Heber et al. 2000). Putative suggested roles for APP include trafficking, neurotrophic signalling, control of cell adhesion, neuritic outgrowth and synaptogenesis, apoptosis and transcription regulation (Zheng and Koo 2006). As APP is proteolysed in the cell, the net effect of full-length APP on cellular activity may be a combination of the function of its proteolytic products, depending on the proportion levels of each of them.

### 2.1 Alpha-secretase

APP is cleaved by α-secretase in the center of Aβ domain, precluding Aβ peptide generation, and a soluble domain of APP is released: sAPPα. Three related proteases, all from the ADAM family, had been suggested to exert the α-secretase activity: ADAM-9, ADAM-10 and ADAM-17 (Asai, et al. 2003). Like full length APP, members of the ADAM family (a desintegrin and metalloprotease family) are type-I transmembrane proteins, possessing both potential adhesion and protease domains. Several studies suggested α-secretase activity for ADAM-9. However, as RNAi of ADAM-9 has no effect in sAPPα generation (Kuhn, et al. 2010), ADAM-9 seems to be involved only in regulated α-cleavage and not in constitutive α-secretase activity. Different studies strongly suggest that ADAM-10 is the main constitutive α-secretase that is active at the cell surface (Lammich, et al. 1999) (Jorissen, et al. 2010), but there may exist some functional redundancy in α-cleavage by the ADAM protease family. ADAM-17 is an 824 amino acid polypeptide containing a secretory signal sequence, a desintegrin domain and a metalloprotease domain, that also seems to be involved in regulated α-secretase activity (Merlos-Suarez, et al. 2001).

sAPPα has important roles in neuronal plasticity/survival, stem cell proliferation in CNS, and is able to rescue the abnormalities of APP deficient mice, indicating that most of APP´s physiological function is mediated by sAPPα (Zhang, et al. 2011).

### 2.2 Beta-secretases: BACEs

β-secretase cleavage is the first critical step in the APP amyloidogenic pathway, and increased β-secretase activity levels have been correlated with brain Aβ deposition in late onset AD patients (Li, et al. 2004). Aβ peptide is generated from APP by a sequential two-step proteolytic process involving β- and γ-secretases (Haass 2004), being BACE 1 (β-site APP cleaving enzyme 1) the major β-secretase in the cell (Vassar, et al. 1999). BACE1 is a member of the pepsin family of aspartyl proteases, and its activity on APP generates the membrane bound C-terminal fragment (CTFβ or C99). BACE1 requires acidic environment for optimal activity and cleaves APP at the known β-site locations, Asp1 and Glu11. Overexpression of BACE1 induces cleavage of APP at β-sites and is mainly found in the early Golgi, late Golgi/early endosomes and endosomes with acidic environment. BACE1 is also found at the cell surface (Huse, et al. 2002; Vassar et al. 1999).

BACE2 is an additional β-secretase, mapped in 21q22.3 region (Solans, et al. 2000), that also cleaves β-secretase substrates. However, BACE2 expression in neurons is lower than BACE1 (Bennett, et al. 2000). BACE1 null mice died in the first weeks and those that survived, were smaller, presented hyperactive behaviour, were affected by hypomyelination of peripheral nerves and had altered neurological behaviours such as elevated pain sensitivity

(Dominguez, et al. 2005). BACE2 KO mice are healthy overall, while a deficiency of both BACE1 and BACE2 enhanced the BACE1 KO lethality phenotype, suggesting functional redundancy (Dominguez et al. 2005).

Cathepsin B has been proposed as another β-secretase. Although its inhibition has been found to reduce Aβ production, its physiological activity is not well established (Hook, et al. 2009).

### 2.3 The gamma secretase complex

γ-secretase is a protein complex, of high molecular weight, responsible for the membrane cleavage of the APP C-terminal remnants after cleavage by either α- or β-secretase (C83 and C99, respectively). The cleavage of C83 and C99 by γ-secretase generates p3 and the Aβ peptide, respectively. In addition to C83 and C99 peptides, several non-APP substracts are cleaved by γ-secretase and all of them are type-I transmembrane proteins that require ectodomain shedding as a prerequisite to γ-secretase cleavage (Haapasalo and Kovacs 2011). γ-secretase complex comprises four core components which include: presenilin (PS1 or PS2), nicastrin, anterior pharynx-defective-1 (APH-1), and presenilin enhancer-2 (PEN2) (Kimberly and Wolfe 2003; Takasugi, et al. 2003). All of these four core components of γ-secretase are necessary for the enzymatic activity of the complex. PS1 and PS2 are two presenilin homologs, and several mutations in the corresponding genes have been described as the major cause of familial AD cases (Bertram et al. 2007). Different kinds of experimental evidences suggest that presenilins are transmembrane proteins with crucial catalytic roles in γ-secretase activity (Zhang et al. 2011). Nicastrin, other component of γ-secretase, is a type-I transmembrane glycoprotein considered the scaffolding protein of the complex (Vassar and Citron 2000). Finally, the other two components of γ-secretase are: APH-1, that interacts with nicastrin to form a stable intermediate in the early assembly stages of the complex and PEN-2, that regulates PS endoproteolysis (Vassar and Citron 2000). Besides the four components of γ-secretase complex, some factors, playing a modulatory role, have been described. Example of that is CD147 that when down regulated increases Aβ production and TMP21/p23 that regulates γ-cleavage (Zhang et al. 2011).

Experimental evidences support the idea that γ-secretase resides in ER, Golgi-TGN, endosomes and intermediate compartments, most of which (except TGN) do not correspond to the main localizations of APP (Cupers, et al. 2001).

## 3. Enzymes and peptides involved in amyloid-beta degradation and clearence

The clearance of Aβ in the human central nervous system (CNS), is roughly 8% of total production per hour. It is controlled by Aβ degradation in the brain and by its efflux from the CNS to the peripheral circulation through the blood-brain barrier or the blood-cerebrospinal fluid barrier (Zlokovic 2004). The high clearance of Aβ is in part due to the presence of cryptidases in several cellular compartments and reduction of Aβ degradation by these enzymes may be implicated in the progression of AD cases. Aβ accumulation, and the concomitant formation of amyloid plaques observed in AD brains occurs in the extracellular space. It is also in this compartment, that Aβ can be degraded by cell surface and/or secreted cryptidases, such as insulin degrading enzyme and neprylisin. The subcellular distribution of Aβ degrading cryptidases is a strong indicator that Aβ degradation can be controlled at multiple subcellular compartments, such as the mitochondria, ER, Golgi, endosomes and lisossomes (Malito, et al. 2008).

In the brain, Aβ metabolism is mainly regulated by the activity of neprilysin (NEP) and insulin-degrading enzyme (IDE), but presequence peptidase, endothelin converting enzyme (ECE), angiotensin-converting enzyme (ACE), the uPA/tPA- plasmin system and matrix metalloproteinases are also involved in the process (Table 1). In addition, some proteins as transthyretin (TTR), gelsolin, alpha2-macroglobulin and apolipoprotein E do also play an important role in Aβ clearance and degradation. Some of them do actually have a direct function in Aβ catabolism such as TTR, plasmin, and gelsolin, which have the capacity to cleave the peptide, others because their interaction with Aβ enable its degradation or prevent its neurotoxicity as it is the case of alpha-2-macroglobulin and apolipoprotein E (Table 2).

| Enzymes | Function | Brain distribution | References |
|---|---|---|---|
| *IDE* | Hydrolises peptide bonds of Aβ40 and Aβ42 | Neurons, microglia, endothelial cells, choroid plexus epithelial cells | (Bora et al. 2010; Bora and Prabhakar 2010; Malito et al. 2008) |
| *NEP* | Hydrolises peptide bonds of Aβ42 | Neurons, microglia, endothelial cells, choroid plexus epithelial cells | (Malito et al. 2008; Meilandt et al. 2009) |
| *PreP* | Hydrolises peptide bonds of Aβ40 and Aβ42 in mitochondria | | (Falkevall et al. 2006) |
| *ECE* | Hydrolises peptide bonds of Aβ40 and Aβ42 | Neurons, astrocytes, endothelial cells | (Miners et al. 2008b) |
| *ACE* | Converts Aβ42 to Aβ40<br>Cleaves Aβ40 | Neurons, endothelial cells, choroid plexus epithelial cells | (Miners et al. 2008a; Zou et al. 2007) |
| *Plasmin* | Degrades aggregated and non-aggregated Aβ40 and Aβ42<br>Inhibits Aβ fibrillogenesis | Neurons, microglia | (Tucker et al. 2002; Tucker et al. 2000b) |
| *MMP-2* | Hydrolises peptide bonds of Aβ40 and Aβ42<br>Beta-secretase activity | Microglia, astrocytes, Schwann cells | (Miners et al. 2008a) |
| *MMP-9* | Hydrolises peptide bonds of Aβ40 and Aβ42 and aggregated Aβ fibrils | Neurons, endothelial cells | (Miners et al. 2008a; Yan et al. 2006) |

Table 1. Functions and brain distribution of key enzymes in Aβ clearance.

| Key players | Function | Brain distribution | References |
|---|---|---|---|
| *TTR* | Hydrolises peptide bonds of Aβ40 and Aβ42, and aggregated Aβ oligomers and fibrils | choroid plexus epithelial cells meninges | (Costa et al. 2008; Schwarzman et al. 1994) |
| *Gelsolin* | Inhibits fibrillization of Aβ and defibrillates preformed fibrils | Oligodendrocytes, microglia, choroid plexus epithelial cells | (Chauhan et al. 2008; Ray et al. 2000) |
| *Alpha-2 macroglobulin* | Aβ carrier, binds Aβ protecting it from proteolysis, reduces Aβ aggregation and fibril formation | astroglia | (Du et al. 1998; Du et al. 1997) |
| *Apo E* | Binds Aβ enhancing the proteolytic activity of NEP, and IDE | Astrocytes, neurons, microglia | (Jiang et al. 2008) |
| *MT-2* | Diminishes Aβ binding to TTR Prevents copper mediated aggregation of Aβ | Cortical neurons | (Chung et al. 2010; Martinho et al. 2010) |
| *MT-3* | Increases Aβ binding to TTR Inhibits formation of Aβ aggregates | Cortical neurons | (Irie and Keung, 2001, 2003; Martinho et al. 2010) |

Table 2. Functions and brain distribution of key proteins in Aβ clearance.

### 3.1 IDE – Insulin degrading enzyme

Insulin degrading enzyme (IDE) is a ~ 110 kDa zinc-containing metalloendopeptidase that degrades monomeric forms of Aβ peptides and insulin, which has also high nanomolar affinity for other substrates with different sequences and structures. The common features of IDE substrates are that they are all amyloidogenic in nature. So, besides Aβ and insulin, IDE also cleaves, insulin-like growth factor 2, atrial natriuretic peptide, bradykinin, endorphin, and glucagon. However, *in vivo* relevance of this degrading activity has only been demonstrated for Aβ and insulin (Malito et al. 2008). Interestingly, patients with type 2 diabetes are under an increased risk of AD. In addition, Aβ is a direct competitive inhibitor of insulin binding and action, and this is a likely justification for the increased levels of Aβ observed in insulin resistant AD patients (Xie, et al. 2002). This dual effect of IDE stresses the importance of the development of inhibitors and activators of its activity for the treatment of diabetes and AD, respectively.

The first evidences of the capacity of IDE to degrade Aβ were reported by Kurochkin and Goto (1994) who identified a protein of 110,000 Da present in cytosol fractions from rat brain and liver that cross-linked to $^{125}$I-labeled synthetic Aβ. A few years later IDE was actually identified as the main soluble Aβ degrading enzyme in human brain and in neuronal cell cultures, where its action takes places in the extracellular milieu (McDermott and Gibson 1997). Besides its ability to degrade Aβ, IDE activity is also associated with oligomerization of synthetic Aβ at physiological levels in the conditioned media of cultured cells (Qiu, et al. 1998). In addition, evidence that membrane-associated and secreted IDE isoforms carry out the degradation and clearance of Aβ secreted by neurons and microglia was provided a couple of years later (Bertram, et al. 2000).

IDE is composed of four homologous domains that share 15–24% sequence similarity. These domains form two functional N- and C-terminal domains that are joined by an extended 28 amino acid residue loop, creating a large catalytic chamber which can accommodate substrates of the order of 6 kDa. Substrate binding is assisted by the C-terminal domain and, its hydrolysis occurs at the N-terminal domain (Li, et al. 2006). The active site of IDE encompasses the His-Glu-aa-aa-His sequence and requires zinc. IDE enzyme hydrolyses several peptide bonds of both Aβ40 and Aβ42, but is particularly efficient at hydrolysing the Lys28-Gly29 peptide bond followed by the Phe19-Phe20 and His14-Gln15 bonds of these substrates (Bora, et al. 2010; Bora and Prabhakar 2010).

IDE is expressed by cortical and subcortical neurons, and has been detected in the cytoplasm of the three major components of the vascular wall: endothelial cells, pericytes and smooth muscle cells (Dorfman, et al. 2010; Gao, et al. 2004). IDE is also expressed towards the apical surface of the choroid plexus tissue where its inhibition leads to disrupted metabolism of Aβ and its concurrent accumulation at the blood-CSF barrier (Behl, et al. 2009). Besides the cytoplasm, IDE is found in endosomes, on the cell surface, and in the extracellular milieu. The type of cell in the nervous system expressing IDE establishes whether it is secreted or associated with the cell surface. Primary mouse microglia and the BV-2 cell line are found to secrete IDE, but in primary hippocampal neurons and differentiated PC12 cells only membrane associated IDE has been found. IDE is also present in mitochondria, and in the dendrites of neurons (Malito et al. 2008).

Evidence that IDE activity in AD brains is reduced compared to age-matched controls has been giving support to the hypothesis that reduced IDE activity may contribute to Aβ accumulation in the brain (Perez, et al. 2000). For example, membrane-bound IDE protein concentrations and activity decrease during the conversion from mild cognitive impairment (MCI) to mild-severe AD in the hippocampus, which correlates negatively with brain Aβ42 content in MCI and in AD brain (Zhao, et al. 2007). Still, other studies indicate that IDE may be less important in the process of Aβ clearance (Wang, et al. 2010). There is also evidence that in transgenic mice brain, Aβ plaques induce cortical mRNA and protein levels of IDE in parallel with increased Aβ40 and Aβ42 production, suggesting a positive feedback regulatory mechanism of Aβ regulation (Vepsalainen, et al. 2008).

### 3.2 NEP – Neprilysin

Neprilysin (NEP) is a 90–110 kDa plasma membrane glycoprotein of the neutral zinc metalloendopeptidase family. It consists of a short N-terminal cytoplasmic tail, a single transmembrane helix and a large C-terminal extracellular ectodomain. The ectodomain of neprilysin is largely made of α-helices with six disulfide bridges and at least three N-glycosylation sites. The ectodomain encompasses the catalytic site, with the conserved HExxH motif necessary for zinc coordination and a proteolytic chamber (Malito et al. 2008). NEP is widely expressed in several tissues such as the brush-border of intestinal and kidney epithelial cells, neutrophils, thymocytes, lung, prostate, testes, and brain. In the brain, it is expressed on the plasma membranes of neurons, pre- and post-synaptically, and is most abundant in the nigrostriatal pathway, and in brain areas vulnerable to amyloid plaque deposition, such as the hippocampus (Wang, et al. 2006). It is also expressed in the tunica media and endothelium of cortical and leptomeningeal blood vessels where it participates in the regulation of the vascular tone, and in pyramidal neurons. NEP is also involved in the regulation of neuropeptide signalling (Dorfman et al. 2010; Miners, et al. 2008b).

NEP has been implicated in the degradation of Aβ. It degrades Aβ42 *in vivo,* and when NEP is inhibited, Aβ degradation in rat hippocampus is blocked with a concomitant increase of Aβ42 plaques in this brain region, and in the cortical region outside the hippocampus. In addition, the capacity to degrade Aβ42 of exogenous origin is severely compromised in NEP knockout homozygote mice in which the levels of Aβ40 and Aβ42 remain very high. These studies are corroborated by correlative studies in patients with sporadic AD and healthy age matched controls. Overexpression of NEP in brains of human amyloid precursor protein (hAPP) transgenic mice decreases overall Aβ levels and amyloid plaque burdens by 50% and effectively prevented early Aβ deposition in the neocortex and hippocampus. However, it did not reduce levels of Aβ oligomers or improved deficits in spatial learning and memory. The differential effect of NEP on plaques and oligomers suggests that NEP-dependent degradation of Aβ affects plaques more than oligomers and that these structures may form through distinct assembly mechanisms (Meilandt, et al. 2009). Moreover, the expression of NEP on the surface of leukocytes, trough lentivirus transplantation of bone marrow cells, reduced soluble brain Aβ levels by ~30% and lowered the accumulation of Aβ peptides by 50–60% when transplantation was performed at both young and early adult age. This peripheral NEP expression reduced amyloid dependent performance deficits of these animals in the Morris Water Maze (Guan, et al. 2009). *Ex-vivo* gene delivery of a soluble form of NEP, via fibroblasts, into transgenic APP mice also demonstrated increased clearance of plaques. Interestingly, mRNA and protein levels of NEP can be induced by intracranial injections of Aβ42, which also reduced the accumulation of amyloid plaques (Malito et al. 2008). Microglia from old PS1-APP mice, but not from younger mice, have a twofold to fivefold decrease in expression of NEP, compared with their littermate controls (Hickman, et al. 2008). Despite all the evidence sustaining the proteolytic action of NEP on Aβ, the molecular basis of the interaction between NEP and Aβ remains largely unexplained because the volume of the proteolytic chamber of NEP is about half the size of Aβ (Malito et al. 2008).

### 3.3 Presequence peptidase

Presequense peptidase (PreP) is a 110 kDa metalloprotease, ubiquitously expressed, but with higher abundance in heart and skeletal muscle. It is responsible for degradation of targeting peptides, which have been cleaved off inside the mitochondrial matrix after protein import, but it also cleaves other unstructured peptides up to 65 amino acids (Stahl, et al. 2002). More recently, PreP was shown to completely degrade Aβ40 and Aβ42, which are present in mitochondria. More relevance is added to this action of PreP as it has been shown that hPreP is actually the only protease responsible for degradation of Aβ in the

mitochondria (Falkevall, et al. 2006) and Aβ-induced mitochondrial toxicity has been associated with AD (Tillement, et al. 2011).
Human PreP consists of 4 domains, creating two halves connected by a hinge region. The two halves can create a large catalytic chamber of 10 000 Å where Aβ fits. The inverted zinc-binding motif is located in the N-terminal region, but also includes residues located in the C-terminal half, about 800 amino acids distant from the zinc-binding motif (Johnson, et al. 2006). Unlike IDE, PreP cannot degrade insulin, making PreP a better therapeutic agent candidate than IDE as its use would preclude deleterious side effects associated with the degradation of insulin. Another interesting feature of PreP is that its proteolytic activity against Aβ is abolished under oxidizing conditions, probably due to the formation of a disulphide bridge between Cys90 and Cys527 that inhibits the substrate from entering the catalytic chamber. These findings indicate a possible inhibition of hPreP under elevated ROS production in mitochondria implicated in AD, and might therefore be relevant in this disease (Alikhani, et al. 2009).

### 3.4 ECE – Endothelin converting enzyme

Endothelin-converting enzymes 1 and 2 (ECE-1 and ECE-2) were originally implicated in the processing of pro-hormone forms of endothelin. They are type II integral membrane zinc metalloendopeptidases that are primarily localized to the endothelium throughout the human vasculature. They share common catalytic substrates and are responsible for cleaving big endothelins to produce potent vasoconstrictor endothelins (Miners, et al. 2008a; Miners et al. 2008b).
ECE sequences and domain organization are similar to NEP's and are also capable of degrading Aβ *in vitro* and *in vivo* (Eckman, et al. 2001). Homozygous knockouts for ECE-1 are lethal and heterozygous animals show an increased amount of Aβ40 and Aβ42 in the brain. Homozygous ECE-2 knockout mice show a gene dose dependent increase of both forms of Aβ in the brain as well (Eckman, et al. 2006; Eckman, et al. 2003).
ECE-1 is present in neurons, specifically in pyramidal neurons of the hippocampus and layer V of the neocortex, and to a less extent in astrocytes (Sluck, et al. 1999). In mice, ECE-2 is largely confined to the brain; in the rat brain, ECE-1 occurs in the cerebrovascular endothelium, whereas ECE-2 is predominantly neuronal, with special incidence on hippocampal pyramidal neurons (Miners et al. 2008a; Miners et al. 2008b).
There is evidence of significant decrease in ECE-2 gene expression in AD patients (Weeraratna, et al. 2007). The contribution of ECE-1 to the accumulation of Aβ or reduction in local microvascular blood flow in AD seems to be detrimental, with abnormal production of ET-1 being more likely to reflect Aβ -mediated upregulation of ECE-2 (Palmer, et al. 2010).

### 3.5 ACE – Angiotensin-converting enzyme

Angiotensin-converting enzyme (ACE) is a membrane-bound zinc metalloprotease expressed in blood vessels throughout the body. ACE is extremely important for the regulation of fluid homeostasis and blood pressure. It converts angiotensin I to the potent vasoconstrictor angiotensin II. Within the brain, ACE has been detected in cortical pyramidal neurons and in the cerebral vasculature. Its highest levels occur in circumventricular organs, such as the subfornical organ, area postrema, and the median eminence but was detected in other areas such as the caudate nucleus, putamen, substantia

nigra pars reticularis, nucleus of the solitary tract, dorsal motor nucleus, median preoptic nucleus, and choroid plexus in rat, human, rabbit, sheep and monkey (Miners et al. 2008a).
ACE has two homologous domains, each having a functional active site. The N-domain of ACE is responsible for converting Aβ42 to Aβ40, whereas the angiotensin-converting activity is found predominantly in the C-domain of ACE. N-linked glycosylation is essential for both Aβ42 to Aβ40 conversion and angiotensin-converting activities and protects ACE from proteolysis (Zou, et al. 2009).
The first correlations between ACE and AD were found in 1985 by Zubenko and colleagues (Zubenko, et al. 1985) who showed that the CSF of patients with moderate degrees of senile dementia of the AD type exhibited about half the ACE activity of age and sex-matched control individuals, raising the possibility that ACE activity in the CSF could be an index of AD. In a posterior study, however, no differences in ACE activity in the CSF were found between AD patients and age matched controls raising some controversy on this issue (Konings, et al. 1993), but other studies reported reduced activity of ACE in the parietal cortex of AD brains (Ichai, et al. 1994).
ACE was found to significantly inhibit Aβ aggregation in 2001 (Hu, et al. 2001). The inhibition of aggregation was specifically blocked by preincubation of ACE with an ACE inhibitor, lisinopril. ACE degraded Aβ by cleaving Aβ40 at the site Asp(7)-Ser(8). Compared with Aβ40, aggregation and cytotoxic effects of the degradation products Aβ-(1-7) and Aβ-(8-40) peptides were reduced or virtually absent. These findings led to the hypothesis that previous associations of ACE genotype with AD susceptibility (Farrer, et al. 2000; Hu, et al. 1999; Isbir, et al. 2001; Yang, et al. 2000) could rely on its capacity to degrade Aβ and prevent the accumulation of amyloid plaques *in vivo*. Besides Aβ40 degradation, cellular expression of ACE also promotes degradation of naturally secreted Aβ42, and leads to the clearance of both species (Hemming and Selkoe 2005). In addition, ACE also converts Aβ42 to Aβ40 which is less neurotoxic (Zou, et al. 2007).
Pharmacological inhibition of ACE with a widely prescribed drug, captopril, promotes the accumulation of cell-derived Aβ in the media of APP expressing cells and questions if prescribed ACE inhibitors against hypertension could elevate cerebral Aβ levels in humans (Hemming and Selkoe 2005). To address this question the ACE inhibitor captopril was administered to two lines of APP transgenic mice presenting low or high levels of Aβ with associated plaque deposition. In both models, captopril did not affect cerebral Aβ levels nor plaque deposition or peripheral Aβ levels (Hemming, et al. 2007).
Epidemiological data obtained from a male population, however, suggests that angiotensin receptor blockers are more efficient in reducing the incidence and progression of AD and dementia compared with ACE inhibitors or other cardiovascular drugs (Li, et al. 2010). However, there are strong indications that ACE inhibitors may reduce the risk for and progression of dementias (Shah, et al. 2009). Still, these effects remain rather controversial, and prescription of ACE inhibitors against hypertension should be regarded with caution (Hajjar, et al. 2008; Kehoe and Wilcock 2007; Shah et al. 2009). Alternatively, ACE inhibitors could be designed to specifically target the angiotensin-converting C-domain, without inhibiting the Aβ42 to Aβ40-converting activity of ACE or increasing neurotoxic Aβ42 (Zou et al. 2009).

### 3.6 uPA/tPA-plasmin system

Plasmin is a serine protease generated from the proteolytic cleavage of inactive plasminogen, by tissue-type (tPA) or by urokinase-type plasminogen activator (uPA). In the brain, plasminogen is synthesized in neurons, whereas uPA and tPA expression can be induced in neurons as well as in microglia. This system is involved in many normal neural functions, such as neuronal plasticity, learning, and memory (Wang et al. 2006; Zhao and Pei 2008).

uPA and tPA are induced by Aβ treatment in primary rat embryonic cortical cultures *in vitro* as well as in a murine model of Aβ accumulation *in vivo* (Tucker, et al. 2000b). In addition, it plasmin degrades both non-aggregated and aggregated Aβ40 (Tucker, et al. 2000a), and also degrades Aβ42, preventing Aβ42 aggregation into beta-pleated sheet structures (Exley and Korchazhkina 2001). Plasmin also inhibits Aβ toxicity, reduces Aβ deposition *in vitro*, and inhibits Aβ fibrillogenesis (Tucker, et al. 2002). The anti-amyloidogenic effect of plasmin is further enhanced by its capacity to increase the processing of human APP, and efficiently degrading secreted amyloidogenic and non-amyloidogenic APP fragments. Consistent with these observations, brains from AD patients contain reduced levels of plasmin (Ledesma, et al. 2000). Moreover, Aβ injected into the hippocampus of mice lacking either tPA or plasminogen persists causing activation of microglial cells and neuronal damage. Conversely, Aβ injected into wild-type mice is rapidly cleared and does not cause neuronal degeneration (Melchor, et al. 2003). Assembly of Aβ42, on the other hand, seems to promote the up-regulation of the tPA/plasminogen proteolytic system, which can modulate the deposition of amyloid plaques *in vivo*, in a negative feedback mechanism (Lee, et al. 2007).

### 3.7 Matrix metalloproteinases

Matrix metalloproteinases (MMPs) are zinc- and calcium dependent endopeptidases, produced by neurons and glial cells. Metalloproteinase 2 (MMP-2) can be detected in the walls of some blood vessels and scattered white matter glia. Metalloproteinase 3 (MMP-3) is present in and around some neurons and within occasional amyloid plaques, and metalloproteinase 9 (MMP-9) is present in many neurons.

MMP-2 and MMP-9 all have Aβ-degrading activity *in vitro*, although the Aβ degrading activity of these MMPs has not received so much attention *in vivo*. However MMP-2 and MMP-9 activity are elevated in homogenates of hippocampal tissue from AD brains, and several cell types (glial, neuronal and vascular) up-regulate endogenous MMP-2 -3 and -9 expression in response to Aβ stimulation (Deb and Gottschall 1996; Miners et al. 2008b; Gottschall 1996).

MMP-2 also known as gelatinase A/type IV collagenase/matrix hydrolyses Aβ40 and Aβ42 peptides at Lys 16-Leu 17, at Leu 34-Met 35, and Met 35-Val 36 peptide bonds (Roher, et al. 1994). Besides its Aβ degrading activity, MMP-2 has also beta-secretase activity (LePage, et al. 1995). In AD brains, MMP-2 is present in the reactive microglia located in the center of senile plaques, and in Schwann cells (Yamada, et al. 1995). Aβ stimulates the expression and activation of MMP-2 to a large extent due to the increased expression of membrane type-1 (MT1)-MMP expression, the primary MMP-2 activator (Jung, et al. 2003).

There seems to be a complex regulation of MMP2 expression by oligomeric Aβ in astrocytes. Oligomeric Aβ directly down-regulates MMP2 expression and activation in astrocytes. However, it also induces the production of pro-inflammatory cytokines which stimulate production of MMP2 (Li, et al. 2011).

Increased MMP-9 immunolabelling has been detected in neurons of AD patients, as well as in neurofibrillary tangles, plaques and blood vessel walls, but not in granular neurons or glial cells. MMP-9 is also detected in the vicinity of extracellular amyloid plaques (Backstrom, et al. 1996). MMP-9, unlike ECE-1, NEP and IDE, is capable of cleaving aggregated Aβ fibrils (Miners et al. 2008b). It cleaves Aβ at several sites, predominantly at Leu34-Met35 within the membrane-spanning domain (Backstrom et al. 1996; Yan, et al. 2006). The presence of the apoE4 significantly dampens Aβ-induced MMP-9 in primary cultures of rat astrocytes. This effect may affect Aβ clearance and promote Aβ deposition in AD brains (Guo, et al. 2006). There is also evidence that reduction of Aβ levels through the action of MMP-9 may also result from the direct processing of cell surface APP with an alpha-secretase like activity, substantially reducing the levels of secreted Aβ peptide (Talamagas, et al. 2007).

Aged APP/presenilin 1 mouse astrocytes surrounding amyloid plaques, showed enhanced expression of MMP-2 and MMP-9. Astrocyte-conditioned medium obtained from these animals degraded Aβ, producing several small fragments. In the brains of MMP-2 and MMP-9 KO mice, significant increases in the Aβ levels were found in comparison to wild-type controls. This study reinforces previous *in vitro* evidences that MMP-2 and -9 may contribute to extracellular brain Aβ clearance through the degradation of Aβ (Yin, et al. 2006).

Several MMPs polymorphisms have been examined in relation to the risk of developing dementia with controversial results (Baig, et al. 2008; Helbecque, et al. 2007; Reitz, et al. 2008; Reitz, et al. 2010). MMPs may also be considered potential plasmatic and cerebrospinal fluid markers of AD as the levels of MMP-3 in the plasma and CSF of AD patients was found higher than in controls, whereas MMP-2 was significantly decreased in CSF but unchanged in plasma (Horstmann, et al. 2010).

### 3.8 Transthyretin

Transthyretin (TTR) is a 55 kDa homotetrameric protein secreted mainly by the liver and choroid plexus into the plasma and CSF, respectively (Soprano, et al. 1985). The name "transthyretin" discloses its dual physiological role as a carrier for thyroid hormones (Woeber and Ingbar 1968) and retinol, the latter through the binding to retinol-binding protein (Goodman 1985). TTR plasma concentration is age dependent and in healthy newborns it is about half of that in adults (Stabilini, et al. 1968; Vahlquist, et al. 1975), varying from 20 to 40 mg/ dL. In spite of the low TTR levels in CSF (~2 mg/ dL), the choroid plexus is presented as the major site of TTR expression, expressed as a ratio of tissue/mass, corresponding to a 30-fold higher than that found in plasma and represents 20% of the total CSF proteins (Weisner and Kauerz 1983).

Over a hundred TTR mutations have been associated with Familial Amyloid Polyneuropathy (FAP), some of which are very common in Portuguese patients, such as the valine at position 30 substituted by a methionine (TTR V30M) (Saraiva, et al. 1984), others provide a very aggressive phenotype, such as the TTR L55P (Jacobson, et al. 1992). Curiously, TTR T119M was described as an example of a non-aggressive mutation that inclusively has a protective role against the disease (Almeida, et al. 2000).

The first report that associates TTR to Aβ and AD as a protective molecule is from Schwarzman et al. who describes the capacity of normal CSF to inhibit amyloid formation and concluded that TTR was the major Aβ binding protein in the CSF, that could also decrease the aggregation state of the peptide and its toxicity (Schwarzman, et al. 1994). Prior to this finding, TTR was found associated to senile plaques, NFTs and microangiopathic lesions (Shirahama, et al. 1982). The sequestration hypothesis was raised suggesting that normally produced Aβ is sequestered by certain extracellular proteins, thereby preventing amyloid formation and Aβ cytotoxicity; when sequestration fails amyloid formation occurs (Schwarzman and Goldgaber 1996). The observation that TTR is reduced in the CSF of AD patients further supported the idea of a TTR protective role in this pathology (Serot, et al. 1997). Authors also observed a decrease in TTR levels with age which could be related to the epithelial atrophy in the choroid plexus. Along time several reports described TTR decrease in CSF of AD patients (Davidsson, et al. 2002; Serot et al. 1997; Gloeckner, et al. 2008; Hansson, et al. 2004) although it remains unclear whether this reduction is restricted to AD, or on the contrary is common to other neurodegenerative disorders (Chiang, et al. 2009). It is also uncertain if the TTR decrease in the CSF happens early in disease development (or even before symptoms appears) or if it is a latter event, and thus studies involving patients with mild cognitive impairment (MCI) and early-staged probable AD patients are needed.

Other studies using a transgenic model of *Caenorhabditis elegans* expressing Aβ42 supported a TTR role in AD as administration of TTR rescued the neurodegeneration observed in this model (Link 1995). Mammalian models used to recapitulate AD features were never completely successful as AD transgenic mice did not show NFTs and demonstrate little or no neuronal cell loss (Holcomb, et al. 1998; Hsiao, et al. 1996; Irizarry, et al. 1997a; Irizarry, et al. 1997b; Stein and Johnson 2002). However, in some of the models, animals showed increased TTR expression in the hippocampus (Stein and Johnson 2002); TTR was then described to be a survival gene (Stein and Johnson 2002) and although this work is controversial because TTR expression is thought to be confined to the choroid plexus and meninges (in the case of the brain), authors further showed that when a chronic infusion of an antibody against TTR was applied into the hippocampus of mice expressing human APP, an increase of Aβ, tau phosphorylation, neuronal loss and apoptosis were observed (Stein, et al. 2004). Underlying these observations is, according to authors, sAPPα that leads to increased expression of protective genes, such as TTR, to confer neuroprotection (Stein et al. 2004). Other studies, using transgenic APP mice hemizigous for endogenous TTR showed accelerated Aβ deposition (Choi, et al. 2007), while double transgenic mice for APP and TTR presented lower deposition (Buxbaum, et al. 2008). However, in other models, TTR was described to have the opposite effect and was associated with increased vascular Aβ deposition (Wati, et al. 2009).

Regarding the nature of TTR/Aβ interaction, different researchers confirmed TTR binding to Aβ (Carro, et al. 2002; Liu and Murphy 2006; Costa, et al. 2008) not only to the monomer but also to Aβ oligomers and fibrils, raising the hypothesis that TTR may be involved in the formation of senile plaques (Costa et al. 2008); TTR was also able to inhibit and to disrupt Aβ fibrils. However, which TTR conformation binds Aβ peptide is still controversial. Du Murphy et al. showed that TTR tetramers interact preferably with Aβ aggregates rather than Aβ monomers enhancing Aβ aggregation, whereas TTR monomers arrest Aβ aggregate growth (Du and Murphy 2010). On the other hand, studies by Costa et al. (Costa et al. 2008) showed that soluble Aβ binds to different TTR variants correlating negatively with the amyloidogenic potential of the TTR mutant. Thus, TTR119M presented the highest affinity to Aβ, contrarily to what was observed by Du and Murphy (Du and Murphy 2010). Other studies also indicated a different relation between TTR variant/amyloidogenic potential and binding to the peptide, with amyloidogenic mutants binding less to Aβ peptide and inhibiting less its aggregation (Schwarzman, et al. 2004). In this work it was also shown that TTRs were functional tetramers. Hence, other studies are necessary to completely understand the nature of the TTR/Aβ interaction, concerning both Aβ and TTR species involved. Structural analysis, obtained from computer-assisted modeling (Schwarzman et al. 2004) predicted the existence of an Aβ binding domain on the surface of each TTR monomer; residues 30-60, especially the 38-42 region of TTR seemed to be the key structure of the Aβ binding domain (Schwarzman and Goldgaber 1996; Schwarzman, et al. 2005). Du and Murphy, identified the A strand, in the inner β-sheet of TTR, as well as the EF helix, as regions of TTR that are involved with Aβ association (Du and Murphy 2010).

The discussion on the TTR interaction with Aβ and consequent inhibition of aggregation and toxicity reduction raised the hypothesis that mutations in the TTR gene or conformational changes in the protein induced by aging, could affect the sequestration properties. A study was conducted with the aim of identifying mutations in the TTR gene in the AD population but no correlation was found (Palha, et al. 1996). Finally, and concerning the mechanism underlying TTR protective role in AD, Costa and colleagues found that TTR is able to proteolytically process Aβ peptide (Costa et al. 2008). Regarding TTR ability to degrade Aβ, several cleavage sites were identified and the newly generated Aβ peptides shown to have decreased amyloidogenic potential, when compared to the full length counterpart (Costa et al. 2008); TTR is also able to degrade aggregated forms of the peptide and inhibition of the TTR activity resulted in increased Aβ fibril formation (Costa et al. 2008).

### 3.9 Gelsolin

Gelsolin can be found both as an intrinsic cytoplasmic protein and as a secreted protein in plasma and CSF (Kwiatkowski, et al. 1985). Intracellular gelsolin regulates actin polymerization by binding to actin, and it also caps and breaks the actin filaments (Janmey, et al. 1985; Matsumoto, et al. 2003). Secreted (plasma/CSF) and intracellular gelsolin originate from the alternative splicing of a single gene, but their disulphide structure is different with recognised functional implications. All of the five cysteine (Cys) residues present in human cytoplasmic gelsolin are free thiols, whereas in plasma/CSF gelsolin, three Cys residues are free thiols and the other two Cys residues are disulfide-linked (Wen, et al. 1996). The five free thiol groups are likely to confer anti-oxidant properties to the molecule. Secreted gelsolin has an extension of 25 amino acids at its N-terminal, which is absent in the cytoplasmic form (Chauhan, et al. 2008).

Gelsolin found in the CSF may originate from oligodendrocytes or microglia (Chauhan et al. 2008). It was also suggested that choroid plexus may be responsible for the presence of gelsolin in CSF (Matsumoto et al. 2003), where it may have also an important function counteracting the neurotoxicity of Aβ (Antequera, et al. 2009; Vargas, et al. 2010).

Plasma and cytosolic gelsolin both bind Aβ and the Aβ -gelsolin complex exists in the plasma and in the cytosol (Chauhan, et al. 1999; Ji, et al. 2008). Both inhibit the fibrillation of Aβ, and defibrillate preformed fibrils (Ray, et al. 2000). In addition it has been demonstrated that when administered to transgenic mouse models of AD reduces the Aβ40/Aβ42 and the amyloid load (Hirko, et al. 2007; Matsuoka, et al. 2003). Therefore, gelsolin may also be looked as a potential therapeutic agent against AD.

### 3.10 Alpha2-macroglobulin

Alpha2-macroglobulin (a2M) is a 720 kDa soluble glycoprotein composed of four identical 180 kDa subunits, each encoded by a single-copy gene on human chromosome 12. Each subunit contains at least five binding sites: the bait region, the internal thiol ester, the receptor binding site, the Aβ binding site, and the zinc binding site. The bait region, the internal thiol ester and the receptor binding site are crucial for the activation and internalization of a2M. The bait region binds any known protease. The four bait regions in the tetramer are in close contact and get cleaved by the bound proteases, triggering activation of a2M. This conformational change results in the exposure of the four thiol esters, and of the four receptor binding sites, to the extracellular environment. The receptor binding site of each monomer, a 27 residue consensus sequence located at their C-terminal tail, will then bind to the receptor and mediate the internalization of the complex. The Aβ binding site is located between the bait and the receptor binding regions of each monomer (Borth 1992; Du, et al. 1997; Hughes, et al. 1998; Kovacs 2000).

Binding to Aβ42 occurs with high affinity (Kd= $3.8 \times 10^{-10}$ M) and protects the peptide from proteolysis by exogenous trypsin, suggesting that a2M may function as a carrier protein for Aβ and may serve to regulate clearance of Aβ from such tissues as the brain (Du et al. 1997; Hughes et al. 1998). a2M co-incubated with Aβ significantly reduces aggregation and fibril formation *in vitro*, and cultured fetal rat cortical neurons are less vulnerable to the toxic actions of Aβ following pretreatment with a2M, being likely that a2M has the capacity to keep Aβ in a soluble state, preventing fibril formation and associated neurotoxicity (Du, et al. 1998). a2M also inhibits both Aβ fibril formation and Aβ -induced cytotoxicity in PC12 cells (Monji, et al. 2000). The inhibition of the formation of amyloid fibrils are probably due to the interaction of a2M with prefibrillar species to maintain the solubility of Aβ (Yerbury, et al. 2009), and therefore their aggregation state in the extracellular milieu. In addition, Qiu et al described a serine protease that binds to a2M to form a stable high molecular weight complex capable of efficiently cleaving Aβ (Qiu, et al. 1996). This serine protease-a2M complex was capable of proteolytically digesting both Aβ40 and Aβ42, resulting in disruption of the central region of the peptide (residues 10–35), which is believed to mediate the conformational change that underlies Aβ self-aggregation (Qiu et al. 1996).

a2M is also a physiological ligand for the low-density lipoprotein receptor-related protein (LRP) abundantly expressed in the CNS. The a2M/Aβ complexes can be degraded by glioblastoma cells and fibroblasts via LRP, but the degradation of free Aβ must be mediated via an LRP-independent pathway. These results suggest that LRP can function as a clearance receptor for Aβ via a2M (Narita, et al. 1997). The effect of self-aggregation and LRP-1 ligands on the elimination of human Aβ 40 from the rat brain across the blood-brain barrier has been investigated recently. In the first instance it was demonstrated that the elimination rate of $^{125}$I hAβ40 dimer was 92.7% decreased compared to the $^{125}$I hAβ40 monomer. When pre-incubated with LRP-1 ligands, such as activated a2M, apolipoprotein E2 (apoE2), apoE3, apoE4, and lactoferrin, the elimination of $^{125}$I hAβ40) was reduced. There seems that dimerization and LRP-1-ligand complex formation prevents the elimination of Aβ40 from the brain across the blood-brain barrier (Ito, et al. 2007).

There is also an over-representation of a common a2M polymorphism, Val1000 (GTC)/Ile1000 (ATC) in AD patients, which correlates with an increase in Aβ burden (Kovacs 2000; Liao, et al. 1998), further sustaining the importance of a2M in Aβ clearance.

### 3.11 Apolipoprotein E

From all the proteins and peptides associated with AD and amyloid beta metabolism, apolipoprotein E (ApoE) is probably the most thoroughly studied, and several recent reviews give excellent and comprehensive overviews about its structure and function (Zhong and Weisgraber 2009a, b), and the pathways in which it is involved in AD (Kim, et al. 2009), either Aβ dependent or Aβ independent (Huang 2010; Mahley, et al. 2006). Therefore, this section will just give a brief overview about ApoE and will focus only on its association with AD via Aβ dependent pathways.

ApoE is a 34,2 kDa glycoprotein containing 299 amino acids. The protein contains two structural domains that are responsible for different functions of apoE. The amino-terminal domain (residues 1-191) contains the lipoprotein receptor binding region (residues 136-150), and the carboxyl-terminal domain (residues 216-299) contains the major lipoprotein (lipid) binding domain.

There are three common isoforms of ApoE, ApoE2, ApoE3 and ApoE4, which are encoded by three alleles (e2, e3 and e4, respectively) of a single gene. Sequence differences among the ApoE isoforms reside only on amino acids 122 or 158 which may be cysteine or arginine, but are sufficient to determine significant functional consequences (Huang 2010; Mahley et al. 2006).

ApoE4 is the major known genetic risk factor for AD and as much as 65–80% of all AD patients are ApoE4 carriers. This allele is over-represented in late-onset familial AD in several populations and in late-onset sporadic AD (Farrer, et al. 1997). In addition, as the number of Apo E alleles increases, the risk of onset of AD also increases while the age of onset decreases; as the number of ApoE4 alleles increases from 0 to 2, the risk of developing late-onset AD increases from 20% to 90%, and the mean age of onset decreases from 84 to 68 years (Corder, et al. 1993; Frangione, et al. 1996). The N and C terminal domains of ApoE interact in ApoE4 (called domain interaction), which is mediated by the formation of a salt bridge between Arg-61 in the N- terminus and Glu-255 in the C- terminus of ApoE4. This interaction might be the molecular basis for the detrimental effects of ApoE4 in AD pathogenesis (Huang 2010).

ApoE is expressed in several organs but is mainly expressed in the liver, followed by the brain. Non-neuronal cells, mainly astrocytes and to some extent microglia, are the major cell types that express apoE in the brain (Boyles, et al. 1985; Pitas, et al. 1987). Neurons also produce ApoE under certain conditions, particularly in response to brain injury (Boschert, et al. 1999) .

ApoE (E2 and E3) are important for the distribution of lipids among cells throughout the body and within the CNS, where the principal apolipoproteins are, and where they transport lipids and cholesterol for cell repair and neurite outgrowth. These properties are not shared by Apo E4 which seems to counteract the features of Apo E2 and ApoE3 with detrimental effects (Mahley et al. 2006).

ApoE is also essential for astrocytes to bind, internalize and degrade Aβ deposits (Koistinaho, et al. 2004). ApoE binds Aβ with high affinity. It was demonstrated that lipid-free ApoE4 and ApoE3 form stable complexes with Aβ, with ApoE4 being more effective in the formation of the complex, but inducing a pathological β-sheet conformational change in Aβ ((Wisniewski and Frangione 1996). This interaction requires the N-terminal and the C-terminal domains, and there are strong indications that the interaction is affected by the lipid content (Weisgraber and Mahley 1996).

ApoE, but not ApoE4 plays a role in facilitating the proteolytic clearance of soluble Aβ from the brain. The endolytic degradation of Aβ peptides within microglia by NEP and related enzymes is dramatically enhanced by ApoE. Similarly, Aβ degradation extracellularly by IDE is facilitated by ApoE. The capacity of ApoE to promote Aβ degradation is dependent upon the ApoE isoform and its lipidation status. The enhanced expression of lipidated ApoE, through the activation of liver X receptors, stimulates Aβ degradation (Jiang, et al. 2008).

In contrast, Apo E4 inhibits Aβ clearance and stimulates Aβ deposition (Huang, et al. 2004). It also enhances Aβ production and potentiates Aβ induced chromosomal leakage and apoptosis (Mahley and Huang 2006). In addition, ApoE4 enhances Aβ42 oligomer induced toxicity (Manelli, et al. 2007). Taken together these observations sustain the effects of ApoE4 in the enhancement of the overall Aβ burden via interaction with the peptide.

### 3.12 Metallothioneins 2 and 3

Metallothioneins (MTs) were discovered as cadmium binding proteins in equine kidney cortex. MTs is a generic name for a superfamily of low molecular weight cysteine- and metal-rich proteins with high affinity for divalent metals, such as zinc, cadmium and copper with four major isoforms, MT-1 to MT-4, identified in humans. They occur in all living organisms from the simplest forms of life, such as prokaryotes to the most complex, such as higher plants and vertebrate animals. It is clear that MTs are multipurpose proteins with unquestionable metal binding and anti-oxidant properties. In addition, there is increasing evidence that MT-1 and MT-2 (MT-1/2), and MT-3 display such diverse physiological actions as inhibition of pro-apoptotic mechanisms, enhancement of cell survival, tissue regeneration, and have anti-inflammatory properties. Concurrent with this wide array of functions, MT-1/2 have been implicated in neuroprotection and neurodegeneration, and particularly in AD (Hidalgo, et al. 2009; Penkowa, et al. 2006).

It is interesting that a considerable body of work has related an increase of MT-1/2 brain levels with aging and AD. In AD patients elevated levels of cytokines and IL-1 may induce MT-1/2 production in astrocytes. Studies in animal models of AD, showed that the MT-1/2 levels were higher, when compared to WT mice, while MT-3 levels were unaltered or reduced, suggesting that these proteins may have a relevant role in providing long term protection against inflammation (Hidalgo et al. 2009). This up-regulation of MT-1/2 in animal models of AD may have detrimental consequences in Aβ clearance as MT-2 diminishes the binding of TTR to Aβ (Martinho, et al. 2010). Considering TTR an Aβ scavenger as explained above, a less efficient removal of Aβ would be expected when MT-2 levels are increased, and this appears to be the case in AD. Furthermore, inhibition of homeodomain interacting protein kinase 2 activity in AD patients, might be involved in p53 misfolding, most likely through MT-2A upregulation (Lanni, et al. 2010). In addition, it was also shown that MT-2A may also prevent copper-mediated Aβ aggregation and neurotoxicity, by a mechanism which primarily involves a specific metal exchange interaction between Zn7.MT-2A and Cu(2).Aβ, and subsequent inhibition of $H_2O_2$ generation (Chung, et al. 2010). Furthermore, a metal swap between Zn7.MT-3 and soluble and aggregated Aβ1–40-Cu(II) abolishes ROS production and related cellular toxicity (Meloni, et al. 2008).

These studies relating metal exchange and Aβ aggregation, conducted to a recent interest in the use of metal-chelation drugs as a potential therapy for AD. For example, the administration of the copper and zinc chelating drug, clioquinol, prevents plaque formation in transgenic AD mice (Hegde, et al. 2009).

Since the discovery of MT-3 as a growth inhibitory factor, with reduced expression levels in AD brains compared to age-matched controls, several studies provide evidence that MT-3 is related to the aetiology of AD. Some studies indicate that MT-3 may potentially promote the clearance of Aβ plaques, while others show an opposite trend or even no differences (Howells, et al. 2010). MT-3 alone antagonizes the toxic effect of Aβ because it inhibits the formation of SDS-resistant Aβ aggregates, thereby protecting cortical neurons from its toxic effects. Both the full-length and the N-terminal domain of MT-3 promote neuron survival at low concentrations but inhibited it at high concentrations. These observations suggest that the anti- Aβ activity of MT-3 is different from its neuronal growth inhibitory activity. Other possible mechanisms underlying the protection of MT-3 from Aβ toxicity may be related to its interaction with TTR by improving its Aβ degrading capacity (Martinho et al. 2010).

## 4. Conclusion

The extracellular neuritic plaque deposits of amyloid found in AD brains contain Aβ, and according to the amyloid cascade hypothesis, the accumulation of Aβ peptide, can trigger gradual synaptic alterations, astrocytic and microglial activation, and modification of the soluble tau protein into insoluble paired helical filaments, with progressive neuronal loss and cognitive failure (Hardy and Selkoe 2002). The cascade hypothesis suggests that stopping or slowing formation of the Aβ plaques would delay the onset of the disease symptoms. Therefore, it is crucial to thoroughly elucidate the regulation of Aβ production and clearance to design new and effective therapies against AD.

APP, takes a central position in AD pathogenesis, as Aβ arises from its proteolytic cleavage through the sequential action of β- and γ-secretase. APP is first cleaved by either α- or β-secretase at the α- or β-sites, respectively, which lie in the extracellular domain of APP. These proteases originate: soluble APPα (sAPPα, for α-secretase) or soluble APPβ (sAPPβ, for β-secretase), which are released to the extracellular space, and a membrane anchored C-terminal end (C83 for α-secretase or C99 for β-secretase). γ-cleavage of C99, generates the Aβ peptide. This pathway is known as the amyloidogenic pathway. Misregulation of all the intervenients in this process may lead to Aβ accumulation. If APP cleavage by β-secretase or γ-cleavage of C99 is more effective than α-secretase, then the all process shifts into the accumulation of Aβ. Also if APP synthesis is enhanced, as it is the case of several mutated forms of APP associated with early onset AD, the production of Aβ is also increased with similar results (Ertekin-Taner 2007). So, alterations in APP synthesis and processing by both secretases, or downstream in the γ-secretase complex action, may account for more severe forms of disease. Another good example of that are the mutations associated with presenilins 1 and 2 , which are part of the γ-secretase complex, known to be responsible for early onset inherited forms of AD (Ertekin-Taner 2007).

Once Aβ has been produced, other important players come into action (Figure 2). These are all the enzymes and proteins that, either by directly cleaving Aβ into less harmful peptides or making them more prone to proteolysis or less susceptible to aggregation through protein-protein interactions, will reduce the Aβ load in vulnerable areas of the brain.

Reduced degradation of Aβ by proteases is generally accepted to enhance plaque pathology in AD brains, and may depend on several factors such as decreased mRNA expression or decreased protein levels or activity, either in the brain cortex, hippocampus or in brain microvessels; and post-translational modifications, such as oxidation and deposition of the enzymes in the diseased brain with consequent loss of its native structure and functionality (Dorfman et al, 2010.).

IDE and NEP are well accepted as Aβ degrading enzymes, but although few studies compare the relative contribution of each of these enzymes to the overall Aβ load, NEP seems to be the major protease involved in Aβ degradation. In transgenic mice models of familial AD, over-expression of IDE or NEP prevents amyloid plaque pathology and consequent early death (Leissring, et al. 2003) indicating that degradation of Aβ by these metalloproteinases may be of high therapeutic interest for AD patients. A recent study carried out in AD patients showed that, NEP mRNA, protein levels, and activity are decreased compared to normal controls without any cognitive impairment. In these patients IDE activity was unchanged, though mRNA levels increased. In the same study ECE-1 expression or activity in AD brains was not different from age-matched controls. Correlation analyses suggested that NEP expression was correlated with Aβ accumulation and clinical diagnosis, being lower in AD than in controls, whereas no correlations of IDE and ECE-1 with Aβ levels or clinical diagnosis has been found. These findings provide additional support for NEP as the major protease involved in Aβ degradation (Wang et al. 2010).

Age is the major risk factor for AD. Aβ -synthesizing enzyme activities increase with age, coinciding with declining soluble Aβ and increasing insoluble Aβ (Miners, et al, 2008b.). In addition, there is an overall ageing-related down regulation of Aβ degrading proteases which is particularly relevant for NEP but not for IDE in transgenic Tg2576 mice brains (Dorfman et al., 2010). Nevertheless further studies assessing the relative contribution of each of these enzymes , IDE, NEP, Prep, ECE, ACE and plasmin are necessary to understand why the system redundancy is not always effective, and which of these enzymes may be more adequate as candidate therapeutic targets.

Regarding proteins with the capacity to degrade Aβ or of interfering in the process, TTR is probably the most promising, with potential as a biomarker of the disease and even as a putative therapeutic agent. The literature shows that TTR plays an important role in the modulation of Aβ aggregation and toxicity. The use of TTR as a sera biomarker for diagnosis purposes in AD patients should also be explored, with obvious advantages, for both patients and researchers, and there are already indications that sera TTR is decreased in AD patients when compared to age-matched controls (Han et al., 2011). Moreover, it is important to investigate the factors that affect TTR/A-Beta binding and/or TTR alterations that lead to its decreased in AD, such as protein oxidation (Biroccio et al., 2006). Further studies are necessary to unravel the mechanism underlying TTR protective role in AD, to establish if TTR decline is a cause or consequence of disease, and the cellular pathways involved.

Other proteins as gelsolin, a2M and Apo E counteract Aβ deposition through interactions with the peptide, but apparently none of them seem to have the capacity to cleave the peptide. In general these proteins bind Aβ and the effects of these interactions translate into preventing Aβ fibrillation, and eventually on disaggregation of pre-existent fibrils (gelsolin and a2M); binding of enzymes conferring them the capacity to degrade Aβ (a2M) or may enhance the capacity of Aβ proteases, as NEP and IDE to cleave Aβ (ApoE). MT ½ and MT3 bind TTR affecting its capacity to cleave Aβ and prevent metal associated Aβ aggregation or inhibit their formation.

The scientific achievements acquired over the past decade on all the pathways and key players involved in the amyloid cascade will hopefully contribute to the development of more adequate therapies against AD in a closer future.

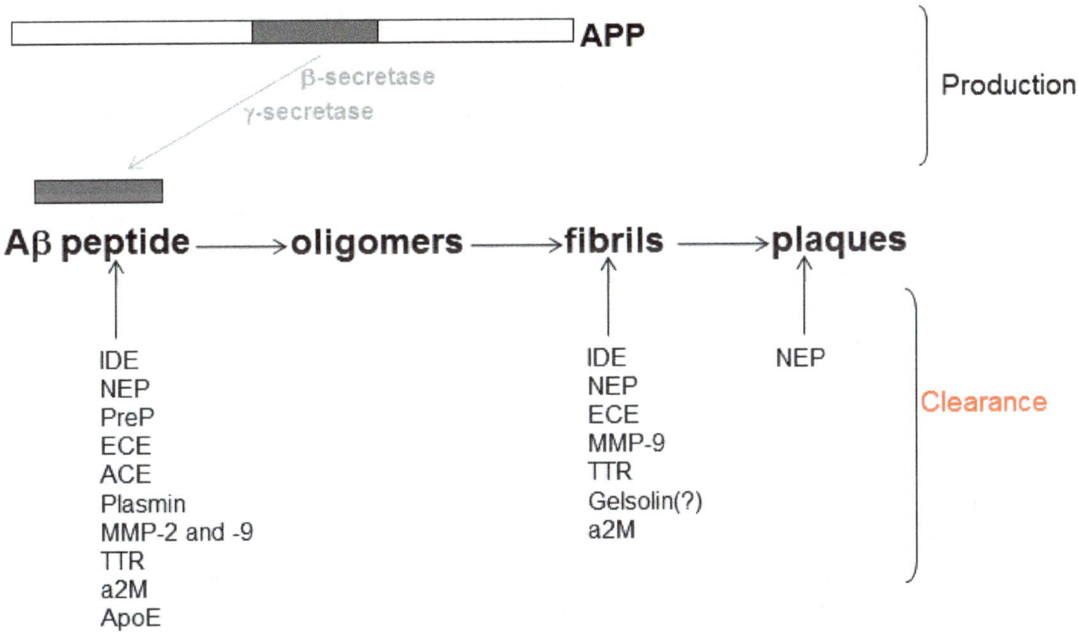


Fig. 2. Schematic diagram depicting APP processing: key proteins in amyloid-beta production and clearance (not drawn in scale). IDE- Insulin degrading enzyme; NEP-Neprilysin; PreP- Presequence peptidase; ECE –Endothelin-converting enzyme; ACE-Angiotensin-converting enzyme; MMP- Matrix metalloproteinase; TTR-Transthyretin; a2M-Alpha2-macroglobulin; ApoE- apolipoprotein E.

## 5. Acknowledgments

Portuguese Foundation for Science and Technology (FCT) research grants PTDC/SAU-NMC/114800/2009 and POCI/SAU-NEU/64593/2006, by COMPETE (Programa operacional Temático Factores de Competitividade) and POCI 2010 (Programa Operacional Ciência e Inovação 2010), respectively, with the participation of the European Communitarian Fund FEDER

## 6. References

Alikhani N, Ankarcrona M & Glaser E 2009 Mitochondria and Alzheimer's disease: amyloid-beta peptide uptake and degradation by the presequence protease, hPreP. *J Bioenerg Biomembr* 41 447-451.

Almeida MR, Alves IL, Terazaki H, Ando Y & Saraiva MJ 2000 Comparative studies of two transthyretin variants with protective effects on familial amyloidotic polyneuropathy: TTR R104H and TTR T119M. *Biochem Biophys Res Commun* 270 1024-1028.

Antequera D, Vargas T, Ugalde C, Spuch C, Molina JA, Ferrer I, Bermejo-Pareja F & Carro E 2009 Cytoplasmic gelsolin increases mitochondrial activity and reduces Abeta burden in a mouse model of Alzheimer's disease. *Neurobiol Dis* 36 42-50.

Asai M, Hattori C, Szabo B, Sasagawa N, Maruyama K, Tanuma S & Ishiura S 2003 Putative function of ADAM9, ADAM10, and ADAM17 as APP alpha-secretase. *Biochem Biophys Res Commun* 301 231-235.

Backstrom JR, Lim GP, Cullen MJ & Tokes ZA 1996 Matrix metalloproteinase-9 (MMP-9) is synthesized in neurons of the human hippocampus and is capable of degrading the amyloid-beta peptide (1-40). *J Neurosci* 16 7910-7919.

Baig S, Kehoe PG & Love S 2008 MMP-2, -3 and -9 levels and activity are not related to Abeta load in the frontal cortex in Alzheimer's disease. *Neuropathol Appl Neurobiol* 34 205-215.

Behl M, Zhang Y & Zheng W 2009 Involvement of insulin-degrading enzyme in the clearance of beta-amyloid at the blood-CSF barrier: Consequences of lead exposure. *Cerebrospinal Fluid Res* 6 11.

Bennett BD, Babu-Khan S, Loeloff R, Louis JC, Curran E, Citron M & Vassar R 2000 Expression analysis of BACE2 in brain and peripheral tissues. *J Biol Chem* 275 20647-20651.

Bertram L, Blacker D, Mullin K, Keeney D, Jones J, Basu S, Yhu S, McInnis MG, Go RC, Vekrellis K, et al. 2000 Evidence for genetic linkage of Alzheimer's disease to chromosome 10q. *Science* 290 2302-2303.

Bertram L, McQueen MB, Mullin K, Blacker D & Tanzi RE 2007 Systematic meta-analyses of Alzheimer disease genetic association studies: the AlzGene database. *Nat Genet* 39 17-23.

Biroccio A, Del Boccio P, Panella M, Bernardini S, Di Ilio C, Gambi D, Stanzione P, Sacchetta P, Bernardi G, Martorana A, Federici G, Stefani A, Urbani A. Differential post-translational modifications of transthyretin in Alzheimer's disease: a study of the cerebral spinal fluid. Proteomics. 2006 Apr;6(7):2305-13.

Biroccio A, Del Boccio P, Panella M, Bernardini S, Di Ilio C, Gambi D, Stanzione P, Sacchetta P, Bernardi G, Martorana A, Federici G, Stefani A, Urbani A. Differential post-translational modifications of transthyretin in Alzheimer's disease: a study of the cerebral spinal fluid. Proteomics. 2006 Apr;6(7):2305-13. Bora RP, Ozbil M & Prabhakar R 2010 Elucidation of insulin degrading enzyme catalyzed site specific hydrolytic cleavage of amyloid beta peptide: a comparative density functional theory study. *J Biol Inorg Chem* 15 485-495.

Bora RP & Prabhakar R 2010 Elucidation of interactions of Alzheimer amyloid beta peptides (Abeta40 and Abeta42) with insulin degrading enzyme: a molecular dynamics study. *Biochemistry* 49 3947-3956.

Borth W 1992 Alpha 2-macroglobulin, a multifunctional binding protein with targeting characteristics. *FASEB J* 6 3345-3353.

Boschert U, Merlo-Pich E, Higgins G, Roses AD & Catsicas S 1999 Apolipoprotein E expression by neurons surviving excitotoxic stress. *Neurobiol Dis* 6 508-514.

Boyles JK, Pitas RE, Wilson E, Mahley RW & Taylor JM 1985 Apolipoprotein E associated with astrocytic glia of the central nervous system and with nonmyelinating glia of the peripheral nervous system. *J Clin Invest* 76 1501-1513.

Buxbaum JN, Ye Z, Reixach N, Friske L, Levy C, Das P, Golde T, Masliah E, Roberts AR & Bartfai T 2008 Transthyretin protects Alzheimer's mice from the behavioral and biochemical effects of Abeta toxicity. *Proc Natl Acad Sci U S A* 105 2681-2686.

Caporaso GL, Takei K, Gandy SE, Matteoli M, Mundigl O, Greengard P & De Camilli P 1994 Morphologic and biochemical analysis of the intracellular trafficking of the Alzheimer beta/A4 amyloid precursor protein. *J Neurosci* 14 3122-3138.

Carro E, Trejo JL, Gomez-Isla T, LeRoith D & Torres-Aleman I 2002 Serum insulin-like growth factor I regulates brain amyloid-beta levels. *Nat Med* 8 1390-1397.

Chauhan V, Ji L & Chauhan A 2008 Anti-amyloidogenic, anti-oxidant and anti-apoptotic role of gelsolin in Alzheimer's disease. *Biogerontology* 9 381-389.

Chauhan VP, Ray I, Chauhan A & Wisniewski HM 1999 Binding of gelsolin, a secretory protein, to amyloid beta-protein. *Biochem Biophys Res Commun* 258 241-246.

Chiang HL, Lyu RK, Tseng MY, Chang KH, Chang HS, Hsu WC, Kuo HC, Chu CC, Wu YR, Ro LS, et al. 2009 Analyses of transthyretin concentration in the cerebrospinal fluid of patients with Guillain-Barre syndrome and other neurological disorders. *Clin Chim Acta* 405 143-147.

Choi SH, Leight SN, Lee VM, Li T, Wong PC, Johnson JA, Saraiva MJ & Sisodia SS 2007 Accelerated Abeta deposition in APPswe/PS1deltaE9 mice with hemizygous deletions of TTR (transthyretin). *J Neurosci* 27 7006-7010.

Chung RS, Howells C, Eaton ED, Shabala L, Zovo K, Palumaa P, Sillard R, Woodhouse A, Bennett WR, Ray S, et al. 2010 The native copper- and zinc-binding protein metallothionein blocks copper-mediated Abeta aggregation and toxicity in rat cortical neurons. *PLoS One* 5 e12030.

Corder EH, Saunders AM, Strittmatter WJ, Schmechel DE, Gaskell PC, Small GW, Roses AD, Haines JL & Pericak-Vance MA 1993 Gene dose of apolipoprotein E type 4 allele and the risk of Alzheimer's disease in late onset families. *Science* 261 921-923.

Costa R, Ferreira-da-Silva F, Saraiva MJ & Cardoso I 2008 Transthyretin protects against A-beta peptide toxicity by proteolytic cleavage of the peptide: a mechanism sensitive to the Kunitz protease inhibitor. *PLoS One* 3 e2899.

Cupers P, Bentahir M, Craessaerts K, Orlans I, Vanderstichele H, Saftig P, De Strooper B & Annaert W 2001 The discrepancy between presenilin subcellular localization and gamma-secretase processing of amyloid precursor protein. *J Cell Biol* 154 731-740.

Davidsson P, Westman-Brinkmalm A, Nilsson CL, Lindbjer M, Paulson L, Andreasen N, Sjogren M & Blennow K 2002 Proteome analysis of cerebrospinal fluid proteins in Alzheimer patients. *Neuroreport* 13 611-615.

Dawson GR, Seabrook GR, Zheng H, Smith DW, Graham S, O'Dowd G, Bowery BJ, Boyce S, Trumbauer ME, Chen HY, et al. 1999 Age-related cognitive deficits, impaired long-term potentiation and reduction in synaptic marker density in mice lacking the beta-amyloid precursor protein. *Neuroscience* 90 1-13.

Deb S & Gottschall PE 1996 Increased production of matrix metalloproteinases in enriched astrocyte and mixed hippocampal cultures treated with beta-amyloid peptides. *J Neurochem* 66 1641-1647.

DeKosky ST & Marek K 2003 Looking backward to move forward: early detection of neurodegenerative disorders. *Science* 302 830-834.

Dominguez D, Tournoy J, Hartmann D, Huth T, Cryns K, Deforce S, Serneels L, Camacho IE, Marjaux E, Craessaerts K, et al. 2005 Phenotypic and biochemical analyses of BACE1- and BACE2-deficient mice. *J Biol Chem* 280 30797-30806.

Dorfman VB, Pasquini L, Riudavets M, Lopez-Costa JJ, Villegas A, Troncoso JC, Lopera F, Castano EM & Morelli L 2010 Differential cerebral deposition of IDE and NEP in sporadic and familial Alzheimer's disease. *Neurobiol Aging* 31 1743-1757.

Du J & Murphy RM 2010 Characterization of the interaction of beta-amyloid with transthyretin monomers and tetramers. *Biochemistry* 49 8276-8289.

Du Y, Bales KR, Dodel RC, Liu X, Glinn MA, Horn JW, Little SP & Paul SM 1998 Alpha2-macroglobulin attenuates beta-amyloid peptide 1-40 fibril formation and associated neurotoxicity of cultured fetal rat cortical neurons. *J Neurochem* 70 1182-1188.

Du Y, Ni B, Glinn M, Dodel RC, Bales KR, Zhang Z, Hyslop PA & Paul SM 1997 alpha2-Macroglobulin as a beta-amyloid peptide-binding plasma protein. *J Neurochem* 69 299-305.

Eckman EA, Adams SK, Troendle FJ, Stodola BA, Kahn MA, Fauq AH, Xiao HD, Bernstein KE & Eckman CB 2006 Regulation of steady-state beta-amyloid levels in the brain by neprilysin and endothelin-converting enzyme but not angiotensin-converting enzyme. *J Biol Chem* 281 30471-30478.

Eckman EA, Reed DK & Eckman CB 2001 Degradation of the Alzheimer's amyloid beta peptide by endothelin-converting enzyme. *J Biol Chem* 276 24540-24548.

Eckman EA, Watson M, Marlow L, Sambamurti K & Eckman CB 2003 Alzheimer's disease beta-amyloid peptide is increased in mice deficient in endothelin-converting enzyme. *J Biol Chem* 278 2081-2084.

Eggert S, Paliga K, Soba P, Evin G, Masters CL, Weidemann A & Beyreuther K 2004 The proteolytic processing of the amyloid precursor protein gene family members APLP-1 and APLP-2 involves alpha-, beta-, gamma-, and epsilon-like cleavages: modulation of APLP-1 processing by n-glycosylation. *J Biol Chem* 279 18146-18156.

Ertekin-Taner N 2007 Genetics of Alzheimer's disease: a centennial review. *Neurol Clin* 25 611-667, v.

Exley C & Korchazhkina OV 2001 Plasmin cleaves Abeta42 in vitro and prevents its aggregation into beta-pleated sheet structures. *Neuroreport* 12 2967-2970.

Falkevall A, Alikhani N, Bhushan S, Pavlov PF, Busch K, Johnson KA, Eneqvist T, Tjernberg L, Ankarcrona M & Glaser E 2006 Degradation of the amyloid beta-protein by the novel mitochondrial peptidasome, PreP. *J Biol Chem* 281 29096-29104.

Farrer LA, Cupples LA, Haines JL, Hyman B, Kukull WA, Mayeux R, Myers RH, Pericak-Vance MA, Risch N & van Duijn CM 1997 Effects of age, sex, and ethnicity on the association between apolipoprotein E genotype and Alzheimer disease. A meta-analysis. APOE and Alzheimer Disease Meta Analysis Consortium. *Jama* 278 1349-1356.

Farrer LA, Sherbatich T, Keryanov SA, Korovaitseva GI, Rogaeva EA, Petruk S, Premkumar S, Moliaka Y, Song YQ, Pei Y, et al. 2000 Association between angiotensin-converting enzyme and Alzheimer disease. *Arch Neurol* 57 210-214.

Frangione B, Castano EM, Wisniewski T, Ghiso J, Prelli F & Vidal R 1996 Apolipoprotein E and amyloidogenesis. *Ciba Found Symp* 199 132-141; discussion 141-135.

Gao W, Eisenhauer PB, Conn K, Lynch JA, Wells JM, Ullman MD, McKee A, Thatte HS & Fine RE 2004 Insulin degrading enzyme is expressed in the human cerebrovascular endothelium and in cultured human cerebrovascular endothelial cells. *Neurosci Lett* 371 6-11.

Glenner GG & Wong CW 1984 Alzheimer's disease and Down's syndrome: sharing of a unique cerebrovascular amyloid fibril protein. *Biochem Biophys Res Commun* 122 1131-1135.

Gloeckner SF, Meyne F, Wagner F, Heinemann U, Krasnianski A, Meissner B & Zerr I 2008 Quantitative analysis of transthyretin, tau and amyloid-beta in patients with dementia. *J Alzheimers Dis* 14 17-25.

Goodman DS 1985 Retinoids and retinoid-binding proteins. *Harvey Lect* 81 111-132.

Gottschall PE 1996 beta-Amyloid induction of gelatinase B secretion in cultured microglia: inhibition by dexamethasone and indomethacin. *Neuroreport* 7 3077-3080.

Greenfield JP, Tsai J, Gouras GK, Hai B, Thinakaran G, Checler F, Sisodia SS, Greengard P & Xu H 1999 Endoplasmic reticulum and trans-Golgi network generate distinct populations of Alzheimer beta-amyloid peptides. *Proc Natl Acad Sci U S A* 96 742-747.

Grundke-Iqbal I, Iqbal K, Tung YC, Quinlan M, Wisniewski HM & Binder LI 1986 Abnormal phosphorylation of the microtubule-associated protein tau (tau) in Alzheimer cytoskeletal pathology. *Proc Natl Acad Sci U S A* 83 4913-4917.

Guan H, Liu Y, Daily A, Police S, Kim MH, Oddo S, LaFerla FM, Pauly JR, Murphy MP & Hersh LB 2009 Peripherally expressed neprilysin reduces brain amyloid burden: a novel approach for treating Alzheimer's disease. *J Neurosci Res* 87 1462-1473.

Guo S, Wang S, Kim WJ, Lee SR, Frosch MP, Bacskai BJ, Greenberg SM & Lo EH 2006 Effects of apoE isoforms on beta-amyloid-induced matrix metalloproteinase-9 in rat astrocytes. *Brain Res* 1111 222-226.

Haapasalo A & Kovacs DM 2011 The Many Substrates of Presenilin/gamma-Secretase. *J Alzheimers Dis.*

Haass C 2004 Take five--BACE and the gamma-secretase quartet conduct Alzheimer's amyloid beta-peptide generation. *EMBO J* 23 483-488.

Haass C & Selkoe DJ 1993 Cellular processing of beta-amyloid precursor protein and the genesis of amyloid beta-peptide. *Cell* 75 1039-1042.

Hajjar IM, Keown M, Lewis P & Almor A 2008 Angiotensin converting enzyme inhibitors and cognitive and functional decline in patients with Alzheimer's disease: an observational study. *Am J Alzheimers Dis Other Demen* 23 77-83.

Han SH, Jung ES, Sohn JH, Hong HJ, Hong HS, Kim JW, N DL, Kim M, Kim H, Ha HJ, Kim YH, Huh N, Jung MW, Mook-Jung I. 2011 Human Serum Transthyretin Levels Correlate Inversely with Alzheimer's Disease. J Alzheimers Dis.

Hansson SF, Puchades M, Blennow K, Sjogren M & Davidsson P 2004 Validation of a prefractionation method followed by two-dimensional electrophoresis - Applied to cerebrospinal fluid proteins from frontotemporal dementia patients. *Proteome Sci* 2 7.

Hardy J & Selkoe DJ 2002 The amyloid hypothesis of Alzheimer's disease: progress and problems on the road to therapeutics. *Science* 297 353-356.

Hardy JA & Higgins GA 1992 Alzheimer's disease: the amyloid cascade hypothesis. *Science* 256 184-185.

Heber S, Herms J, Gajic V, Hainfellner J, Aguzzi A, Rulicke T, von Kretzschmar H, von Koch C, Sisodia S, Tremml P, et al. 2000 Mice with combined gene knock-outs reveal essential and partially redundant functions of amyloid precursor protein family members. *J Neurosci* 20 7951-7963.

Hegde ML, Bharathi P, Suram A, Venugopal C, Jagannathan R, Poddar P, Srinivas P, Sambamurti K, Rao KJ, Scancar J, et al. 2009 Challenges associated with metal chelation therapy in Alzheimer's disease. *J Alzheimers Dis* 17 457-468.

Helbecque N, Cottel D, Hermant X & Amouyel P 2007 Impact of the matrix metalloproteinase MMP-3 on dementia. *Neurobiol Aging* 28 1215-1220.

Hemming ML & Selkoe DJ 2005 Amyloid beta-protein is degraded by cellular angiotensin-converting enzyme (ACE) and elevated by an ACE inhibitor. *J Biol Chem* 280 37644-37650.

Hemming ML, Selkoe DJ & Farris W 2007 Effects of prolonged angiotensin-converting enzyme inhibitor treatment on amyloid beta-protein metabolism in mouse models of Alzheimer disease. *Neurobiol Dis* 26 273-281.

Hickman SE, Allison EK & El Khoury J 2008 Microglial dysfunction and defective beta-amyloid clearance pathways in aging Alzheimer's disease mice. *J Neurosci* 28 8354-8360.

Hidalgo J, Chung R, Penkowa M, Vašák M. 2009 Structure and function of vertebrate metallothioneins, in"Metallothioneins and Related Chelators", Vol. 5 of 'Metal Ions in

Life Sciences'; Sigel, A., Sigel, H., Sigel, R.K.O., Eds. (2009) The Royal Society of Chemistry, Cambridge, UK, pp 279-317.

Hirko AC, Meyer EM, King MA & Hughes JA 2007 Peripheral transgene expression of plasma gelsolin reduces amyloid in transgenic mouse models of Alzheimer's disease. *Mol Ther* 15 1623-1629.

Holcomb L, Gordon MN, McGowan E, Yu X, Benkovic S, Jantzen P, Wright K, Saad I, Mueller R, Morgan D, et al. 1998 Accelerated Alzheimer-type phenotype in transgenic mice carrying both mutant amyloid precursor protein and presenilin 1 transgenes. *Nat Med* 4 97-100.

Hook VY, Kindy M, Reinheckel T, Peters C & Hook G 2009 Genetic cathepsin B deficiency reduces beta-amyloid in transgenic mice expressing human wild-type amyloid precursor protein. *Biochem Biophys Res Commun* 386 284-288.

Horstmann S, Budig L, Gardner H, Koziol J, Deuschle M, Schilling C & Wagner S 2010 Matrix metalloproteinases in peripheral blood and cerebrospinal fluid in patients with Alzheimer's disease. *Int Psychogeriatr* 22 966-972.

Howells C, West AK & Chung RS 2010 Neuronal growth-inhibitory factor (metallothionein-3): evaluation of the biological function of growth-inhibitory factor in the injured and neurodegenerative brain. *Febs J* 277 2931-2939.

Hsiao K, Chapman P, Nilsen S, Eckman C, Harigaya Y, Younkin S, Yang F & Cole G 1996 Correlative memory deficits, Abeta elevation, and amyloid plaques in transgenic mice. *Science* 274 99-102.

Hu J, Igarashi A, Kamata M & Nakagawa H 2001 Angiotensin-converting enzyme degrades Alzheimer amyloid beta-peptide (A beta ); retards A beta aggregation, deposition, fibril formation; and inhibits cytotoxicity. *J Biol Chem* 276 47863-47868.

Hu J, Miyatake F, Aizu Y, Nakagawa H, Nakamura S, Tamaoka A, Takahash R, Urakami K & Shoji M 1999 Angiotensin-converting enzyme genotype is associated with Alzheimer disease in the Japanese population. *Neurosci Lett* 277 65-67.

Huang Y 2010 Abeta-independent roles of apolipoprotein E4 in the pathogenesis of Alzheimer's disease. *Trends Mol Med* 16 287-294.

Huang Y, Weisgraber KH, Mucke L & Mahley RW 2004 Apolipoprotein E: diversity of cellular origins, structural and biophysical properties, and effects in Alzheimer's disease. *J Mol Neurosci* 23 189-204.

Hughes SR, Khorkova O, Goyal S, Knaeblein J, Heroux J, Riedel NG & Sahasrabudhe S 1998 Alpha2-macroglobulin associates with beta-amyloid peptide and prevents fibril formation. *Proc Natl Acad Sci U S A* 95 3275-3280.

Huse JT, Liu K, Pijak DS, Carlin D, Lee VM & Doms RW 2002 Beta-secretase processing in the trans-Golgi network preferentially generates truncated amyloid species that accumulate in Alzheimer's disease brain. *J Biol Chem* 277 16278-16284.

Ichai C, Chevallier N, Delaere P, Dournaud P, Epelbaum J, Hauw JJ, Vincent JP & Checler F 1994 Influence of region-specific alterations of neuropeptidase content on the catabolic fates of neuropeptides in Alzheimer's disease. *J Neurochem* 62 645-655.

Irie, Y., and Keung, W. M. (2001) Metallothionein-III antagonizes the neurotoxic and neurotrophic effects of amyloid beta peptides. Biochem Biophys Res Commun 282, 416-420

Irie, Y., and Keung, W. M. (2003) Anti-amyloid beta activity of metallothionein-III is different from its neuronal growth inhibitory activity: structure-activity studies. Brain research 960, 228-234

Irizarry MC, McNamara M, Fedorchak K, Hsiao K & Hyman BT 1997a APPSw transgenic mice develop age-related A beta deposits and neuropil abnormalities, but no neuronal loss in CA1. *J Neuropathol Exp Neurol* 56 965-973.

Irizarry MC, Soriano F, McNamara M, Page KJ, Schenk D, Games D & Hyman BT 1997b Abeta deposition is associated with neuropil changes, but not with overt neuronal loss in the human amyloid precursor protein V717F (PDAPP) transgenic mouse. *J Neurosci* 17 7053-7059.

Isbir T, Agachan B, Yilmaz H, Aydin M, Kara I, Eker D & Eker E 2001 Interaction between apolipoprotein-E and angiotensin-converting enzyme genotype in Alzheimer's disease. *Am J Alzheimers Dis Other Demen* 16 205-210.

Ito S, Ohtsuki S, Kamiie J, Nezu Y & Terasaki T 2007 Cerebral clearance of human amyloid-beta peptide (1-40) across the blood-brain barrier is reduced by self-aggregation and formation of low-density lipoprotein receptor-related protein-1 ligand complexes. *J Neurochem* 103 2482-2490.

Jacobson DR, McFarlin DE, Kane I & Buxbaum JN 1992 Transthyretin Pro55, a variant associated with early-onset, aggressive, diffuse amyloidosis with cardiac and neurologic involvement. *Hum Genet* 89 353-356.

Janmey PA, Chaponnier C, Lind SE, Zaner KS, Stossel TP & Yin HL 1985 Interactions of gelsolin and gelsolin-actin complexes with actin. Effects of calcium on actin nucleation, filament severing, and end blocking. *Biochemistry* 24 3714-3723.

Ji L, Chauhan A & Chauhan V 2008 Cytoplasmic gelsolin in pheochromocytoma-12 cells forms a complex with amyloid beta-protein. *Neuroreport* 19 463-466.

Jiang Q, Lee CY, Mandrekar S, Wilkinson B, Cramer P, Zelcer N, Mann K, Lamb B, Willson TM, Collins JL, et al. 2008 ApoE promotes the proteolytic degradation of Abeta. *Neuron* 58 681-693.

Johnson KA, Bhushan S, Stahl A, Hallberg BM, Frohn A, Glaser E & Eneqvist T 2006 The closed structure of presequence protease PreP forms a unique 10,000 Angstroms3 chamber for proteolysis. *EMBO J* 25 1977-1986.

Jorissen E, Prox J, Bernreuther C, Weber S, Schwanbeck R, Serneels L, Snellinx A, Craessaerts K, Thathiah A, Tesseur I, et al. 2010 The disintegrin/metalloproteinase ADAM10 is essential for the establishment of the brain cortex. *J Neurosci* 30 4833-4844.

Jung SS, Zhang W & Van Nostrand WE 2003 Pathogenic A beta induces the expression and activation of matrix metalloproteinase-2 in human cerebrovascular smooth muscle cells. *J Neurochem* 85 1208-1215.

Kang J & Muller-Hill B 1990 Differential splicing of Alzheimer's disease amyloid A4 precursor RNA in rat tissues: PreA4(695) mRNA is predominantly produced in rat and human brain. *Biochem Biophys Res Commun* 166 1192-1200.

Kehoe PG & Wilcock GK 2007 Is inhibition of the renin-angiotensin system a new treatment option for Alzheimer's disease? *Lancet Neurol* 6 373-378.

Kim J, Basak JM & Holtzman DM 2009 The role of apolipoprotein E in Alzheimer's disease. *Neuron* 63 287-303.

Kimberly WT & Wolfe MS 2003 Identity and function of gamma-secretase. *J Neurosci Res* 74 353-360.

Koistinaho M, Lin S, Wu X, Esterman M, Koger D, Hanson J, Higgs R, Liu F, Malkani S, Bales KR, et al. 2004 Apolipoprotein E promotes astrocyte colocalization and degradation of deposited amyloid-beta peptides. *Nat Med* 10 719-726.

Konings CH, Kuiper MA, Scheltens P, Grijpma AM, van Pelt W & Wolters EC 1993 Re-evaluation of cerebrospinal fluid angiotensin-converting enzyme activity in patients with 'probable' Alzheimer's disease. *Eur J Clin Chem Clin Biochem* 31 495-497.

Korenberg JR, Pulst SM, Neve RL & West R 1989 The Alzheimer amyloid precursor protein maps to human chromosome 21 bands q21.105-q21.05. *Genomics* 5 124-127.

Kovacs DM 2000 alpha2-macroglobulin in late-onset Alzheimer's disease. *Exp Gerontol* 35 473-479.

Kowalska A 2003 Amyloid precursor protein gene mutations responsible for early-onset autosomal dominant Alzheimer's disease. *Folia Neuropathol* 41 35-40.

Kuhn PH, Wang H, Dislich B, Colombo A, Zeitschel U, Ellwart JW, Kremmer E, Rossner S & Lichtenthaler SF 2010 ADAM10 is the physiologically relevant, constitutive alpha-secretase of the amyloid precursor protein in primary neurons. *EMBO J* 29 3020-3032.

Kurochkin IV & Goto S 1994 Alzheimer's beta-amyloid peptide specifically interacts with and is degraded by insulin degrading enzyme. *FEBS Lett* 345 33-37.

Kwiatkowski DJ, Janmey PA, Mole JE & Yin HL 1985 Isolation and properties of two actin-binding domains in gelsolin. *J Biol Chem* 260 15232-15238.

Lammich S, Kojro E, Postina R, Gilbert S, Pfeiffer R, Jasionowski M, Haass C & Fahrenholz F 1999 Constitutive and regulated alpha-secretase cleavage of Alzheimer's amyloid precursor protein by a disintegrin metalloprotease. *Proc Natl Acad Sci U S A* 96 3922-3927.

Lanni C, Nardinocchi L, Puca R, Stanga S, Uberti D, Memo M, Govoni S, D'Orazi G & Racchi M 2010 Homeodomain interacting protein kinase 2: a target for Alzheimer's beta amyloid leading to misfolded p53 and inappropriate cell survival. *PLoS One* 5 e10171.

Ledesma MD, Da Silva JS, Crassaerts K, Delacourte A, De Strooper B & Dotti CG 2000 Brain plasmin enhances APP alpha-cleavage and Abeta degradation and is reduced in Alzheimer's disease brains. *EMBO Rep* 1 530-535.

Lee JY, Kweon HS, Cho E, Byun HR, Kim DH, Kim YH, Han PL & Koh JY 2007 Upregulation of tPA/plasminogen proteolytic system in the periphery of amyloid deposits in the Tg2576 mouse model of Alzheimer's disease. *Neurosci Lett* 423 82-87.

Leissring MA, Farris W, Chang AY, Walsh DM, Wu X, Sun X, Frosch MP & Selkoe DJ 2003 Enhanced proteolysis of beta-amyloid in APP transgenic mice prevents plaque formation, secondary pathology, and premature death. *Neuron* 40 1087-1093.

LePage RN, Fosang AJ, Fuller SJ, Murphy G, Evin G, Beyreuther K, Masters CL & Small DH 1995 Gelatinase A possesses a beta-secretase-like activity in cleaving the amyloid protein precursor of Alzheimer's disease. *FEBS Lett* 377 267-270.

Li NC, Lee A, Whitmer RA, Kivipelto M, Lawler E, Kazis LE & Wolozin B 2010 Use of angiotensin receptor blockers and risk of dementia in a predominantly male population: prospective cohort analysis. *BMJ* 340 b5465.

Li P, Kuo WL, Yousef M, Rosner MR & Tang WJ 2006 The C-terminal domain of human insulin degrading enzyme is required for dimerization and substrate recognition. *Biochem Biophys Res Commun* 343 1032-1037.

Li R, Lindholm K, Yang LB, Yue X, Citron M, Yan R, Beach T, Sue L, Sabbagh M, Cai H, et al. 2004 Amyloid beta peptide load is correlated with increased beta-secretase activity in sporadic Alzheimer's disease patients. *Proc Natl Acad Sci U S A* 101 3632-3637.

Li W, Poteet E, Xie L, Liu R, Wen Y & Yang SH 2011 Regulation of matrix metalloproteinase 2 by oligomeric amyloid beta protein. *Brain Res.*

Liao A, Nitsch RM, Greenberg SM, Finckh U, Blacker D, Albert M, Rebeck GW, Gomez-Isla T, Clatworthy A, Binetti G, et al. 1998 Genetic association of an alpha2-macroglobulin (Val1000lle) polymorphism and Alzheimer's disease. *Hum Mol Genet* 7 1953-1956.

Link CD 1995 Expression of human beta-amyloid peptide in transgenic Caenorhabditis elegans. *Proc Natl Acad Sci U S A* 92 9368-9372.

Liu L & Murphy RM 2006 Kinetics of Inhibition of beta-Amyloid Aggregation by Transthyretin. *Biochemistry* 45 15702-15709.

Mahley RW & Huang Y 2006 Apolipoprotein (apo) E4 and Alzheimer's disease: unique conformational and biophysical properties of apoE4 can modulate neuropathology. *Acta Neurol Scand Suppl* 185 8-14.

Mahley RW, Weisgraber KH & Huang Y 2006 Apolipoprotein E4: a causative factor and therapeutic target in neuropathology, including Alzheimer's disease. *Proc Natl Acad Sci U S A* 103 5644-5651.

Malito E, Hulse RE & Tang WJ 2008 Amyloid beta-degrading cryptidases: insulin degrading enzyme, presequence peptidase, and neprilysin. *Cell Mol Life Sci* 65 2574-2585.

Manelli AM, Bulfinch LC, Sullivan PM & LaDu MJ 2007 Abeta42 neurotoxicity in primary co-cultures: effect of apoE isoform and Abeta conformation. *Neurobiol Aging* 28 1139-1147.

Martinho A, Goncalves I, Cardoso I, Almeida MR, Quintela T, Saraiva MJ & Santos CR 2010 Human metallothioneins 2 and 3 differentially affect amyloid-beta binding by transthyretin. *Febs J* 277 3427-3436.

Matsumoto N, Kitayama H, Kitada M, Kimura K, Noda M & Ide C 2003 Isolation of a set of genes expressed in the choroid plexus of the mouse using suppression subtractive hybridization. *Neuroscience* 117 405-415.

Matsuoka Y, Saito M, LaFrancois J, Gaynor K, Olm V, Wang L, Casey E, Lu Y, Shiratori C, Lemere C, et al. 2003 Novel therapeutic approach for the treatment of Alzheimer's disease by peripheral administration of agents with an affinity to beta-amyloid. *J Neurosci* 23 29-33.

McDermott JR & Gibson AM 1997 Degradation of Alzheimer's beta-amyloid protein by human and rat brain peptidases: involvement of insulin-degrading enzyme. *Neurochem Res* 22 49-56.

Meilandt WJ, Cisse M, Ho K, Wu T, Esposito LA, Scearce-Levie K, Cheng IH, Yu GQ & Mucke L 2009 Neprilysin overexpression inhibits plaque formation but fails to reduce pathogenic Abeta oligomers and associated cognitive deficits in human amyloid precursor protein transgenic mice. *J Neurosci* 29 1977-1986.

Melchor JP, Pawlak R & Strickland S 2003 The tissue plasminogen activator-plasminogen proteolytic cascade accelerates amyloid-beta (Abeta) degradation and inhibits Abeta-induced neurodegeneration. *J Neurosci* 23 8867-8871.

Meloni G, Sonois V, Delaine T, Guilloreau L, Gillet A, Teissie J, Faller P & Vasak M 2008 Metal swap between Zn7-metallothionein-3 and amyloid-beta-Cu protects against amyloid-beta toxicity. *Nat Chem Biol* 4 366-372.

Merlos-Suarez A, Ruiz-Paz S, Baselga J & Arribas J 2001 Metalloprotease-dependent protransforming growth factor-alpha ectodomain shedding in the absence of tumor necrosis factor-alpha-converting enzyme. *J Biol Chem* 276 48510-48517.

Miners JS, Ashby E, Van Helmond Z, Chalmers KA, Palmer LE, Love S & Kehoe PG 2008a Angiotensin-converting enzyme (ACE) levels and activity in Alzheimer's disease, and relationship of perivascular ACE-1 to cerebral amyloid angiopathy. *Neuropathol Appl Neurobiol* 34 181-193.

Miners JS, Baig S, Palmer J, Palmer LE, Kehoe PG & Love S 2008b Abeta-degrading enzymes in Alzheimer's disease. *Brain Pathol* 18 240-252.

Monji A, Yoshida I, Tashiro K, Hayashi Y, Matsuda K & Tashiro N 2000 Inhibition of A beta fibril formation and A beta-induced cytotoxicity by senile plaque-associated proteins. *Neurosci Lett* 278 81-84.

Narita M, Holtzman DM, Schwartz AL & Bu G 1997 Alpha2-macroglobulin complexes with and mediates the endocytosis of beta-amyloid peptide via cell surface low-density lipoprotein receptor-related protein. *J Neurochem* 69 1904-1911.

Palha JA, Moreira P, Wisniewski T, Frangione B & Saraiva MJ 1996 Transthyretin gene in Alzheimer's disease patients. *Neurosci Lett* 204 212-214.

Palmer JC, Kehoe PG & Love S 2010 Endothelin-converting enzyme-1 in Alzheimer's disease and vascular dementia. *Neuropathol Appl Neurobiol* 36 487-497.

Penkowa M, Tio L, Giralt M, Quintana A, Molinero A, Atrian S, Vasak M & Hidalgo J 2006 Specificity and divergence in the neurobiologic effects of different metallothioneins after brain injury. *J Neurosci Res* 83 974-984.

Perez A, Morelli L, Cresto JC & Castano EM 2000 Degradation of soluble amyloid beta-peptides 1-40, 1-42, and the Dutch variant 1-40Q by insulin degrading enzyme from Alzheimer disease and control brains. *Neurochem Res* 25 247-255.

Pitas RE, Boyles JK, Lee SH, Foss D & Mahley RW 1987 Astrocytes synthesize apolipoprotein E and metabolize apolipoprotein E-containing lipoproteins. *Biochim Biophys Acta* 917 148-161.

Qiu WQ, Borth W, Ye Z, Haass C, Teplow DB & Selkoe DJ 1996 Degradation of amyloid beta-protein by a serine protease-alpha2-macroglobulin complex. *J Biol Chem* 271 8443-8451.

Qiu WQ, Walsh DM, Ye Z, Vekrellis K, Zhang J, Podlisny MB, Rosner MR, Safavi A, Hersh LB & Selkoe DJ 1998 Insulin-degrading enzyme regulates extracellular levels of amyloid beta-protein by degradation. *J Biol Chem* 273 32730-32738.

Ray I, Chauhan A, Wegiel J & Chauhan VP 2000 Gelsolin inhibits the fibrillization of amyloid beta-protein, and also defibrillizes its preformed fibrils. *Brain Res* 853 344-351.

Reitz C, van Rooij FJ, de Maat MP, den Heijer T, Hofman A, Witteman JC & Breteler MM 2008 Matrix metalloproteinase 3 haplotypes and dementia and Alzheimer's disease. The Rotterdam Study. *Neurobiol Aging* 29 874-881.

Reitz C, van Rooij FJ, Soares HD, de Maat MP, Hofman A, Witteman JC & Breteler MM 2010 Matrix metalloproteinase 3 haplotypes and plasma amyloid beta levels: the Rotterdam Study. *Neurobiol Aging* 31 715-718.

Roher AE, Kasunic TC, Woods AS, Cotter RJ, Ball MJ & Fridman R 1994 Proteolysis of A beta peptide from Alzheimer disease brain by gelatinase A. *Biochem Biophys Res Commun* 205 1755-1761.

Saraiva MJ, Birken S, Costa PP & Goodman DS 1984 Family studies of the genetic abnormality in transthyretin (prealbumin) in Portuguese patients with familial amyloidotic polyneuropathy. *Ann N Y Acad Sci* 435 86-100.

Schochet SS, Jr., Lampert PW & McCormick WF 1973 Neurofibrillary tangles in patients with Down's syndrome: a light and electron microscopic study. *Acta Neuropathol* 23 342-346.

Schwarzman AL & Goldgaber D 1996 Interaction of transthyretin with amyloid beta-protein: binding and inhibition of amyloid formation. *Ciba Found Symp* 199 146-160; discussion 160-144.

Schwarzman AL, Gregori L, Vitek MP, Lyubski S, Strittmatter WJ, Enghilde JJ, Bhasin R, Silverman J, Weisgraber KH, Coyle PK, et al. 1994 Transthyretin sequesters amyloid beta protein and prevents amyloid formation. *Proc Natl Acad Sci U S A* 91 8368-8372.

Schwarzman AL, Tsiper M, Gregori L, Goldgaber D, Frakowiak J, Mazur-Kolecka B, Taraskina A, Pchelina S & Vitek MP 2005 Selection of peptides binding to the amyloid b-protein reveals potential inhibitors of amyloid formation. *Amyloid* 12 199-209.

Schwarzman AL, Tsiper M, Wente H, Wang A, Vitek MP, Vasiliev V & Goldgaber D 2004 Amyloidogenic and anti-amyloidogenic properties of recombinant transthyretin variants. *Amyloid* 11 1-9.

Serot JM, Christmann D, Dubost T & Couturier M 1997 Cerebrospinal fluid transthyretin: aging and late onset Alzheimer's disease. *J Neurol Neurosurg Psychiatry* 63 506-508.

Seubert P, Vigo-Pelfrey C, Esch F, Lee M, Dovey H, Davis D, Sinha S, Schlossmacher M, Whaley J, Swindlehurst C, et al. 1992 Isolation and quantification of soluble Alzheimer's beta-peptide from biological fluids. *Nature* 359 325-327.

Shah K, Qureshi SU, Johnson M, Parikh N, Schulz PE & Kunik ME 2009 Does use of antihypertensive drugs affect the incidence or progression of dementia? A systematic review. *Am J Geriatr Pharmacother* 7 250-261.

Shirahama T, Skinner M, Westermark P, Rubinow A, Cohen AS, Brun A & Kemper TL 1982 Senile cerebral amyloid. Prealbumin as a common constituent in the neuritic plaque, in the neurofibrillary tangle, and in the microangiopathic lesion. *Am J Pathol* 107 41-50.

Sluck JM, Lin RC, Katolik LI, Jeng AY & Lehmann JC 1999 Endothelin converting enzyme-1-, endothelin-1-, and endothelin-3-like immunoreactivity in the rat brain. *Neuroscience* 91 1483-1497.

Solans A, Estivill X & de La Luna S 2000 A new aspartyl protease on 21q22.3, BACE2, is highly similar to Alzheimer's amyloid precursor protein beta-secretase. *Cytogenet Cell Genet* 89 177-184.

Soprano DR, Herbert J, Soprano KJ, Schon EA & Goodman DS 1985 Demonstration of transthyretin mRNA in the brain and other extrahepatic tissues in the rat. *J Biol Chem* 260 11793-11798.

Stabilini R, Vergani C, Agostoni A & Agostoni RP 1968 Influence of age and sex on prealbumin levels. *Clin Chim Acta* 20 358-359.

Stahl A, Moberg P, Ytterberg J, Panfilov O, Brockenhuus Von Lowenhielm H, Nilsson F & Glaser E 2002 Isolation and identification of a novel mitochondrial metalloprotease (PreP) that degrades targeting presequences in plants. *J Biol Chem* 277 41931-41939.

Stein TD, Anders NJ, DeCarli C, Chan SL, Mattson MP & Johnson JA 2004 Neutralization of transthyretin reverses the neuroprotective effects of secreted amyloid precursor protein (APP) in APPSW mice resulting in tau phosphorylation and loss of hippocampal neurons: support for the amyloid hypothesis. *J Neurosci* 24 7707-7717.

Stein TD & Johnson JA 2002 Lack of neurodegeneration in transgenic mice overexpressing mutant amyloid precursor protein is associated with increased levels of transthyretin and the activation of cell survival pathways. *J Neurosci* 22 7380-7388.

Takasugi N, Tomita T, Hayashi I, Tsuruoka M, Niimura M, Takahashi Y, Thinakaran G & Iwatsubo T 2003 The role of presenilin cofactors in the gamma-secretase complex. *Nature* 422 438-441.

Talamagas AA, Efthimiopoulos S, Tsilibary EC, Figueiredo-Pereira ME & Tzinia AK 2007 Abeta(1-40)-induced secretion of matrix metalloproteinase-9 results in sAPPalpha release by association with cell surface APP. *Neurobiol Dis* 28 304-315.

Tang BL 2009 Neuronal protein trafficking associated with Alzheimer disease: from APP and BACE1 to glutamate receptors. *Cell Adh Migr* 3 118-128.

Tillement L, Lecanu L & Papadopoulos V 2011 Alzheimer's disease: effects of beta-amyloid on mitochondria. *Mitochondrion* 11 13-21.

Tucker HM, Kihiko-Ehmann M & Estus S 2002 Urokinase-type plasminogen activator inhibits amyloid-beta neurotoxicity and fibrillogenesis via plasminogen. *J Neurosci Res* 70 249-255.

Tucker HM, Kihiko-Ehmann M, Wright S, Rydel RE & Estus S 2000a Tissue plasminogen activator requires plasminogen to modulate amyloid-beta neurotoxicity and deposition. *J Neurochem* 75 2172-2177.

Tucker HM, Kihiko M, Caldwell JN, Wright S, Kawarabayashi T, Price D, Walker D, Scheff S, McGillis JP, Rydel RE, et al. 2000b The plasmin system is induced by and degrades amyloid-beta aggregates. *J Neurosci* 20 3937-3946.

Vahlquist A, Rask L, Peterson PA & Berg T 1975 The concentrations of retinol-binding protein, prealbumin, and transferrin in the sera of newly delivered mothers and children of various ages. *Scand J Clin Lab Invest* 35 569-575.

Vargas T, Antequera D, Ugalde C, Spuch C & Carro E 2010 Gelsolin restores A beta-induced alterations in choroid plexus epithelium. *J Biomed Biotechnol* 2010 805405.

Vassar R, Bennett BD, Babu-Khan S, Kahn S, Mendiaz EA, Denis P, Teplow DB, Ross S, Amarante P, Loeloff R, et al. 1999 Beta-secretase cleavage of Alzheimer's amyloid precursor protein by the transmembrane aspartic protease BACE. *Science* 286 735-741.

Vassar R & Citron M 2000 Abeta-generating enzymes: recent advances in beta- and gamma-secretase research. *Neuron* 27 419-422.

Vepsalainen S, Hiltunen M, Helisalmi S, Wang J, van Groen T, Tanila H & Soininen H 2008 Increased expression of Abeta degrading enzyme IDE in the cortex of transgenic mice with Alzheimer's disease-like neuropathology. *Neurosci Lett* 438 216-220.

Vigo-Pelfrey C, Lee D, Keim P, Lieberburg I & Schenk DB 1993 Characterization of beta-amyloid peptide from human cerebrospinal fluid. *J Neurochem* 61 1965-1968.

von Koch CS, Zheng H, Chen H, Trumbauer M, Thinakaran G, van der Ploeg LH, Price DL & Sisodia SS 1997 Generation of APLP2 KO mice and early postnatal lethality in APLP2/APP double KO mice. *Neurobiol Aging* 18 661-669.

Wang DS, Dickson DW & Malter JS 2006 beta-Amyloid degradation and Alzheimer's disease. *J Biomed Biotechnol* 2006 58406.

Wang S, Wang R, Chen L, Bennett DA, Dickson DW & Wang DS 2010 Expression and functional profiling of neprilysin, insulin-degrading enzyme, and endothelin-converting enzyme in prospectively studied elderly and Alzheimer's brain. *J Neurochem* 115 47-57.

Wati H, Kawarabayashi T, Matsubara E, Kasai A, Hirasawa T, Kubota T, Harigaya Y, Shoji M & Maeda S 2009 Transthyretin accelerates vascular Abeta deposition in a mouse model of Alzheimer's disease. *Brain Pathol* 19 48-57.

Weeraratna AT, Kalehua A, Deleon I, Bertak D, Maher G, Wade MS, Lustig A, Becker KG, Wood W, 3rd, Walker DG, et al. 2007 Alterations in immunological and neurological gene expression patterns in Alzheimer's disease tissues. *Exp Cell Res* 313 450-461.

Weisgraber KH & Mahley RW 1996 Human apolipoprotein E: the Alzheimer's disease connection. *FASEB J* 10 1485-1494.

Weisner B & Kauerz U 1983 The influence of the choroid plexus on the concentration of prealbumin in CSF. *J Neurol Sci* 61 27-35.

Wen D, Corina K, Chow EP, Miller S, Janmey PA & Pepinsky RB 1996 The plasma and cytoplasmic forms of human gelsolin differ in disulfide structure. *Biochemistry* 35 9700-9709.

Wisniewski T & Frangione B 1996 Molecular biology of brain aging and neurodegenerative disorders. *Acta Neurobiol Exp (Wars)* 56 267-279.

Woeber KA & Ingbar SH 1968 The contribution of thyroxine-binding prealbumin to the binding of thyroxine in human serum, as assessed by immunoadsorption. *J Clin Invest* 47 1710-1721.

Xie L, Helmerhorst E, Taddei K, Plewright B, Van Bronswijk W & Martins R 2002 Alzheimer's beta-amyloid peptides compete for insulin binding to the insulin receptor. *J Neurosci* 22 RC221.

Yamada T, Yoshiyama Y, Sato H, Seiki M, Shinagawa A & Takahashi M 1995 White matter microglia produce membrane-type matrix metalloprotease, an activator of gelatinase A, in human brain tissues. *Acta Neuropathol* 90 421-424.

Yan P, Hu X, Song H, Yin K, Bateman RJ, Cirrito JR, Xiao Q, Hsu FF, Turk JW, Xu J, et al. 2006 Matrix metalloproteinase-9 degrades amyloid-beta fibrils in vitro and compact plaques in situ. *J Biol Chem* 281 24566-24574.

Yang JD, Feng G, Zhang J, Lin ZX, Shen T, Breen G, St Clair D & He L 2000 Association between angiotensin-converting enzyme gene and late onset Alzheimer's disease in Han chinese. *Neurosci Lett* 295 41-44.

Yerbury JJ, Kumita JR, Meehan S, Dobson CM & Wilson MR 2009 alpha2-Macroglobulin and haptoglobin suppress amyloid formation by interacting with prefibrillar protein species. *J Biol Chem* 284 4246-4254.

Yin KJ, Cirrito JR, Yan P, Hu X, Xiao Q, Pan X, Bateman R, Song H, Hsu FF, Turk J, et al. 2006 Matrix metalloproteinases expressed by astrocytes mediate extracellular amyloid-beta peptide catabolism. *J Neurosci* 26 10939-10948.

Zhang YW, Thompson R, Zhang H & Xu H 2011 APP processing in Alzheimer's disease. *Mol Brain* 4 3.

Zhao J & Pei G 2008 Evoking plasmin for beta-amyloid clearance. *Cell Res* 18 803-804.

Zhao Z, Xiang Z, Haroutunian V, Buxbaum JD, Stetka B & Pasinetti GM 2007 Insulin degrading enzyme activity selectively decreases in the hippocampal formation of cases at high risk to develop Alzheimer's disease. *Neurobiol Aging* 28 824-830.

Zheng H & Koo EH 2006 The amyloid precursor protein: beyond amyloid. *Mol Neurodegener* 1 5.

Zhong N & Weisgraber KH 2009a Understanding the association of apolipoprotein E4 with Alzheimer disease: clues from its structure. *J Biol Chem* 284 6027-6031.

Zhong N & Weisgraber KH 2009b Understanding the basis for the association of apoE4 with Alzheimer's disease: opening the door for therapeutic approaches. *Curr Alzheimer Res* 6 415-418.

Zlokovic BV 2004 Clearing amyloid through the blood-brain barrier. *J Neurochem* 89 807-811.

Zou K, Maeda T, Watanabe A, Liu J, Liu S, Oba R, Satoh Y, Komano H & Michikawa M 2009 Abeta42-to-Abeta40- and angiotensin-converting activities in different domains of angiotensin-converting enzyme. *J Biol Chem* 284 31914-31920.

Zou K, Yamaguchi H, Akatsu H, Sakamoto T, Ko M, Mizoguchi K, Gong JS, Yu W, Yamamoto T, Kosaka K, et al. 2007 Angiotensin-converting enzyme converts amyloid beta-protein 1-42 (Abeta(1-42)) to Abeta(1-40), and its inhibition enhances brain Abeta deposition. *J Neurosci* 27 8628-8635.

Zubenko GS, Volicer L, Direnfeld LK, Freeman M, Langlais PJ & Nixon RA 1985 Cerebrospinal fluid levels of angiotensin-converting enzyme in Alzheimer's disease, Parkinson's disease and progressive supranuclear palsy. *Brain Res* 328 215-221.

# 6

# Structural and Toxic Properties of Protein Aggregates: Towards a Molecular Understanding of Alzheimer's Disease

Lei Wang and Silvia Campioni
*Swiss Federal Institute of Technology (ETH) Zurich*
*Switzerland*

## 1. Introduction

Alzheimer's disease (AD) is an age-related irreversible brain disorder that progresses over 10 to 20 years. AD gradually destroys human memory and thinking skills, leads to severe loss of mental function, and eventually causes death (Querfurth and LaFerla, 2010). Normally, AD symptoms first appear after age 65. It is estimated that AD affected 36 million people globally in 2009, and the number will be more than doubled by 2050. Currently, there is no cure for AD, except few medications that can relieve AD symptoms (Brunden et al., 2009; Citron, 2004).

AD is accompanied by a significant shrunk of brain tissue, which is a result of brain neuron degeneration. In the brains of AD patients, neurons are found to have lost their synaptic connections with other neurons and are unable to survive (Wenk, 2003). The synaptic failure is indeed the earliest event associated with the cognitive impairment caused by the disease (Selkoe, 2002). In addition, the brains of AD patients are characterized by the presence of two types of hystopathological hallmark lesions: amyloid plaques and neurofibrillary tangles (NFTs), which are composed of aggregated proteinaceous material (Tiraboschi et al., 2004). Although both amyloid plaques and NFTs are also present in brains of healthy individuals, the amount of these aggregates in the brains of AD patients is significantly higher. Early studies correlated neuron degeneration in AD with the formation of these insoluble protein aggregates. However, recent studies suggest that soluble protein aggregates of the same protein composition are more toxic to neurons (Rahimi et al., 2008). It has also been suggested that the insoluble aggregates actually play a beneficial role in that they sequester the toxic soluble aggregates into less toxic or non-toxic insoluble aggregates (Greenwald and Riek, 2010).

At current stage, we are still trying to understand how different protein aggregates in the brain mediate neuron degeneration and lead to AD. Like any other protein activity, the neurotoxicity of protein aggregates must be associated with their specific molecular structures. Therefore, investigating the high-resolution structures of amyloid plaques, NFTs and soluble aggregates would greatly facilitate the development of diagnostic and therapeutic strategies. Here, in this chapter, we review current knowledge about the structure and toxicity of the aggregates involved in AD.

## 2. Structure and toxicity of different protein aggregates involved in AD

### 2.1 Amyloid-β peptides, tau protein and their relation to AD

Amyloid plaques are extracellular deposits mainly composed of full length and truncated fragments of amyloid-β (Aβ) peptides. Aβ peptides are produced upon cleavage of the amyloid precursor protein (APP) by β- and γ- secretases (Hooper, 2005). APP is an integral membrane protein expressed in many tissues and concentrated in the neuronal synapses (Turner et al., 2003). The γ-secretase protease cleaves APP at different positions, thus producing different Aβ fragments composed by 36 to 43 amino-acid-residues (Kang et al., 1987; Masters et al., 1985). Among those, the Aβ fragments having 40 ($A\beta_{40}$) or 42 ($A\beta_{42}$) amino-acid-residues are the most common (Hartmann et al., 1997). The amino-acid sequences of $A\beta_{40}$ and $A\beta_{42}$ are:

$A\beta_{40}$ : DAEFRHDSGYEVHHQKLVFFAEDVGSNKGAIIGLMVGGVV
$A\beta_{42}$ : DAEFRHDSGYEVHHQKLVFFAEDVGSNKGAIIGLMVGGVVIA

In the amyloid plaques, Aβ peptides form highly-ordered insoluble fibrillar aggregates, termed amyloid fibrils (Ohnishi and Takano, 2004). Besides, in the brain of AD patients, Aβ peptides can also form different types of soluble aggregates, such as small spherical aggregates, large spherical aggregates and small curved fibrils that are different from mature amyloid fibrils found in amyloid plaques (Dahlgren et al., 2002). An important role for of Aβ peptides in AD pathogenesis is also suggested by the fact that many mutations related to early-onset familial forms of AD increase total Aβ peptides levels and/or the relative concentration of $A\beta_{40}$ and $A\beta_{42}$, which is an important factor for AD since the latter peptide is more hydrophobic and hince aggregation prone (Borchelt et al., 1996; Eckman et al., 1997).

Neurofibrillary tangles (NFTs) are intracellular deposits mainly composed of the tau protein. Normally, tau interacts with tubulins and facilitates their assembly into microtubules, which act as cell skeleton and are important for cell health (Hernandez and Avila, 2007). Tau sequence can be divided into two major domains: a projection domain and a C-terminal microtubules binding domain. The latter contains similar but not identical repeats of 31-32 residues responsible for tubulin binding (Kosik, 1990). Six isoforms of tau are present in the brain, with 352 to 441 amino-acid-residues (Goedert et al., 1992). They differ from each other in the number of tubulin binding domains. Tau can undergo multiple types of post-translational modification. Its most important modification in AD is phosphorylation. When tau is hyperphosphorylated, it looses binding affinity to the microtubules, and starts to self-assemble into paired helical filaments (PHFs), which in turn deposit into NFTs (Alonso et al., 2001). Tau deposition as NFTs is also a characteristics of a subset of frontotemporal dementia. The fact that mutations in the gene encoding for tau are related to familial forms of frontotemporal dementia indicate an important role for tau in neurodegeneration (Heutink, 2000).

In early reports, spreading of NFTs in the brain had been observed to correlate with the progression of AD, suggesting a central role for tau in AD, but later studies rather led to the dominant idea that the aggregation of Aβ peptides in the brain is the primary event in AD and occurs before tau aggregation (Hardy and Selkoe, 2002). The amyloid cascade hypothesis for AD proposes that the imbalance between the production and clearance of Aβ peptides leads to Aβ aggregation and plaques formation, initiating a complex cascade of

events, such as synaptic failure, tau hyperphosphorylation and inflammation, that finally lead to AD (Tanzi and Bertram, 2005). So far, the correlation between Aβ amyloid fibrils and AD onset remains weak (Schmitz et al., 2004), wheareas soluble Aβ aggregates are believed to play the most important role in AD (Rahimi et al., 2008).
Despite the primary role of Aβ aggregates in AD, Aβ and tau have been demonstrated to interact with each other and most likely they cause AD through synergic effects. Indeed, the presence of Aβ peptides in transgenic mice influences the aggregation of tau into NFTs and, on the other hand, tau protein mediates Aβ toxicity (Lewis et al., 2001; Rapoport et al., 2002). Recently, a novel hypothesis linking Aβ and tau has been proposed on the basis of the observation that tau can also have a dendritic localization under physiological conditions and that tau-mediated postsynaptic targeting of the tyrosine protein kinase FYN confers Aβ toxicity (Ittner et al., 2010).

### 2.2 Structure of $A\beta_{42}$ amyloid fibrils

$A\beta_{42}$ amyloid fibrils are the most abundant aggregates in amyloid plaques (Roher et al., 1993). Under electron microscope, they look like unbranched filaments with a diameter of ~ 10 nm, and their length can reach up to several micrometer (Antzutkin et al., 2002) (Figure 1A). The X-ray diffraction pattern of aligned $A\beta_{42}$ amyloid fibrils shows two characteristic bands: one sharp band at ~ 4.7 Å position, and another diffused orthogonal band at ~ 10 Å (Kirschner et al., 1986) (Figure 1B).
Two structural models of $A\beta_{42}$ amyloid fibrils are available. In the first model, the structural information was obtained by using solid-state nuclear magnetic resonance (ssNMR) and solution NMR combined with the hydrogen/deuterium exchange (H/D-exchange) method. The ssNMR techinque provides distance restraints within amyloid fibrils while H/D-exchange monitored with solution NMR allows the identification of the regions of the protein sequence involved in the core structure of amyloid fibrils (Hoshino et al., 2002; Wang et al., 2008; Wang et al., 2010). The obtained model shows that: (a) in amyloid fibrils, amino-acid-residues 1-10 of $A\beta_{42}$ are unstructured, residues 11-22 and 31-42 form two β-strands (β1 and β2), and residues 23-30 form a bend (Figure 1C) (Ahmed et al., 2010; Olofsson et al., 2006); (b) through backbone hydrogen bonds, β1- and β2-strands interact with β1- and β2-strands in other $A\beta_{42}$ molecules and form two parallel β-sheets. All β-strands are perpendicular to the fibril axis, and both β-sheets are parallel to the fibril axis. This structure is called the cross-β-sheet structure (Figure 1E) (Balbach et al., 2002; Kirschner et al., 1986; Tycko, 2004); (c) the two β-sheets are connected by the intramolecular side chain interaction between Phe19 and Leu34, the salt bridge between Asp23 and Lys28, and the intermolecular side chain interaction between Gln15 and Gly37 (Figure 1C & 1F) (Ahmed et al., 2010). The distance between two adjacent β-strands is ~ 4.7 Å, and the distance between two β-sheets is ~ 10 Å, corresponding to the two characteristic bands observed in X-ray diffraction of amyloid fibrils.
In the second model, ${}^{35Mox}A\beta_{42}$ was used to produce amyloid fibrils. ${}^{35Mox}A\beta_{42}$ contains a methionine sulfoxide at position 35. This structural model was obtained by using solution NMR combined with H/D-exchange method and pairwise mutagenesis experiments. The resulting structure shows that: (a) in the fibrils, amino-acid-residues 1-17 of ${}^{35Mox}A\beta_{42}$ are unstructured, residues 18-26 and 31-42 form two β-strands (β1 and β2), and residues 27-30 form a bend (Figure 1D) (Luhrs et al., 2005); (b) β1- and β2-strands in different

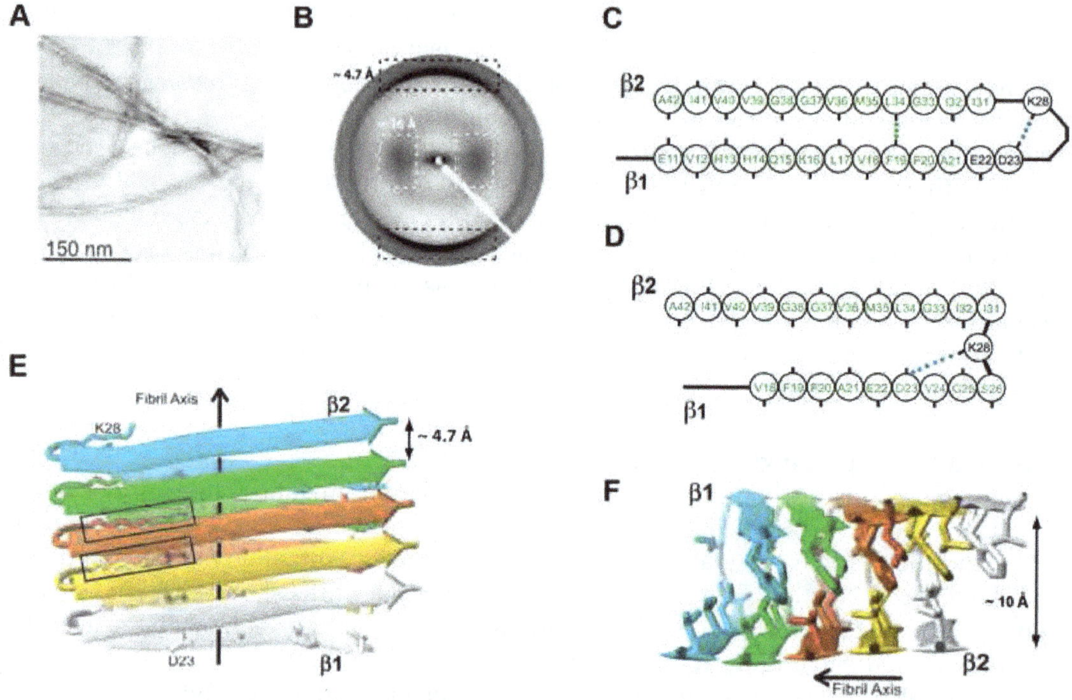


Fig. 1. Structural model of $A\beta_{42}$ amyloid fibrils. (A)Electron microscope image of $A\beta_{42}$ amyloid fibrils. (B) X-ray diffraction pattern of amyloid fibrils. (C) Illustration of $A\beta_{42}$ in amyloid fibrils. (D) Illustration of ${}^{Mox}A\beta_{42}$ in amyloid fibrils. (E) The cross-β-sheet structure of amyloid fibrils. (F) The side chain arrangement in amyloid fibrils. This figure is adapted from Fig 4 (Antzutkin et al., 2002), Fig 1 (Ahmed et al., 2010) and Fig 4 (Luhrs et al., 2005).

${}^{35Mox}A\beta_{42}$ molecules interconnect and form the cross-β-sheet structure (Figure 1E); (c) the two β-sheets are connected by the intermolecular side chain interactions between Phe19 and Gly38, Ala21 and Val36, and the salt bridge between Asp23 and Lys28 (Figure 1D & 1F) (Luhrs et al., 2005). Compared to the structure of $A\beta_{42}$ amyloid fibrils, the structural difference of ${}^{35Mox}A\beta_{42}$ amyloid fibrils may reflect the effect of Met35 modification, or, it may reflect the a structural polymorphism of $A\beta_{42}$ amyloid fibrils.

## 2.3 Structure of $A\beta_{40}$ amyloid fibrils

$A\beta_{40}$ can form at least three types of amyloid fibrils with distinct morphology, which include striated-ribbon fibrils (Figure 2A), twisted-pair fibrils (Figure 2B) and brain-seeded fibrils (Figure 2C) (Paravastu et al., 2009; Petkova et al., 2005). The polymorphism of the fibrils is induced by the different conditions used to form them. In particular, incubation of $A\beta_{40}$ under agitation leads to the formation of straight-rod shaped protofilaments with a width of 6 nm, and these protofilaments associate laterally to form striated-ribbon fibrils. Quiescent growth rather leads to the formation of twisted-pair fibrils that are composed of single protofilaments (Petkova et al., 2005). Seeding $A\beta_{40}$ aggregation with purified fibrils from brain tissue of AD patients leads to the formation of curved and untwisted fibrils (Paravastu et al., 2009). All three $A\beta_{40}$ fibrils have different underlying molecular structures.

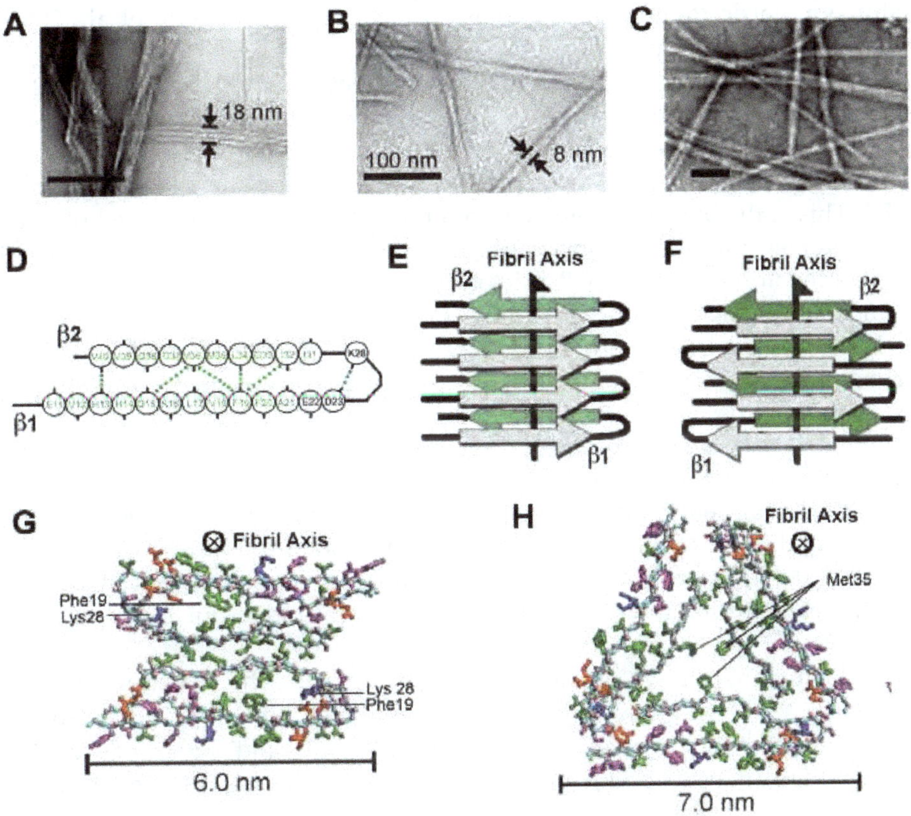


Fig. 2. Structural model of $A\beta_{40}$ amyloid fibrils. (A-C) Electron microscope images of striated-ribbon fibrils (A), twisted-pair fibrils (B) and brain-seeded (C) amyloid fibrils of $A\beta_{40}$. Scale bar = 100 nm. (D) Illustration of $A\beta_{40}$ in amyloid fibrils. (E) The parallel cross-β-sheet structure of $A\beta_{40}$ amyloid fibrils. (F) The antiparallel cross-β-sheet structure of $A\beta_{40}$–D23N amyloid fibrils. (G) One protofilament in the striated-ribbon fibrils is composed of two cross-β-sheet units. (H) One protofilament in the twisted-pair fibrils is composed of three cross-β-sheet units. This figure is adapted from Fig 4 (Paravastu et al., 2008), Fig 1 (Paravastu et al., 2009), and Fig 4 (Sawaya et al., 2007).

A structural model for striated-ribbon fibrils of $A\beta_{40}$ was obtained using solid-state NMR spectroscopy and electron microscopy. It shows that: (a) in amyloid fibrils, amino-acid-residues 1-9 of $A\beta_{40}$ are unstructured, residues 10-22 and 30-40 form two β-strands (β1 and β2), and residues 23-29 form a bend (Figure 2D) (Petkova et al., 2006); (b) through backbone hydrogen bonds, β1- and β2-strands interact with β1- and β2-strands in other $A\beta_{40}$ molecules and form two parallel β-sheets. All β-strands are perpendicular to the fibril axis, and both β-sheets are parallel to the fibril axis. This structure is considered as one cross-β-sheet unit (Figure 2E); (c) the two β-sheets are connected by side chain interactions, including the intermolecular interaction between Phe19 in one molecule and Leu34 in the neighboring molecule, and the intramolecular salt bridge between Asp23 and Lys28 (Petkova et al., 2006) (Figure 2D); (d) the individual protofilament in the striated-ribbon fibrils is composed of two cross-β-sheet units, which are two-fold rotationally symmetric to each other along the fibril axis (Sciarretta et al., 2005; Tycko, 2010) (Figure 2G).

The structural model for twisted-pair fibrils of $A\beta_{40}$ contains similar cross-β-sheet unit as in striated-ribbon fibrils (Petkova et al., 2006) (Figure 2D & 2E). But the individual protofilament in the twisted-pair fibrils is composed of three cross-β-sheet units, which are three-fold rotationally symmetric to each other along the fibril axis (Sciarretta et al., 2005) (Figure 2H). This is the biggest difference from the protofilament composed of two cross-β-sheet units obtained for striated-ribbon fibrils. Other structural differences in twisted-pair fibrils include the absence of the salt bridge between Asp23 and Lys28, and different side chain interactions among cross-β-sheet units.

Brain-seeded fibrils have been produced to mimic amyloid fibrils of $A\beta_{40}$ formed *in vivo*. Due to experimental limit, currently it is not possible to measure the structure of fibrils directly from human tissue. As an alternative, fibrils extracted from the brain tissue of AD patients were used as seeds to produce large amount of isotopically labeled brain-seeded fibrils for structural study (Paravastu et al., 2009). These fibrils are thus likely to represent the amyloid fibrils formed *in vivo*. It has been shown that the ssNMR spectra of the brain-seeded fibrils are different from that of the striated-ribbon or twisted-pair fibrils, suggesting that brain-seeded fibrils have a different structure than previous identified structures of $A\beta_{40}$ fibrils (Tycko, 2010). However, a detailed structural model for brain-seeded fibrils is not yet available.

Disease-related mutants of $A\beta_{40}$ also form amyloid fibrils. The structure of the amyloid fibrils formed by the Iowa mutant ($A\beta_{40}$-D23N), associated with early-onset familial AD, is composed of a different cross-β-sheet unit, in which β1- and β2-strands of $A\beta_{40}$-D23N molecules are interconnected and form two antiparallel β-sheets (Tycko et al., 2009) (Figure 2F).

### 2.4 Structure of paired helical filaments of tau

As mentioned before, neurofibrillary tangles (NFTs) deposits are composed of paired helical filaments (PHFs) of tau protein (Wischik et al., 1988) (Figure 3A). Although the high-resolution structure of tau PHFs has not been solved yet, several structural models are available based on various experimental data. Fourier transform infrared (FT-IR) spectroscopy experiments show that tau PHFs are composed of a large amount of random coil structure together with some α-helical and β-sheet structure (Sadqi et al., 2002). It has also been found that the residues 265-338 in PHFs (PHF43) are protected against proteases digestion, and PHF43 alone can also form amyloid fibrils (von Bergen et al., 2000). Further investigation shows that the amino-acid-residues 306-311 (sequence: VQIVYK) (PHF6) within PHF43 are responsible for PHF43 amyloid fibrils formation. PHF6 alone forms amyloid fibrils that resemble tau PHFs (von Bergen et al., 2005; von Bergen et al., 2000). X-ray microcrystallography data show that PHF6 forms parallel β-sheets in amyloid fibrils, and the β-sheets are connected by side chains that form steric zippers (Sawaya et al., 2007) (Figure 3B & 3C).

One structural model of tau PHFs suggests that they contain one cross-β sheet composed of PHF6 while the rest of the sequence is structurally disordered or contains some α-helical structure (von Bergen et al., 2005) (Figure 3D). Another structural model suggests that PHFs may contain an additional cross-β sheet, which is composed of amino-acid-residues 272-289 (S2) (Figure 3E). This model is based on the finding that isolated S2 can also form amyloid fibrils under certain conditions (Margittai and Langen, 2006).

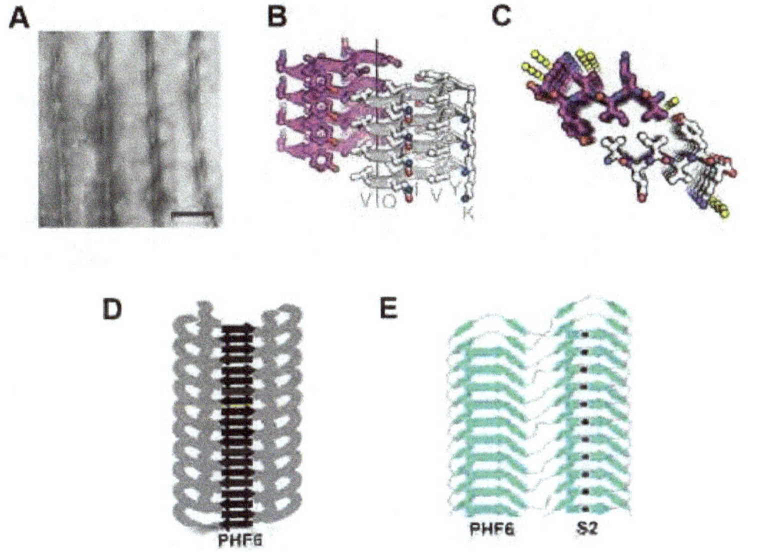


Fig. 3. Structural model of paired helical filaments (PHFs) of tau. (A) Electron microscope image of tau PHFs. Scale bar = 100 nm. (B-C) The side and top view of the cross-β-sheet structure of PHF6 amyloid fibrils. (D) The proposed structural model for tau PHFs, in which PHF6 form the cross-β-sheet structure, and the rest of tau PHFs is not/least structured. (E) Another proposed structural model for tau PHFs, in which PHF6 and S2 form two cross-β-sheet structures. This figure is adapted from Fig 1B (Wischik et al., 1988), Fig 2 & 3 (Sawaya et al., 2007), Fig 6 (von Bergen et al., 2005) and Fig 4A (Margittai and Langen, 2006).

### 2.5 Soluble Aβ aggregates: Mechanism of toxicity and structure

Increasing evidence suggest that the pathogenic agents in amyloid-related diseases are the transient, pre-fibrillar Aβ assemblies preceding the formation of mature fibrils, whereas amyloid fibrils rather represent the protective end state of the protein misfolding event (Sakono and Zako, 2010; Rahimi et al., 2008; Chiti and Dobson, 2006). This is particularly valid in the case of AD, where a weak correlation exists between cognitive impairment and amyloid plaques formation (Terry et al., 1991) and, in transgenic mouse lines used to model AD, synaptotoxicity is observed before and/or independently of amyloid plaque formation (Mucke et al., 2000). Instead, the levels of soluble Aβ oligomers in AD patients correlate much better with the onset of neurodegeneration (for a review on the oligomer-toxicity hypothesis see Klein et al., 2001). Remarkably, a mutated form of Aβ showing enhanced oligomerization but no fibrillation was identified in a Japanese pedigree of AD patients with little deposition of fibrillar amyloid (Tomiyama et al., 2008).

Despite their relevance to disease, a detailed structural and functional characterization of amyloid pre-fibrillar species is considerably hampered by their transient and heterogeneous nature. In addition, in the case of Aβ pre-fibrillar species, further complications arise due to the various methods used to produce the synthetic peptide/s used in the experiments and the fact that the $A\beta_{40}$ and $A\beta_{42}$ are more aggregation prone than other amyloidogenic peptides and protein and form ensembles of oligomeric species already upon dissolution of the lyophilized peptides in aqueous buffer (Teplow, 2006). Describing in detail all types of Aβ oligomers reported in the literature up to date would be beyond the scopes of this book chapter; we will

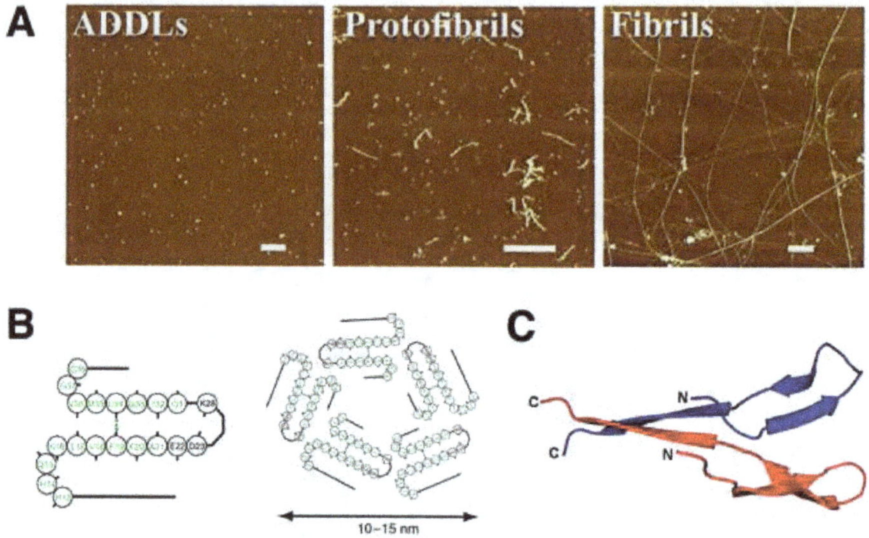


Fig. 4. Morphology and conformation of different aggregates formed by Aβ$_{42}$ under different incubation conditions. (A) Atomic force microscopy images of ADDLs (left), protofibrils (middle) and mature fibrils (right). (B) Schematic model of Aβ$_{42}$ monomer within a spherical pentameric aggregated from solid-state magic angle spinning data. Light blue squares connect Phe19 and Leu34. The areas showing little protection from hydrogen-deuterium exchange are coloured in green. (C) Model for the structure of Aβ$_{42}$ preglobulomers obtained from solution state NMR. According to this model, preglobulomers are formed by dimer units adopting mixed parallel and antiparallel structure. This figure is adapted from Fig 2 & 4 (Klein et al., 2001), and Fig 3 (Yu et al., 2009).

thus limit our description to a summary of the most consolidated and recent information on the species thought to play an important role in AD disease. Although all these species are generally referred to as "Aβ oligomers", the readers should keep in mind that they may differ in structure, pathway of formation and mechanism of toxicity as well.

### 2.5.1 Aβ pre-fibrillar aggregates formed in vitro

In studies performed *in vitro*, Aβ peptides have been found to form various types of aggregates having spherical morphology. Cross-linking experiments show that Aβ$_{40}$ and Aβ$_{42}$ preparations differ in their oligomers distributions, with the former peptide forming roughly equimolar mixtures of aggregates ranging from dimers to tetramers, whereas the latter preferentially forms pentamers/hexamers (termed paranuclei), which self-associate into dodecamers and octadecamers (Bitan et al., 2001; Bitan et al., 2003). These larger species appear not to be artifacts of the cross-linking technique since Aβ$_{42}$ stable dodecamers formed by stacked hexamer units have been detected also in the absence of any cross-linking (Bernstein et al., 2009). Here we will summarize present information on the toxic effect and the conformational properties of the most investigated oligomeric species.

Aβ-derived diffusible ligands (ADDLs) are slowly sedimenting aggregates observed only in preparations of synthetic Aβ$_{42}$ peptides; they appear as globular species with 3-8 nm height (Figure 4A) and they are believed to be composed of 3-24 monomers (Oda et al., 1995;

Lambert et al., 1998; Klein et al., 2002; Chromy et al., 2003). Their pathological relevance is supported by the detection of aggregates (in particular dodecamers) immunoreactive to anti-ADDLs antibodies in the brain and cerebrospinal fluid of AD patients (Gong et al., 2003; Georganopoulou et al., 2005). ADDLs are potent neurotoxins: they induce the death of principal neurons of the hippocampus and, in rat hippocampal brain slices, they inhibit long-term potentiation (LTP) but not long-term depression (LTD), two forms of synaptic plasticity implicated in learning and memory (Lambert et al., 1998; Wang et al., 2002). Binding of ADDLs to hippocampal neurons appears to occur at the postsynaptic termini of excitatory synapses and stimulates aberrant expression of the activity-regulated cytoskeletal-associated (Arc) protein (implicated in long-term memory formation), tau hyperphosphorylation, synapses deterioration and loss, and enhanced formation of reactive oxygen species (ROS) thought to play a major role in the pathogenesis of AD (Lacor et al., 2004; Guzowski 2002; Hsieh et al., 2006; De Felice et al., 2007a; De Felice et al., 2007b; Lacor et al., 2007; Shankar et al., 2007). Monoclonal antibodies targeting ADDLs can prevent their aberrant binding and synaptotoxicity (Lambert et al., 2007). *In vivo*, insulin signaling and the cellular prion protein ($PrP^C$) have been suggested to mediate the toxicity of ADDLs, even if in the latter case an effective involvement in AD is currently under debate (De Felice et al., 2009; Laurén et al., 2009; Gimbel et al., 2010; Calella et al., 2010; Caetano et al., 2011). Despite the large amount of data on the toxic effect of ADDLs, still little is known about their structure; mainly because they are heterogeneous mixtures of oligomers of different sizes. The structure of neurotoxic $A\beta_{42}$ pentamers has been recently investigated (Figure 4B). Hydrogen-deuterium exchange measurements indicate that the first nine residues are solvent exposed, as well as residues 13-15, 25-29 and 37-38 that presumably form solvent-accessible turns (Ahmed et al., 2010). Solid-state magic angle spinning measurements show the lack of parallel, in-register β-sheets, but the C-terminal regions of the constituting monomers are packed together and adopt a conformation similar to that observed in the mature fibrils (U-shaped hairpin structure), with Phe19 in contact with Leu34 (Ahmed et al., 2010).

Globular oligomers having a size of 4-5 nm, composed of twelve monomeric units and forming independently from fibril formation have been obtained from $A\beta_{42}$ samples incubated at high concentration (400 μM) in the presence of sodium dodecyl sulfate (SDS) or fatty acids; such species are known as Aβ globulomers (Barghorn et al., 2005; Gellermann et al., 2008; Yu et al., 2009). Similarly to ADDLs, globulomers selectively bind to neuronal cells, inhibit LTP in hippocampal brain slices and their toxicity can be rescued with a globulomer-specific antibody (Barghorn et al., 2005; Hillen et al., 2010). Moreover, antibodies against globulomers detect immunoreactive species in tissue sections from the brains of AD patients and human APP transgenic mice (Barghorn et al., 2005). In contrast to ADDLs preparations, globulomer samples are stable and homogeneous; thus can be used for structural studies. Protease digestion, cross-linking and antibody binding data suggest that residues 1-20 of $A\beta_{42}$ are accessible to the solvent while the rest of the sequence forms the core of the aggregates. Solution NMR data on smaller pre-globulomeric species (tetramers) indicate that they are composed of dimer repeating units (Figure 4C) with residues 18-23 and 28-40 forming β-structure in mixed parallel and antiparallel β-sheets (Yu et al., 2009). Finally, hydrogen-deuterium exchange measurements indicate that globulomers and pre-globulomers have similar secondary structures and that the former species result from association of pre-globulomeric units.

A$\beta_{40}$ and A$\beta_{42}$ can also form, off-pathway from fibril formation, large globular aggregates with little or no cross-β structure (they do not bind the amyloid-specific dye thioflavin T) termed amylospheroids (ASPDs) (Hoschi et al., 2003; Matsumura et al., 2011). ASPDs of 10-15 nm diameter are potent neurotoxins to primary cultures from rat septum regions; the most toxic species being 32-mers (Hoschi et al., 2003; Matsumura et al., 2011). Antibodies generated to recognize ASPDs stain AD brains and have been used to immunoisolate ASPDs directly from AD and dementia with Lewy bodies brains (Noguchi et al., 2009). Levels of ASPDs in AD patients correlate with the severity of disease and the immunoprecipitated species induce degeneration on neurons *in vitro* (Noguchi et al., 2009). Chimon et al. investigated the structure of globular A$\beta_{40}$ aggregates formed by at least 150 monomers that impair the viability of cultured PC-12 cells and have a diameter similar to that of ASPDs, but, in contrast to ASPDs, they are rich in β-sheet structure and are on-pathway intermediates of fibril formation (Chimon and Ishii, 2005; Chimon et al., 2007). Solid-state NMR spectra show that these assemblies have ordered parallel, in regisister, β-stucture, extremely similar to that of mature A$\beta_{40}$ fibrils, particularly in the hydrophobic core and C-terminal regions (Chimon and Ishii, 2005; Chimon et al., 2007).

Aβ protofibrils (Figure 4A) also belong to the wide range of possible Aβ pre-fibrillar aggregates. These are soluble aggregates formed by both A$\beta_{40}$ and A$\beta_{42}$ *via* association of smaller globular units, with an apparent mass higher than 100 kDa and appearing as curved fibril-like structures of 3-8 nm diameter and less than 200 nm length (Harper et al., 1997; Walsh et al., 1997; Walsh et al., 1999; Harper et al., 1999). PFs formed *in vitro* alter the viability of cultured rat primary cortical neurons and induce neuronal injury, impaired electrophysiological activities and neuronal loss (Walsh et al., 1999; Hartley et al., 1999). The fact that the early-onset AD-related Arctic mutation enhances PF formation suggests that these species might be relevant for the disease (Nilsberth et al., 2001). Moreover, 4-hydroxy-2-nonenal (HNE), a metabolite of oxidative stress found to exist at increased concentrations in AD patients and to co-localize with Aβ deposits, causes *in vitro* accumulation of A$\beta_{40}$ PFs and prevents their conversion into mature fibrils, thus leading to sustained neurotoxicity to cultured cells (Sayre et al., 1997; Siegel et al., 2007; Johansson et al., 2007). PFs appear transiently and are considered to be the direct precursors of long and rigid amyloid fibrils (Harper et al., 1997; Walsh et al., 1997). Indeed, they already possess a high content of β-sheet structure and the capability to bind the WO1 amyloid fibrils-specific antibody (Williams et al., 2005). Nonetheless, they are still metastable and can dissociate into low molecular weight oligomers (Walsh et al., 1999; Harper et al., 1999). A$\beta_{40}$ PFs possess a stable structural core (Kheterpal et al., 2003). Proline substitution and hydrogen-deuterium exchange experiments on A$\beta_{40}$ PFs stabilized by a small molecule show that the first N-terminal 14-19 residues and the C-terminal 3-5 residues are not involved in the formation of their structural core and that, in comparison to mature fibrils, PFs are less structured in the fragment spanning residues 20-34 (Williams et al., 2005; Kheterpal et al., 2006).

Protofibrillar aggregates formed by the E22G (Arctic mutation) mutant of A$\beta_{40}$ can also adopt annular structures (Lashuel et al., 2002). These species have a pore-like appearance with an outer diameter of 7-10 nm and an inner diameter of 1.5-2.0 nm, and appear to be composed of 40-60 peptide molecules (Lashuel et al., 2002). Structures similar to annular PFs have been observed upon incorporation of different Aβ peptides into artificial and natural membranes and have been hypothesized to serve as calcium channels that mediate Aβ-induced toxicity in AD (Arispe et al., 2007). However, the formation of Aβ pores is still debated since spherical Aβ aggregates can increase membrane permeability and intracellular calcium levels without any evidence of discrete channel of pore formation (Kayed et al., 2004; Demuro et al., 2005). Antibodies specific for annular protofibrils, but not spherical oligomers and fibrils, also recognize heptameric alpha-hemolysin pores, suggesting that the antibody recognizes an epitope that is specific for a β barrel structural motif (Kayed et al., 2009).

### 2.5.2 Cell-derived pre-fibrillar aggregates

Oligomerization studies performed *in vitro* with synthetic peptides have various limitations: 1) the usually employed peptide concentrations are in the micromolar range, whereas Aβ concentration *in vivo* is rather in the nanomolar or even subnanomolar range (Seubert et al., 1992; Suzuki et al., 1994; Tabaton et al., 1994); 2) *in vitro*, peptides of specified lengths are used, whereas numerous Aβ species, with extensive amino and carboxyl terminal heterogeneity, are usually present *in vivo* (reviewed in Golde and Younkin, 1996); 3) aggregation is usually examined under non-physiological conditions, with the peptides solubilized in organic solvents and then diluted in water or aqueous buffers free of other proteins, macromolecules or small molecules. These limitations imply that pathologically relevant aggregates may differ substantially from those produced *in vitro*. Thus, considerable effort has been recently spent in isolating and characterizing Aβ oligomers formed *in vivo*. Detailed structural characterization of cell-derived oligomers is lacking due to their low concentration, but their ability to cause toxicity and cognitive impairment has been deeply investigated.

Small SDS-stable oligomers have been isolated at nanomolar concentration from the medium of caltured cells, human cerebrospinal fluid, APP transgenic mouse brain and human brain (reviewed in Selkoe 2008; Rahimi et al., 2008). Aβ dimers have been detected and proved to form intracellularly in primary human neurons and in both neuronal and non-neural cell lines (Walsh et al., 2000). Stable dimers and trimers of Aβ isolated from the neuritic plaques of AD patients and leptomeningeal vessels compromise the viability of cultured rat hippocampal neuron glia cells through a microglia-dependent mechanism and Aβ dimers from the cerebral cortex of AD patients can also impair synaptic plasticity and memory in rats (Roher et al., 1996; Shankar et al., 2008). Synaptic dysfunction is also caused by dimers from *ex vivo* human cerebrospinal fluid (Klyubin et al., 2008).

Oligomers (in particular trimers) secreted in the medium of Chinese Hamster Ovary cells over-expressing the β-amyloid precursor protein inhibit hippocampal LTP, decrease the density of dendritic spines, impair cognitive function in rats and inhibit the remodeling of synapses, a prerequisite for memory consolidation (Walsh et al., 2002; Cleary et al., 2005; Townsend et al., 2006; Shankar et al., 2007; Poling et al., 2008; Freir et al., 2010). Compounds that inhibit oligomers formation or antibodies that bind to the oligomers rescue their toxic effects (Walsh et al., 2005a; Walsh et al., 2005b).

A soluble, SDS-stable dodecamer termed Aβ*56 was found in the brain of middle-aged APP transgenic mice carrying a familial AD-linked double mutation (Lesné et al., 2006). Levels of Aβ*56 dodecamers in middle-aged APP transgenic mice correlate with cognitive deficits and administration of purified Aβ*56 to young rats disrupts their memory (Lesné et al., 2006). In a recent study, synthetic $A\beta_{42}$-derived oligomers, cell- and brain-derived low molecular weight oligomers, and Aβ*56 have been compared for their ability to produce deficits in learned behavior of rats, finding that dimers derived from the culture medium of APP transgenic cells are the most potent neurotoxins (Reed et al., 2009).

Oligomers of modified forms of N-terminally truncated Aβ peptides having pyroglutamate as first residue in the sequence (pE-Aβ) have also been detected in the cerebral cortex of AD patients (Piccini et al., 2005). pE-Aβ peptides are believed to play an important role in the pathogenesis of AD because they are highly abundant in the brains of AD patients and they are major constituents of the amyloid plaques (for a recent review, see Gunn et al., 2010). *In vitro* studies indicate that pE-Aβ peptides are more aggregation prone and neurotoxic than full length Aβ (Harigaya et al., 2000; Russo et al., 2002). When a novel mouse monoclonal antibody specifically targeting low molecular weights oligomers of pE-Aβ is used to passively immunize transgenic mice, plaque load and Aβ levels are reduced and behavioral deficits are normalized, suggesting that pE-Aβ oligomers are valuable targets for AD diagnosis and therapeutic intervention (Wirths et al., 2010).

## 3. Conclusion

In this chapter, we reviewed current knowledge of the structure and toxicity of different protein aggregates that are involved in Alzheimer's disease (AD). Currently, two structural models are available for $A\beta_{42}$ amyloid fibrils. Both models show a parallel cross-β-sheet structure. But in the first model, amino-acid-residues 11-22 and 31-42 adopt β-strand conformation ($A\beta_{42}$); wheareas in the second model, residues 18-26 and 31-42 adopt β-strand conformation ($^{35Mox}A\beta_{42}$). For $A\beta_{40}$ amyloid fibrils, structural polymorphism has been observed. The striated-ribbon fibrils, twisted-pair fibrils and brain-seeded fibrils of $A\beta_{40}$ all have different morphology and molecular structure. Tau PHFs also contain a cross-β-sheet structure, in which amino-acid-residues 306-311 and possibly 272-289 adopt the β-strand conformation. The rest of tau is either disordered or contains small amount of α-helical structure.

Recent studies suggest that the soluble Aβ aggregates (pre-fibrillar aggregates), instead of Aβ amyloid fibrils and tau PHFs, correlate more closelly with neuron degeneration in AD. Several types of Aβ pre-fibrillar aggregates have been described. Their common toxicity may be due to multiple reasons such as the heterogeneity of Aβ aggregates preparations, most likely containing different amounts of monomeric, oligomeric and fibrillar Aβ rather than single species, and the fact that all these species may share a "misfolded" nature, meaning that they most likely expose on their surfaces repetitive clusters and/or arrays of groups that enable their interaction with different targets. It has been recently suggested that it's the ongoing Aβ polymerization process involving the elongation and growth of pre-fibrillar aggregates such as protofibrils, rather than the formation of a specific toxic oligomeric species to be responsible for Aβ toxicity in AD (Jan et al., 2011). Similarly to what has been proposed for another amyloid forming peptide, the cooperative binding of Aβ peptides to cell membranes, and the growth and elongation of Aβ aggregates at the level of the membrane could result in changes in membrane curvature and weakened lipid packing, leading to membrane permeabilization and toxicity (Engel et al., 2008; Friedman et al., 2009). Further studies are therefore necessary to clearly elucidate the structural properties and mechanism of toxicity of Aβ aggregates in order to develop efficient therapeutic strategies for AD.

## 4. Acknowledgment

We would like to thank Prof. Roland Riek for his helpful comments and suggestions.

## 5. References

Ahmed, M., Davis, J., Aucoin, D., Sato, T., Ahuja, S., Aimoto, S., Elliott, J.I., Van Nostrand, W.E., & Smith, S.O. (2010). Structural conversion of neurotoxic amyloid-$\beta_{1-42}$ oligomers to fibrils. *Nat Struct Mol Biol.*, 17, 561-567.

Alonso, A., Zaidi, T., Novak, M., Grundke-Iqbal, I., & Iqbal, K. (2001). Hyperphosphorylation induces self-assembly of tau into tangles of paired helical filaments/straight filaments. *Proc Natl Acad Sci U S A*, 98, 6923-6928.

Antzutkin, O.N., Leapman, R.D., Balbach, J.J., & Tycko, R. (2002). Supramolecular structural constraints on Alzheimer's beta-amyloid fibrils from electron microscopy and solid-state nuclear magnetic resonance. *Biochemistry*, 41, 15436-15450.

Arispe, N., Diaz, J.C., & Simakova, O. (2007). Abeta ion channels. Prospects for treating Alzheimer's disease with Abeta channel blockers. *Biochim Biophys Acta.*, 1768, 1952-1965.

Balbach, J.J., Petkova, A.T., Oyler, N.A., Antzutkin, O.N., Gordon, D.J., Meredith, S.C., & Tycko, R. (2002). Supramolecular structure in full-length Alzheimer's beta-amyloid fibrils: evidence for a parallel beta-sheet organization from solid-state nuclear magnetic resonance. *Biophys J.*, 83, 1205-1216.

Barghorn, S., Nimmrich, V., Striebinger, A., Krantz, C., Keller, P., Janson, B., Bahr, M., Schmidt, M., Bitner, R.S., Harlan, J., Barlow, E., Ebert, U., & Hillen, H. (2005). Globular amyloid beta-peptide oligomer - a homogeneous and stable neuropathological protein in Alzheimer's disease. *J Neurochem.*, 95, 834-847.

Bernstein, S.L., Dupuis, N.F., Lazo, N.D., Wyttenbach, T., Condron, M.M., Bitan, G., Teplow, D.B., Shea, J.E., Ruotolo, B.T., Robinson, C.V., & Bowers, M.T. (2009). Amyloid-β protein oligomerization and the importance of tetramers and dodecamers in the aetiology of Alzheimer's disease. *Nat Chem.*, 1, 326-331.

Bitan, G., Lomakin, A., & Teplow, D.B. (2001). Amyloid beta-protein oligomerization: prenucleation interactions revealed by photo-induced cross-linking of unmodified proteins. *J Biol Chem.*, 276, 35176-35184.

Bitan, G., Kirkitadze, M.D., Lomakin, A., Vollers, S.S., Benedek, G.B., & Teplow, D.B. (2003). Amyloid beta -protein (Abeta) assembly: Abeta 40 and Abeta 42 oligomerize through distinct pathways. *Proc Natl Acad Sci USA*, 100, 330-335.

Borchelt, D.R., Thinakaran, G., Eckman, C.B., Lee, M.K., Davenport, F., Ratovitsky, T., Prada, C.M., Kim, G., Seekins, S., Yager, D., Slunt, H.H., Wang, R., Seeger, M., Levey, A.I., Gandy, S.E., Copeland, N.G., Jenkins, N.A., Price, D.L., Younkin, S.G., & Sisodia, S.S. (1996). Familial Alzheimer's disease-linked presenilin 1 variants elevate Abeta1-42/1-40 ratio in vitro and in vivo. *Neuron*, 17, 1005-1013.

Braak, H., & Braak, E. (1995) Staging of Alzheimer's disease-related neurofibrillary changes. *Neurobiol Aging*, 16, 271–278.

Brunden, K.R., Trojanowski, J.Q., & Lee, V.M. (2009). Advances in tau-focused drug discovery for Alzheimer's disease and related tauopathies. *Nat Rev Drug Discov*, 8, 783-793.

Caetano, F.A., Beraldo, F.H., Hajj, G.N., Guimaraes, A.L., Jürgensen, S., Wasilewska-Sampaio, A.P., Hirata, P.H., Souza, I., Machado, C.F., Wong, D.Y., De Felice, F.G., Ferreira, S.T., Prado, V.F., Rylett, R.J., Martins, V.R., & Prado, M.A. (2011). Amyloid-beta oligomers increase the localization of prion protein at the cell surface. *J Neurosci.*, 117, 538-553.

Calella, A.M., Farinelli, M., Nuvolone, M., Mirante, O., Moos, R., Falsig, J., Mansuy, I.M., & Aguzzi, A. (2010). Prion protein and Abeta-related synaptic toxicity impairment. *EMBO Mol Med.*, 2, 306-314.

Chimon, S., & Ishii, Y. (2005). Capturing intermediate structures of Alzheimer's b-amyloid, Abeta (1-40), by solid-state NMR spectroscopy. *J Am Chem Soc.*, 127, 13472-13473.

Chimon, S., Shaibat, M.A., Jones, C.R., Calero, D.C., Aizezi, B., & Ishii, Y. (2007). Evidence of fibril-like beta-sheet structures in a neurotoxic amyloid intermediate of Alzheimer's beta-amyloid. *Nat Struct Mol Biol.*, 14, 1157-1164.

Chiti, F., & Dobson, C.M. (2006). Protein misfolding, functional amyloid, and human disease. *Annu Rev Biochem.*, 75, 333-366.

Chromy, B.A., Nowak, R.J., Lambert, M.P., Viola, K.L., Chang, L., Velasco, P.T., Jones, B.W., Fernandez, S.J., Lacor, P.N., Horowitz, P., Finch, C.E., Krafft, G.A., & Klein, W.L. (2003). Self-assembly of Abeta(1-42) into globular neurotoxins. *Biochemistry*, 42, 12749-12760.

Cleary, J.P., Walsh, D.M., Hofmeister, J.J., Shankar, G.M., Kuskowski, M.A., Selkoe, D.J., Ashe, K.H. (2005). Natural oligomers of the amyloid-beta protein specifically disrupt cognitive function. *Nat Neurosci.*, 8, 79-84.

Citron, M. (2004). Strategies for disease modification in Alzheimer's disease. *Nat Rev Neurosci* 5, 677-685.

Dahlgren, K.N., Manelli, A.M., Stine, W.B., Jr., Baker, L.K., Krafft, G.A., & LaDu, M.J. (2002). Oligomeric and fibrillar species of amyloid-beta peptides differentially affect neuronal viability. *J Biol Chem.*, 277, 32046-32053.

De Felice, F.G., Velasco, P.Y., Lambert, M.P., Viola, K., Fernandez, S.J., Ferreira, S.T., & Klein, W.L. (2007a) Abeta oligomers induce neuronal oxidative stress through an N-methyl-D-aspartate receptor-dependent mechanism that is blocked by the Alzheimer drug memantine. *J Biol Chem.*, 282, 11590-11601.

De Felice, F.G., Wu, D., Lambert, M.P., Fernandez, S.J., Velasco, P.T., Lacor, P.N., Bigio, E.H., Jerecic, J., Acton, P.J., Shughrue, P.J., Chen-Dodson, E., Kinney, G.G., & Klein, W.L. (2007b) Alzheimer's disease-type neuronal tau hyperphosphorylation induced by Abeta oligomers. *Neurobiol Aging.*, 29, 1334-1347.

De Felice, F.G., Vieira, M.N.N., Bomfim, T.R., Decker, H., Velasco, P.T., Lambert, M.P., Viola, K.L., Zhao, W.Q., Ferreira, S.T., Klein, W.L. (2009) Protection of synapses against Alzheimer's-linked toxins: insulin signaling prevents the pathogenic binding of Abeta oligomers. *Proc Natl Acad Sci U S A*, 106, 1971-1976.

Demuro, A., Mina, E., Kayed, R., Milton, S.C., Parker, I., & Glabe, C.G. (2005). Calcium dysregulation and membrane disruption as a ubiquitous neurotoxic mechanism of soluble amyloid oligomers. *J Biol Chem.*, 280, 17294-17300.

Dovey, H.F., Suomonsaari-Chrysler, S., Lieberburg, I., Sinha, S., & Keim, P.S. (1993). Cells with a familial Alzheimer's disease mutation produce authentic beta-peptide. *Neuroreport.*, 4, 1039-1042.

Eckman, C.B., Mehta, N.D., Crook, R., Perez-tur, J., Prihar, G., Pfeiffer, E., Graff-Radford, N., Hinder, P., Yager, D., Zenk, B., Refolo, L.M., Prada, C.M., Younkin, S.G., Hutton, M., Hardy, J. (1997). A new pathogenic mutation in the APP gene (I716V) increases the relative proportion of A beta 42(43). *Hum Mol Genet.*, 6, 2087-2089.

Engel, M.F.M., Khemtemourian, L., Kleijer, C., Meeldijk, H.J.D., Jacobs, J., Verkleij, A.J., de Kruijff, B., Killian, J.A., & Höppener, J.W. (2008). Membrane damage by human islet amyloid polypeptide through fibril growth at the membrane. *Proc Natl Acad Sci U S A*, 105, 6033-6038.

Freir, D.B., Fedriani, R., Scully, D., Smith, I.M., Selkoe D.J., Walsh, D.M., & Regan, C.M. (2010) Abeta oligomers inhibit synapse remodeling necessary for memory consolidation. *Neurobiol Aging*. Epub ahead of print.

Friedman, R., Pellarin, R., & Caflisch, A. (2009) Amyloid aggregation on lipid bilayers and its impact on membrane permeability. *J Mol Biol.*, 387, 407-415.

Gellermann, G.P., Byrnes, H., Striebinger, A., Ullrich, K., Mueller, R., Hillen, H., & Barghorn, S. (2008). Abeta-globulomers are formed independently of the fibril pathway. Neurobiol Dis., 30, 212-220.

Georganopoulou, D.G., Chang, L., Nam, J-M., Thaxton, C.S., Mufson, E.J., Klein, W.L., & Mirkin, C.A. (2005). Nanoparticle-based detection in cerebral spinal fluid of a soluble pathogenic biomarker for Alzheimer's disease. *Proc Natl Acad Sci U S A*, 102, 2273-2276.

Gimbel, D.A., Nygaard, H.B., Coffey, E.E., Gunther, E.C., Laurén, J., Gimbel, Z.A., & Strittmatter, S.M. (2010). Memory impairment in transgenic Alzheimer mice requires cellular prion protein. *J Neurosci.*, 30, 6367-6374.

Golde, T.E., & Younkin, S.G. (1996) in *Pathology of Alzheimer's Disease*, Goate A. (Ed.), p. 113, Academic press, New York.

Gong, Y., Chang, L., Viola, K.L., Lacor, P.N., Lambert, M.P., Finch, C.E., Krafft, G.A., & Klein, W.L. (2003). Alzheimer's disease-affected brain: presence of oligomeric Abeta ligands (ADDLs) suggests a molecular basis for reversible memory loss. *Proc Natl Acad Sci U S A*, 100, 10417-10422.

Gunn, A.P., Masters, C.L., & Cherny, R.A. (2010) Pyroglutamate-Aβ: Role in the natural history of Alzheimer's disease. *Int J Biochem Cell Biol.*, 42, 1915-1918.

Guzowski, J.F. (2002). Insights into immediate-early gene function in hippocampal memory consolidation using antisense oligonucleotide and fluorescent imaging approaches. *Hippocampus*, 12, 86-104.

Goedert, M., Spillantini, M.G., Cairns, N.J., & Crowther, R.A. (1992). Tau proteins of Alzheimer paired helical filaments: abnormal phosphorylation of all six brain isoforms. *Neuron*, 8, 159-168.

Greenwald, J., & Riek, R. (2010). Biology of amyloid: structure, function, and regulation. *Structure*, 18, 1244-1260.

Hardy, J., & Selkoe, D.J. (2002). The amyloid hypothesis of Alzheimer's disease: progress and problems on the road to therapeutics. *Science*, 297, 353-356.

Hartmann, T., Bieger, S.C., Bruhl, B., Tienari, P.J., Ida, N., Allsop, D., Roberts, G.W., Masters, C.L., Dotti, C.G., Unsicker, K., & Beyreuther, K. (1997). Distinct sites of intracellular production for Alzheimer's disease A beta40/42 amyloid peptides. *Nat Med.*, 3, 1016-1020.

Hernandez, F., & Avila, J. (2007). Tauopathies. *Cell Mol Life Sci.*, 64, 2219-2233.

Heutink, P. (2000). Untangling tau-related dementia. *Hum Mol Genet.*, 9, 979-986.

Hooper, N.M. (2005). Roles of proteolysis and lipid rafts in the processing of the amyloid precursor protein and prion protein. *Biochem Soc Trans.*, 33, 335-338.

Hoshino, M., Katou, H., Hagihara, Y., Hasegawa, K., Naiki, H., & Goto, Y. (2002). Mapping the core of the beta(2)-microglobulin amyloid fibril by H/D exchange. *Nat Struct Biol.*, 9, 332-336.

Haass, C., Schlossmacher, M.G., Hung, A.Y., Vigo-Pelfrey, C., Mellon, A., Ostaszewski, B.L., Lieberburg, I., Koo, E.H., Schenk, D., Teplow, D.B. et al. (1992). Amyloid beta-peptide is produced by cultured cells during normal metabolism. *Nature*, 359, 322-325.

Hardy, J., & Selkoe, D.J. (2002). The amyloid hypothesis of Alzheimer's disease: progress and problems on the road to therapeutics. *Science*, 297, 353-356.

Harigaya, Y., Saido, T.C., Eckman, C.B., Prada, C.M., Shoji, M., & Younkin, S.G. (2000). Amyloid beta protein starting pyroglutamate at position 3 is a major component of the amyloid deposits in the Alzheimer's disease brain. *Biochem Biophys Res Commun.*, 276, 422-427.

Harper, J.D., Wong, S.S., Lieber, C.M., & Lansbury, P.T. (1997) Observation of metastable Aβ amyloid protofibrils by atomic force microscopy. *Chem Biol.*, 4, 119-125.

Harper, J.D., Wong, S.S., Lieber, C.M., & Lansbury, P.T. (1999) Assembly of Abeta amyloid protofibrils: an *in vitro* model for a possible early event in Alzheimer's disease. *Biochemistry*, 38, 8972-8980.

Hartley, D.M., Walsh, D.M., Ye, C.P., Diehl, T., Vasquez, S., Vassilev, P.M., Teplow, D.B., & Selkoe, D.J. (1999). Protofibrillar intermediates of amyloid β-protein induce acute electrophysiological changes and progressive neurotoxicity in onrtical neurons. *J Neurosci.*, 19, 8876-8884.

Hillen, H., Barghorn, S., Striebinger, A., Labkovsky, B., Müller, R., Nimmrich, V., Nolte, M.W., Perez-Cruz, C., van der Auwera, I., van Leuven, F., van Gaalen, M., Bespalov, A.Y., Schoemaker, H., Sullivan, J.P., & Ebert, U. (2010). Generation and therapeutic efficacy of highly oligomer-specific beta-amyloid antibodies. *J Neurosci.*, 30, 10369-10379.

Hoshi, M., Sato, M., Matsumoto, S., Noguchi, A., Yasutake, K., Yoshida, N., & Sato, K. (2003). Spherical aggregates of beta-amyloid (amylospheroid) show high neurotoxicity and activate tau protein kinase I/glycogen synthase kinase-3b. *Proc Natl Acad Sci U S A*, 100, 6370-6375.

Hsieh, H., Boehm, J., Sato, C., Iwatsubo, T., Tomita, T., Sisodia, S., & Malinow, R. (2006). AMPAR removal underlies Abeta-induced synaptic depression and dendritic spine loss. *Neuron*, 52, 831-43.

Ittner, L.M., Ke, Y.D., Delerue, F., Bi, M., Gladbach, A., van Eersel, J., Wolfing, H., Chieng, B.C., Christie, M.J., Napier, I.A., Eckert, A., Staufenbiel, M., Hardeman, E., & Götz, J. (2010). Dendritic function of tau mediates amyloid-beta toxicity in Alzheimer's disease mouse models. *Cell*, 142, 387-397.

Johansson, A.S., Garlind, A., Berlind-Dehlin, F., Karlsson, G., Edwards, K., Gellerfors, P., Ekholm-Pettersson, F., Palmblad, J., & Lannfelt, L. (2007). Docosahexaenoic acid stabilizes soluble amyloid-beta protofibrils and sustains amyloid-β-induced neurotoxicity in vitro. *FEBS J.*, 274, 990-1000.

Kayed, R., Head, E., Thompson, J.L., McIntire, T.M., Milton, S.C., Cotman, C.W., & Glabe, C.G. (2003). Common structure of soluble amyloid oligomers implies common mechanism of pathogenesis. *Science*, 300, 486-489.

Kayed, R., Sokolov, Y., Edmonds, B., McIntire, T.M., Milton, S.C., Hall, J.E., & Glabe, C.G. (2004). Permeabilization of lipid bilayers is a common conformation-dependent activity of soluble amyloid oligomers in protein misfolding diseases. J Biol Chem., 279, 46363-46366.

Kayed, R., Pensalfini, A., Margol, L., Sokolov, Y., Sarsoza, F., Head, E., Hall, J., & Glabe, C. (2009). Annular protofibrils are a structurally and functionally distinct type of amyloid oligomer. *J Biol Chem.*, 284, 4230-4237.

Kheterpal, I., Lashuel, H.A., Hartley, D.M., Walz, T., Lansbury, P.T.Jr., & Wetzel, R. (2003). Abeta protofibrils possess a stable core structure resistant to exchange. *Biochemistry*, 42, 4092-4098.

Kheterpal, I., Chen, M., Cook, K.D., & Wetzel, R. (2006). Structural differences in Aβ amyloid protofibrils and fibrils mapped by hydrogen exchange--mass spectrometry with on-line proteolytic fragmentation. *J Mol Biol.*, 361, 785-795.

Klein, W.L., Krafft, G.A., & Finch, C.E. (2001). Targeting small Abeta oligomers: the solution to an Alzheimer's disease conundrum? *Trends Neurosci.*, 24, 219-224.

Klein, W.L. (2002) Abeta toxicity in Alzheimer's disease: globular oligomers (ADDLs) as new vaccine and drug targets. *Neurochem Int.*, 41, 345-352.

Klyubin, I., Betts, V., Wetzel, A.T., Blennow, K., Zetterberg, H., Wallin, A., Lemere, C.A., Cullen, W.K., Peng, Y., Wisniewski, T., Selkoe, D.J., Anwyl, R., Walsh, D.M., & Rowan, M.J. (2008). Amyloid beta protein dimer-containing human CSF disrupts synaptic plasticity: prevention by systemic passive immunization. *J Neurosci.*, 28, 4231-4237.

Kang, J., Lemaire, H.G., Unterbeck, A., Salbaum, J.M., Masters, C.L., Grzeschik, K.H., Multhaup, G., Beyreuther, K., & Muller-Hill, B. (1987). The precursor of Alzheimer's disease amyloid A4 protein resembles a cell-surface receptor. *Nature*, 325, 733-736.

Kosik, K.S. (1990). Tau protein and Alzheimer's disease. *Curr Opin Cell Biol.*, 2, 101-104.

Kirschner, D.A., Abraham, C., & Selkoe, D.J. (1986). X-ray diffraction from intraneuronal paired helical filaments and extraneuronal amyloid fibers in Alzheimer disease indicates cross-beta conformation. *Proc Natl Acad Sci U S A*, 83, 503-507.

Lewis, J., Dickson, D.W., Lin, W.L., Chisholm, L., Corral, A., Jones, G., Yen, S.H., Sahara, N., Skipper, L., Yager, D., Eckman, C., Hardy, J., Hutton, M., & McGowan, E. (2001). Enhanced neurofibrillary degeneration in transgenic mice expressing mutant tau and APP. *Science*, 293, 1487-1491.

Luhrs, T., Ritter, C., Adrian, M., Riek-Loher, D., Bohrmann, B., Dobeli, H., Schubert, D., & Riek, R. (2005). 3D structure of Alzheimer's amyloid-beta(1-42) fibrils. *Proc Natl Acad Sci U S A*, 102, 17342-17347.

Lacor, P.N, Buniel, M.C, Chang, L., Fernandez, S.J., Gong, Y., Viola, K.L., Lambert, M.P., Velasco, P.T., Bigio, E.H., Finch, C.E., Krafft, G.A., & Klein, W.L. (2004) Synaptic targeting by Alzheimer's-related amyloid b oligomers. J Neurosci., 24, 10191-10200.

Lacor, P.N., Buniel, M.C., Furlow, P.W., Clemente, A.S., Velasco, P.T., Wood, M., Viola, K.L., & Klein, W.L. (2007) Abeta oligomer-induced aberrations in synapse composition, shape, and density provide a molecular basis for loss of connectivity in Alzheimer's disease. *J Neurosci.*, 27, 796-807.

Lambert, M.P., Barlow, A.K., Chomy, B.A., Edwards, C, Freed, R., Liosatos, M., Morgan, T.E., Rozovsky, I., Trommer, B., Viola, K.L., Wals, P., Zhang, C., Finch, C.E., Krafft, G.A., & Klein, W.L. (1998) Diffusible, nonfibrillar ligands derived from $A\beta_{1-42}$ are potent central nervous system neurotoxins. *Proc Natl Acad Sci U S A*, 95, 6448-6453.

Lambert, M.P., Velasco, P.T., Chang, L., Viola, K.L., Fernandez, S., Lacor, P.N., Khuon, D., Gong, Y., Bigio, E.H., Shaw, P., De felice, F.G., Krafft, G.A., & Klein, W.L. (2007) Monoclonal antibodies that target pathological assemblies of Abeta. *J Neurochem.*, 199, 23-35.

Lashuel, H.A., Hartley, D., Petre, B.M., Walz, T., & Lansbury, P.T.Jr. (2002) Neurodegenerative disease: amyloid pores from pathogenic mutations. *Nature*, 418, 291.

Laurén, J., Gimbel, D.A., Nygaard, H.B., Gilbert, J.W., & Strittmatter, S.M. (2009) Cellular prion protein mediates impairment of synaptic plasticity by amyloid-beta oligomers. *Nature*, 457, 1128-1132.

Lesné, S., Koh, M.T., Kotilinek, L., Kayed, R., Glabe, C.G., Yang, A., Gallagher, M., & Ashe, K.H. (2006) A specific amyloid-beta protein assembly in the brain impairs memory. *Nature*, 440, 352-357.

Lewis, J., Dickson, D.W., Lin, W.L., Chisholm, L., Corral, A., Jones, G., Yen, S.H., Sahara, N., Skipper, L., Yager, D., Eckman, C., Hardy, J., Hutton, M., & McGowan, E. (2001). Enhanced neurofibrillary degeneration in transgenic mice expressing mutant tau and APP. *Science*, 293, 1487-1491.

Margittai, M., & Langen, R. (2006). Side chain-dependent stacking modulates tau filament structure. *J Biol Chem.*, 281, 37820-37827.

Masters, C.L., Simms, G., Weinman, N.A., Multhaup, G., McDonald, B.L., & Beyreuther, K. (1985). Amyloid plaque core protein in Alzheimer disease and Down syndrome. *Proc Natl Acad Sci U S A*, 82, 4245-4249.

Matsumura, S., Shinoda, K., Yamada, M., Yokojima, S., Inoue, M., Ohnishi, T., Shimada, T., Kikuchi, K., Masui, D., Hashimoto, S., Sato, M., Ito, A., Akioka, M., Takagi, S., Nakamura, Y., Nemoto, K., Hasegawa, Y., Takamoto, H., Inoue, H., Nakamura, S., Nabeshima, Y., Teplow, D.B., Kinjo, M., & Hoshi, M. (2011). Two distinct amyloid beta-protein (Abeta) assembly pathways leading to oligomers and fibrils identified by combined fluorescence correlation spectroscopy, morphology and toxicity analyses. *J Biol Chem.*, 286, 11555-11562.

Mori, H., Takio, K., Ogawara, M., & Selkoe, D.J. (1992). Mass spectrometry of purified amyloid beta protein in Alzheimer's disease. *J Biol Chem.*, 267, 17082-17086.

Nilsberth, C., Westlind-Danielsson, A., Eckman, C.B., Condron, M.M., Axelman, K., Forsell, C., Stenh, C., Luthman, J., Teplow, D.B., Younkin, S.G., Naslund, J., & Lannfelt, L. (2001). The 'Arctic' APP mutation (E693G) causes Alzheimer's disease by enhanced Ab protofibril formation. *Nat Neurosci.*, 4, 887-893.

Noguchi, A., Matsumura, S., Dezawa, M., Tada, M., Yanazawa, M., Ito, A., Akloka, M., Kikuchi, S., Sato, M., Ideno, S., Noda, M., Fukunari, A., Maramatsu, S., Itokazu, Y., Sato, K., Takahashi, H., Teplow, D.B., Nabeshima, Y., Kakita, A., Imahori, K., & Hoshi, M. (2009). Isolation and characterization of patient-derived, toxic, high mass amyloid beta-protein (Abeta) assembly from Alzheimer disease brains. *J Biol Chem.*, 284, 32895-32905.

Oda, T., Wals, P., Osterburg, H.H., Johnson, S.A., Pasinetti, G.M., Morgan, T.E., Rozovsky, I., Stine, W.B., Snyder, S.W., Holzman, T.F. *et al.* (1995). Clusterin (apoJ) alters the aggregation of amyloid beta-peptide (A beta 1-42) and forms slowly sedimenting A beta complexes that cause oxidative stress. *Exp Neurol.*, 136, 22-31.

Ohnishi, S., & Takano, K. (2004). Amyloid fibrils from the viewpoint of protein folding. *Cell Mol Life Sci.*, 61, 511-524.

Olofsson, A., Sauer-Eriksson, A.E., & Ohman, A. (2006). The solvent protection of alzheimer amyloid-beta-(1-42) fibrils as determined by solution NMR spectroscopy. *J Biol Chem.*, 281, 477-483.

Paravastu, A.K., Qahwash, I., Leapman, R.D., Meredith, S.C., & Tycko, R. (2009). Seeded growth of beta-amyloid fibrils from Alzheimer's brain-derived fibrils produces a distinct fibril structure. *Proc Natl Acad Sci U S A*, 106, 7443-7448.

Paravastu, A.K., Leapman, R.D., Yau, W.M., & Tycko, R. (2008). Molecular structural basis for polymorphism in Alzheimer's beta-amyloid fibrils. *Proc Natl Acad Sci U S A*, 105, 18349-18354.

Petkova, A.T., Leapman, R.D., Guo, Z., Yau, W.M., Mattson, M.P., & Tycko, R. (2005). Self-propagating, molecular-level polymorphism in Alzheimer's beta-amyloid fibrils. *Science*, 307, 262-265.

Petkova, A.T., Yau, W.M., & Tycko, R. (2006). Experimental constraints on quaternary structure in Alzheimer's beta-amyloid fibrils. *Biochemistry*, 45, 498-512.

Piccini, A., Russo, C., Gliozzi, A., Relini, A.,Vitali, A., Borghi, R., Giliberto, L., Armirotti, A., D'Arrigo, C., Bachi, A., Cattaneo, A., Canale, C., Torrassa, S., Saldo, T.C., Markesbery, W., Gambetti, P., & Tabaton, M. (2005). beta-Amyloid is different in normal aging and in Alzheimer disease. *J Biol Chem.*, 280, 34186-34192.

Poling, A., Morgan-Paisley, K., Panos, J.J., Kim, E.M., O'Hare, E., Cleary, J.P., Lesné, S., Ashe, K.H., Porritt, M., & Baker, L.E. (2008). Oligomers of the amyloid-beta protein disrupt working memory: confirmation with two behavioral procedures. *Behav Brain Res.*, 193, 230-234.

Portelius, E., Bogdanovic, N., Gustavsson, M.K., Volkmann, I., Brinkmalm, G., Zetterberg, H., Winblad, B., & Blennow, K. (2010). Mass spectrometric characterization of brain amyloid beta isoform signatures in familial and sporadic Alzheimer's disease. *Acta Neuropathol.*, 120, 185-193.

Querfurth, H.W., & LaFerla, F.M. (2010). Alzheimer's disease. *N Engl J Med.*, 362, 329-344.

Rahimi, F., Shanmugam, A., & Bitan, G. (2008). Structure-function relationships of pre-fibrillar protein assemblies in Alzheimer's disease and related disorders. *Curr Alzheimer Res.*, 5, 319-341.

Rapoport, M., Dawson, H.N., Binder, L.I., Vitek, M.P., & Ferreira, A. (2002). Tau is essential to beta -amyloid-induced neurotoxicity. *Proc Natl Acad Sci U S A*, 99, 6364-6369.

Roher, A.E., Lowenson, J.D., Clarke, S., Woods, A.S., Cotter, R.J., Gowing, E., & Ball, M.J. (1993). beta-Amyloid-(1-42) is a major component of cerebrovascular amyloid deposits: implications for the pathology of Alzheimer disease. *Proc Natl Acad Sci U S A*, 90, 10836-10840.

Reed, M.N., Hofmeister, J.J., Jungbauer, L., Welzel, A.T., Yu, C., Sherman, M.A., Lesné, S., Ladu, M.J., Walsh, D.M., Ashe, K.H., & Cleary, J.P. (2009). Cognitive effects of cell-derived and synthetically derived Abeta oligomers. Neurobiol Aging., Ebup ahead of print.

Roher, A.E., Chaney, M.O., Kuo, Y.M., Webster, S.D., Stine, W.B., Haverkamp, L.J., Woods, A.S., Cotter, R.J., Tuohy, J.M., Krafft, G.A., Bonnell, B.S., & Emmerling, M.R. (1996). Morphology and toxicity of Abeta-(1-42) dimer derived from neuritic and vascular amyloid deposits of Alzheimer's disease. *J Biol Chem.*, 271, 20631-20635.

Russo, C., Violani, E., Salis, S., Venezia, V., Dolcini, V., Damonte, G., Benatti, U., D'Arrigo, C., Patrone, E., Carlo, P., & Schettini, G. (2002). Pyroglutamate-modified amyloid beta-peptides - AbetaN3(pE) - strongly affects cultured neuron and astrocyte survival. *J Neurochem.*, 82, 1480-1489.

Sakono, M., & Zako, T. (2010). Amyloid oligomers: formation and toxicity of Abeta oligomers. *FEBS J.*, 277, 1348-1358.

Saido, T.C., Iwatsubo, T., Mann, D.M., Shimada, H., Ihara, Y., & Kawashima, S. (1995). Dominant and differential deposition of distinct beta-amyloid peptide species, A beta N3(pE), in senile plaques. *Neuron*, 14, 457-466.

Sayre, L.M., Zelasko, D.A., Harris, P.L., Perry, G., Salomon, R.G., & Smith, M.A. (1997). 4-Hydroxynonenal-derived advanced lipid peroxidation end products are increased in Alzheimer's disease. J Neurochem., 68, 2092-2097.

Selkoe, D.J. (2008). Soluble oligomers of the amyloid beta-protein impair synaptic plasticity and behavior. *Behav Brain Res.*, 192, 106-113.

Seubert, P., Vigo-Pelfrey, C., Esch, F., Lee, M., Dovey, H., Davis, D., Sinha, S., Schlossmacher, M., Whaley, J., Swindlehurst, C. et al. (1992). Isolation and quantification of soluble Alzheimer's beta-peptide from biological fluids. *Nature*, 359, 325-327.

Shankar, G.M., Bloodgood, B.L., Townsend, M., Walsh, D.M., Selkoe, D.J., & Sabatini, B.L. (2007). Natural oligomers of the Alzheimer amyloid-beta peptide induce reversible synapse loss by modulating an NMDA-type glutamate receptor-dependent signaling pathway. *J Neurosci.*, 27, 2866-2875.

Shankar G.M., Li S., Mehta T.H., Garcia-Munoz A., Shepardson N.E., Smith, I., Brett, F.M., Farrell, M.A., Rowan, M.J., Lemere, C.A., Regan, C.M., Walsh, D.M., Sabatini, B.L., & Selkoe, D.J. (2008). Amyloid-beta protein dimers isolated directly from Alzheimer's brains impair synaptic plasticity and memory. *Nat Med.*, 14, 837-842.

Siegel, S.J., Bieschke, J., Powers, E.T., & Kelly, J.W. (2007). The oxidative stress metabolite 4-hydroxynonenal promotes Alzheimer protofibril formation. *Biochemistry*, 46, 1503-1510.

Suzuki, N., Cheung, T.T., Cai, X.D., Odaka, A., Otvos, L.Jr., Eckman, C., Golde, T.E., & Younkin, S.G. (1994). An increased percentage of long amyloid beta protein secreted by familial amyloid beta protein precursor (beta APP717) mutants. *Science*, 264, 1336-1340.

Sadqi, M., Hernandez, F., Pan, U., Perez, M., Schaeberle, M.D., Avila, J., & Munoz, V. (2002). Alpha-helix structure in Alzheimer's disease aggregates of tau-protein. *Biochemistry*, 41, 7150-7155.

Sawaya, M.R., Sambashivan, S., Nelson, R., Ivanova, M.I., Sievers, S.A., Apostol, M.I., Thompson, M.J., Balbirnie, M., Wiltzius, J.J., McFarlane, H.T., *et al.* (2007). Atomic structures of amyloid cross-beta spines reveal varied steric zippers. *Nature*, 447, 453-457.

Schmitz, C., Rutten, B.P., Pielen, A., Schafer, S., Wirths, O., Tremp, G., Czech, C., Blanchard, V., Multhaup, G., Rezaie, P., *et al.* (2004). Hippocampal neuron loss exceeds amyloid plaque load in a transgenic mouse model of Alzheimer's disease. *Am J Pathol.*, 164, 1495-1502.

Sciarretta, K.L., Gordon, D.J., Petkova, A.T., Tycko, R., & Meredith, S.C. (2005). Abeta40-Lactam(D23/K28) models a conformation highly favorable for nucleation of amyloid. *Biochemistry*, 44, 6003-6014.

Selkoe, D.J. (2002). Alzheimer's disease is a synaptic failure. *Science*, 298, 789-791.

Tanzi, R.E., & Bertram, L. (2005). Twenty years of the Alzheimer's disease amyloid hypothesis: a genetic perspective. *Cell*, 120, 545-555.

Tiraboschi, P., Hansen, L.A., Thal, L.J., & Corey-Bloom, J. (2004). The importance of neuritic plaques and tangles to the development and evolution of AD. *Neurology*, 62, 1984-1989.

Turner, P.R., O'Connor, K., Tate, W.P., & Abraham, W.C. (2003). Roles of amyloid precursor protein and its fragments in regulating neural activity, plasticity and memory. *Prog Neurobiol.*, 70, 1-32.

Tycko, R. (2004). Progress towards a molecular-level structural understanding of amyloid fibrils. *Curr Opin Struct Biol.*, 14, 96-103.

Tycko, R. (2010). Solid-State NMR Studies of Amyloid Fibril Structure. Annu Rev Phys Chem.

Tycko, R., Sciarretta, K.L., Orgel, J.P., & Meredith, S.C. (2009). Evidence for novel beta-sheet structures in Iowa mutant beta-amyloid fibrils. *Biochemistry*, 48, 6072-6084.

Tabaton, M., Nunzi, M.G., Xue, R., Usiak, M., Autilio-Gambetti, L., & Gambetti, P. (1994). Soluble amyloid beta-protein is a marker of Alzheimer amyloid in brain but not in cerebrospinal fluid. *Biochem Biophys Res Commun.*, 200, 1598-1603.

Teplow, D.B. (2006). Preparation of amyloid beta-protein for structural and functional studies. *Methods Enzymol.*, 413, 20-33.

Terry, R.D., Masliah, E., Salmon, D.P., Butters, N., De Teresa, R., Hill, R., Hansen, L.A., & Katzman, R. (1991). Physical basis of cognitive alterations in Alzheimer's disease: synapse loss is the major correlate of cognitive impairment. *Ann Neurol.*, 30, 572-580.

Tomiyama, T., Nagata, T., Shimada, H., Teraoka, R., Fukushima, A., Kanemitsu, H., Takuma, H., Kuwano, R., Imagawa, M., Ataka, S., Wada, Y., Yoshioka, E., Nishizaki, T., Watanabe, Y., & Mori, H. (2008). A new amyloid beta variant favoring oligomerization in Alzheimer's-type dementia. *Ann. Neurol.*, 63, 377-387.

Townsend, M., Shankar, G.M., Mehta, T., Walsh, D.M., & Selkoe, D.J. (2006). Effects of secreted oligomers of amyloid beta-protein on hyppocampal synaptic plasticity: a potent role for trimers. *J Physiol.*, 572, 477-492.

Vigo-Pelfrey, C., Lee, D., Keim, P., Lieberburg, I., & Schenk, D.B. (1993). Characterization of beta-amyloid peptide from human cerebrospinal fluid. *J Neurochem.*, 61, 1965-1968.

von Bergen, M., Barghorn, S., Biernat, J., Mandelkow, E.M., & Mandelkow, E. (2005). Tau aggregation is driven by a transition from random coil to beta sheet structure. *Biochim Biophys Acta*, 1739, 158-166.

von Bergen, M., Friedhoff, P., Biernat, J., Heberle, J., Mandelkow, E.M., & Mandelkow, E. (2000). Assembly of tau protein into Alzheimer paired helical filaments depends on a local sequence motif ((306)VQIVYK(311)) forming beta structure. *Proc Natl Acad Sci U S A*, 97, 5129-5134.

Walsh, D.M., Lomakin, A., Benedeck, G.B., Condron, M.M., & Teplow, D.B. (1997). Amyloid-beta protein fibrillogenesis. Detection of a protofibrillar intermediate. *J Biol Chem.*, 292, 22364-22372.

Walsh, D.M., Hartley, D.M., Kusumoto, Y., Fezoui, Y., Condron, M.M., Lomakin, A., Benedek, G.B., Selkoe, D.J., & Teplow, D.B. (1999). Amyloid-beta protein fibrillogenesis. Structure and biological activity of protofibrillar intermediates. *J Biol Chem.*, 274, 25945-25952.

Walsh, D.M., Tseng, B.P., Rydel, R.E., Podlisny, M.B., & Slekoe, D.J. (2000). The oligomerization of amyloid beta-protein begins intracellularly in cells derived from human brain. *Biochemistry*, 39, 10831-10839.

Walsh, D.M., Klyubin, I., Fadeeva, J., Cullen, W.K., Anwyl, R., Wolfe, M.S., Rowan, M.J., & Selkoe, D.J. (2002). Naturally secreted oligomers if the Alzheimer amiloid beta-protein potently inhibit hippocampal long-term potentiation in vivo. *Nature*, 416, 535-539.

Walsh, D.M., Townsend, M., Podlisny, M.B., Shankar, G.M. Fadeeva, J.V., El Agnaf, O., Hartley, D.M., & Selkoe, D.J. (2005a). Certain inhibitors of synthetic amyloid beta-peptide (Abeta) fibrillogenesis block oligomerization of natural Abeta and thereby rescue long-term potentiation. *J Neurosci.*, 25, 2455-2462.

Walsh, D.M., Klyubin, I., Shankar, G.M., Townsend, M., Fadeeva, J.V., Betts, V., Podlisny, M.B., Cleary, J.P., Ashe, K.H., Rowan, M.J., & Selkoe, D.J. (2005b). The role of cell-derived oligomers of Abeta in Alzheimer's disease and avenues for therapeutic intervention. *Biochem Soc Trans.*, 33, 1087-1090.

Wang, H.W., Pasternak, J.F., Kuo, H., Ristic, H., Lambert, M.P., Chromy, B., Viola, K.L., Klein, W.L., Stine, W.B., Krafft, G.A., & Trommer, B.L. (2002). Soluble oligomers of beta amyloid (1-42) inhibit long-term potentiation but not long-term depression in rat dentate gyratus. *Brain Res.*, 924, 133-140.

Wang, L., Maji, S.K., Sawaya, M.R., Eisenberg, D., & Riek, R. (2008). Bacterial inclusion bodies contain amyloid-like structure. *PLoS Biol.*, 6, e195.

Wang, L., Schubert, D., Sawaya, M.R., Eisenberg, D., & Riek, R. (2010). Multidimensional structure-activity relationship of a protein in its aggregated states. *Angew Chem Int Ed Engl.*, 49, 3904-3908.

Westlind-Danielsson, A., & Arnerup, G. (2001). Spontaneous in vitro formation of supramolecula b-amyloid structures, "betaamy balls", by beta-amyloid 1-40 peptide. *Biochemistry*, 40, 14736-14743.

Wenk, G.L. (2003). Neuropathologic changes in Alzheimer's disease. *J Clin Psychiatry*, 64 Suppl 9, 7-10.

Wischik, C.M., Novak, M., Edwards, P.C., Klug, A., Tichelaar, W., & Crowther, R.A. (1988). Structural characterization of the core of the paired helical filament of Alzheimer disease. *Proc Natl Acad Sci U S A*, 85, 4884-4888.

Williams, A.D., Sega, M., Chen, M., Kheterpal, I., Geva, M., Berthelier, V., Kaleta, D.T., Cook, K.D., & Wetzel, R. (2005). Structural properties of Abeta protofibrils stabilized by a small molecule. *Proc Natl Acad Sci U S A*, 102, 7115-7120.

Wirths, O., Erck, C., Martens, H., Harmeier, A., Geumann, C., Jawhar, S., Kumar, S., Multhauo, G., Walter, J., Ingelsson, M., Degerman-Gunnarsson, M. *et al.* (2010). Identification of low molecular weight pyroglutamate Abeta oligomers in Alzheimer disease: a novel tool for therapy and diagnosis. *J Biol Chem.*, 285, 41517-41524.

Yu, L., Edalji, R., Harlan, J.E., Holzman, T.F., Lopez, A.P., Labkovsky, B., Hillen, H., Barghorn, S., Ebert, U., Richardson, P.L. *et al.* (2009). Structural characterization of a soluble amyloid b-peptide oligomer. *Biochemistry*, 48, 1870-1877.

# 7

# Alzheimer´s Disease – The New Actors of an Old Drama

Mario Álvarez Sánchez, Carlos A. Sánchez Catasús,
Ivonne Pedroso Ibañez, Maria L. Bringas and Arnoldo Padrón Sánchez
*International Center of Neurological Restoration*
*Cuba*

## 1. Introduction

Alzheimer's Disease is the most common neurodegeneration and the prototype of this group of diseases. Now threatens to become an epidemy with a predictable and profound impact.

In 1906 Alois Alzheimer brilliantly defined the clinicopathologic syndrome that now bears his name to relate the progression of cognitive impairment to pathological anatomic findings wich remains as the markers of the disease: amyloid plaques and neurofibrillary tangles. After more than a hundred years since its description, especially in the last two decades new interesting clues have been revealed to understanding the basic mechanisms of disease. This research highlights the discovery of genes in familial and sporadic forms, the description in detail of the beta amyloid cascade and tau protein metabolism and a better understanding of the role of vascular factors, inflammation, brain resistance to insulin and the recent and intriguing findings about the role of the prion receptors and prion like mechanisms in the development of disease. Thus, new actors earn role in the pathophysiology of an ancient drama: Alzheimer's disease.

This chapter discusses these topics with the assurance that in the coming years will be the basis for the development of new diagnostic tools and more effective treatments.

## 2. Pathology

### 2.1 Macroscopic

Alzheimer's disease (AD) is characterized by a global involvement, bilateral and symmetrical in both hemispheres with cortical predominance. There is reduced transparency and fibrosis of the leptomeninges and subarachnoid large gaps remains in the spaces left between the cerebral sulci. When the meninges are removed we can see a pale brain with weight decrease of approximately 800 to 1000g from 1300 to 1700g in the normal adult. There is greater involvement of the association areas (fronto temporal and parietal) and to a lesser degree of primary motor and sensory areas. The most affected region is the mesial temporal lobe and especially the entorhinal cortex. The increase of the ventricles is secondary to parenchymal loss. A recent neuroimage-based quantitative meta-analysis revealed that early AD affects structurally the hippocampal regions (figures 1.A and 1.B), while functionally affects the inferior parietal lobules (figures 1.C and 1.D), which might be caused by regional amyloid deposits and by disconnection from the hippocampus through disruption of the cingulum bundle (Schroeter et al., 2009).

Although not define the disease, there is usually involvement of the subcortical white matter leukoaraiosis as well as small infarcts and atherosclerotic changes in large arteries.

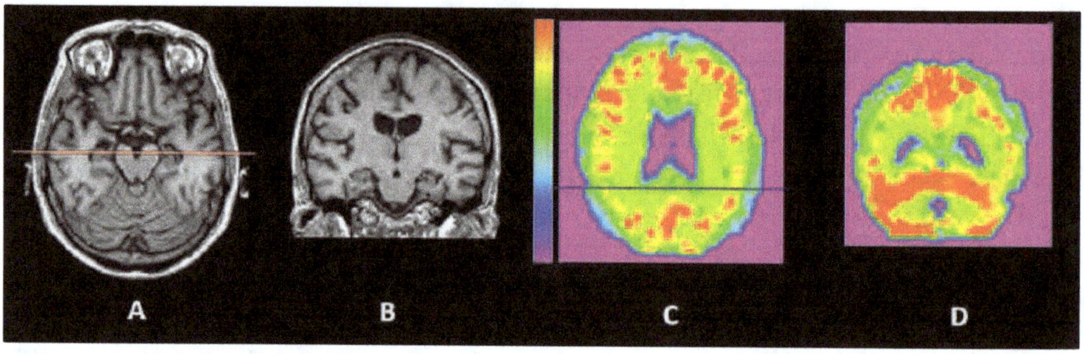


Fig. 1. Brain MRI (Magnetic Resonance Imaging) and perfusion SPECT (Single Photon Emission Computed Tomography) images of a patient with AD in early stage examined in our institution (female, age= 66 years, Mini Mental State Examination (MMSE)=22); all images are oriented in the radiological convention. A) Axial view of high resolution MRI image (T1) showing brain atrophy, particularly in the hippocampus bilaterally; B) Coronal slice at the level of the red line show in the axial view; C) $^{99m}$Tc-ECD SPECT image using a double-head system and corrected for partial volume effect (corrected for atrophy), showing regional hypoperfusion in the parietal regions, particularly in the angular gyrus bilaterally; and D) Coronal slice at the level of the blue line show in the axial view C. For comparison see figure 2 with similar images of a clinically healthy subject.

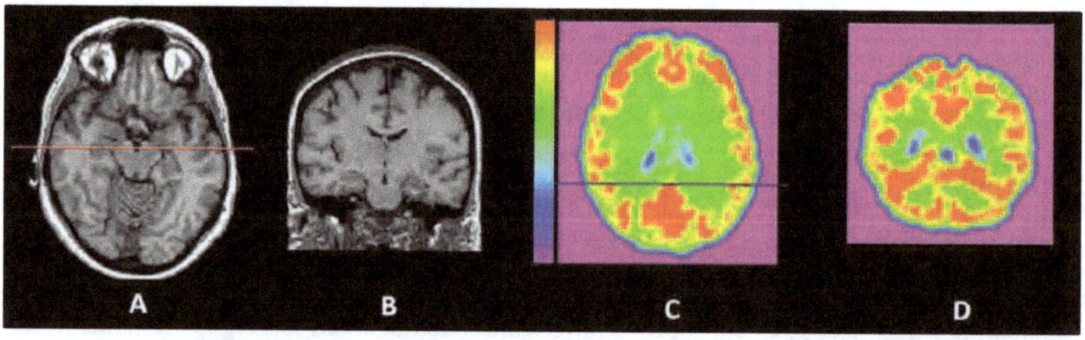


Fig. 2. Brain MRI and perfusion SPECT images of a clinically healthy subject (female, age= 64 years, MMSE=30). A) to D) are similar images show in figure 1.

There are atypical or asymmetric forms where the degeneration and atrophy is restricted to one lobe or cerebral hemisphere. A series of cases shows that these phenotypes are not as infrequent as it is supposed (Alladi et al., 2007). The pathology of AD is a common substrate in the Posterior Cortical Atrophy, Non Fluent Progressive Aphasia and Cortico Basal Degeneration although is rare in others such as Semantic Dementia and Fronto Temporal Dementia. In the case of Non Fluent Progressive Aphasia most cases corresponds with typical findings of AD.

### 2.2 Microscopic

Corroborate the findings described above. It were also observed important changes such as subcortical neuronal depopulation of the nucleus basalis of Meynert, raphe nuclei, the nucleus ceruleus, amygdala, and white matter lesions. The two typical lesions that define AD are senile plaques and neurofibrillary tangles:

#### 2.2.1 Senile Plaques (SP)

Observed in the interstice, between neurons. They measure between 20 and 100 microns and consist of a core which principal component is beta amyloid (βA). This core is surrounded by a nest formed by degenerating neurites, activated microglia and astrocytes. Other substances that conform the SP are the alpha-synuclein (principal not amyloid component), alpha 1 antichymotrypsin, alpha 2 macroglobulin, apolipoprotein E, ubiquitin and the presenilins. Degenerative neurons are also distinguished around but not in contact with the plaques. According his appearance they are classified as:

a. Difuse. Formed by a delicate network of fine filaments of amyloid fibrils without degenerate neurites. Center and its boundaries are not well defined.
b. Primitive. Are the most common. They are characterized by disordered extracellular Aβ deposits wich are poorly or not fibrillar. Center is not well defined but the borders are more accurate.
c. Classic. Also called neuritic plaques, amyloid have a center surrounded by a crown composed of reactive astrocytes, microglia and dystrophic neurites corresponding to dendrites and degenerate axons.
d. Burns. Present only a condensed central amyloid. It has no cellular components.

These forms represent different developmental stages of the plaques, beginning with the accumulation of diffuse amyloid, then it is organized and defined, by associating the immune response. Finally, the cellular elements disappear.

The SP are relatively rare in limbic structures and neocortex and are more visible in frontal temporal and occipital regions, while respecting the primary sensorimotor areas. They can be found in the brains of people without cognitive deficits, but to a lesser extent (Table 1). Higher concentrations are criteria for pathological diagnosis of AD.

| Age (years) | Amount |
|---|---|
| Less than 50 | Less than 5 |
| Between 50 and 65 | Less than 9 |
| Between 66 and 75 | Less than 11 |
| More than 75 | Less than 16 |

Table 1. Amount of Senile Plaques (SP) per mm3 with 200x augmentation.

We can now follow the progression of βA in vivo deposits using Carbon-11-Pittsburgh Compound B Positron Emission Tomography (PIB-PET) which correlates with the number of SP. This technique shows a broader distribution in both normal subjects and patients with AD. One study (Engler et al., 2006) compared the PIB-PET signal between healthy controls and patients with AD found that was higher in patients. Unexpectedly, the most notable difference was found in the striatum. Other regions with significant differences were the frontal, temporal and occipital lobes. By repeating the test after two years, there was only one significant difference in the occipital cortex of patients with AD. The PIB-PET signal change did not correlate with the progression of cognitive impairment suggesting that, after an initial period, βA deposits stabilizes.

Some familiar forms as mutations of presenilin 1 that cause variant-AD have atypical SP that coexists with the usual. There are Cotton Wool plaques, non cored and devoid of dystrophic neurites. The distribution is also uncommon, presenting high concentrations in the interhemispheric motor cortex representing the lower extremities, which is consistent with early-onset spasticity that often accompanies memory and visuospatial disorders (Koivunen et al., 2008).

### 2.2.2 Neuro-fibrillary tangles (NFT)

Neurons present an accumulation of flame-shaped inclusions and sometimes form a elongated basket around the nucleus. The inclusions are basophils to the hematoxylin and eosin and strongly stained with silver stains. The inclusions fill the cytoplasm, particularly in the soma and apical dendrite causing neuronal death mainly by apoptosis. Finally there are only remnants of the cytoskeleton, such as ghosts´ nodules.

Development of new staining techniques to visualize phosphorylated Tau protein (Tau-p) while they are soluble, in early states called pre-fibrillar, is the basis for classification according to the developmental stages of Braak, which suggested changes in the pathological diagnostic criteria (figure 3).

The NFT is distributed in very characteristics areas as the entorhinal and perirhinal allocortex, CA1 region of hippocampus and the amygdala. Also found in the nucleus basalis of Meynert, Temporal isocortex (areas 20 and 21 of Brodmann) and the rest of the hippocampal structures. The NFT coincide with the SP in fronto temporal regions but their presence is lower in not limbic structures.

Recent studies in patients with AD show that less than one third of cases had a "pure" disease, being more frequent association of SP and NFT with vascular lesions (50%) or Lewy bodies (20 %).

### 2.2.3 Vascular changes

Over 80% of patients have cerebral amyloid angiopathy, which affects the pial vessels of the brain and especially the capillaries, which become refined, atrophic, fragmented and distorted. Endothelial basement membrane is thickened and disrupted, with amyloid deposits and collagen which is associated with an inflammatory response that includes the vascular endothelium, perivascular microglia, pericytes and astrocytes, interfering with the functioning of the blood-brain barrier (BBB) (Bowman et al., 2007).

The muscular layer shows segmentary contractions and peripheral vascular plexus is impaired or absent. Often these changes are accompanied by ischemic or hemorrhagic lesions.

A meta-analysis included 5 studies and 450 patients (Cordonnier and van der Flier, 2011) finds that in 23% of cases are characterized by microbleeding with focal leakage of hemosiderin from small abnormal blood vessels. Microbleedings prevalence is higher in AD patients than in subjects with mild cognitive impairment, while in the general population is rare. The microbleedings are distributed in cortico-subcortical regions predominantly in the occipital lobe, a pattern shared with amyloid angiopathy (Zlokovic, 2008).

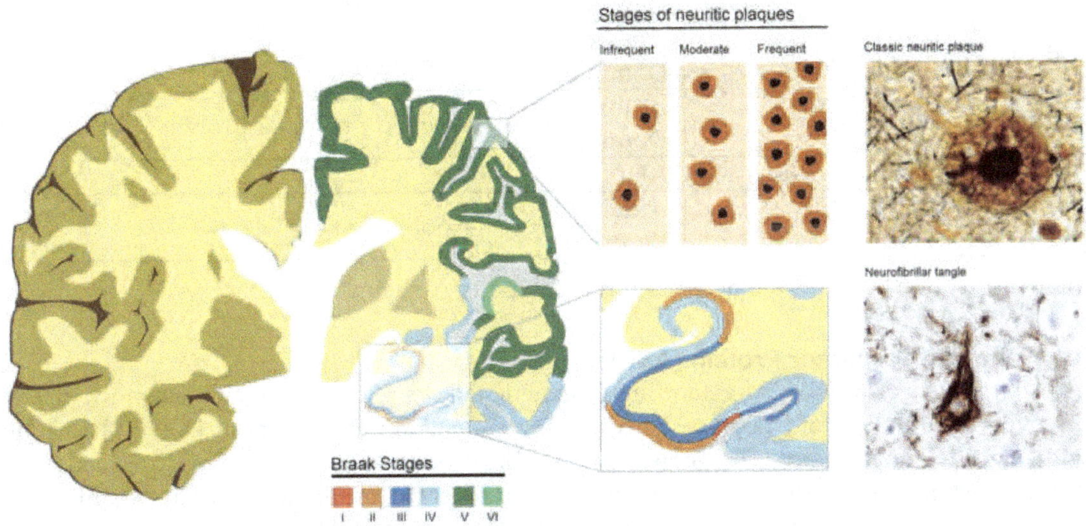


Fig. 3. Schematic representation of a hemisphere of a normal subject (left) and a hemisphere of a person with AD (right). A scale of colors represent the Braak´s NFT stages. The first stages are entorhinal (I and II) with absent or mild symptoms. Stages III and IV are called limbic and are associated with memory deficit (which influences the intellectual reserve) and subtle changes of personality. In cortical stages (V and VI) adding further deterioration in neocortical regions with the reverse pattern of myelination, affecting primarily the association areas and finally the primary areas. The stages of senile plaques are represented in the top.

### 2.2.4 Other less specific findings include

- Inclusions and pigments: Lipofuscin, Hirano bodies (actin) and Lewy bodies (alpha synuclein).
- Granulovacuolar degeneration: The presence of intra-neuronal vacuoles (3 to 5 microns) that can be associated or not with NFT. It is mostly found in the hippocampus.
- Other: satellitosis, neuronofagia and fragmentation are stages of neuronal death mediated by glia.

## 3. Genetics

The AD is an entity with genetic and clinical heterogeneity. There are familial and sporadic forms (Table 2).

### 3.1 Familial AD

The familial AD forms are relatively rare, less than 10% and have an autosomal dominant pattern. The debut occur at an early age (Early Onstet AD or EAOD), characterized by cognitive impairment associated with other neurological signs such as spasticity, motor control disorders, ataxia and seizures.

| Debut | Chromosome | Herency | Product |
|---|---|---|---|
| Early Onset Alzheimer Disease (EOAD) | | | |
| 28-50 | 14 | Autosomal Dominant | Presenilin 1 |
| 40-50 | 1 | Autosomal Dominant | Presenilin 2 |
| 55-65 | 21 | Autosomal Dominant | amyloid precursor protein (APP) |
| Late Onset Alzheimer Disease (LOAD) | | | |
| Later or never | 19 | Autosomal Recesive | Apolipoprotein E4 |

Table 2. Relation between genotype and phenotype in Alzheimer´s Disease (AD)

#### 3.1.1 Amyloid Precursor Protein (APP)

The first advances in the understanding of genetic factors related to the AD began with the discovery of the Amyloid Precursor Protein (APP) in brain of carriers of Down syndrome with cognitive impairment. The gene encoding this protein is located in the 21q21 locus and is inherited in an autosomal dominant pattern of early onset. More than 32 missense mutations have now been described in 85 families.

The APP gene encodes by alternative splicing. The larger form is a polypeptide of 770 amino acids. Alternative splicing of exon 7 encoding the Kurnitz domain and exon 8 encoding the OX-2 antigen wich is a polypeptide of 695 amino acids that predominate and other of 751, less frequent. So far their function is unknown, although presumably involved in the regulation of neuronal plasticity and signal transduction.

#### 3.1.2 Presenilin 1 (PSEN1)

Presenilin (PSEN) is the major component of the gamma-secretase. The Locus of PSEN1 was found on chromosome 14q24.2. The PSEN1 is a polytopic membrane protein that forms the catalytic center of the gamma-secretase complex. Other functions independent of βA are the acidification of vacuoles by the addition of ATPase, required for autophagy, calcium regulation and stimulation of neuronal growth and survival (Pimplikar et al., 2010).

Depending on the PSEN1 mutation type may be an increase or decrease in the production of beta-amyloid. Missense mutations of PSEN1 have full penetrance and are the most common cause of early-onset familial AD, between 25-65 years, causing the more severe clinical forms.

#### 3.1.3 Presenilin 2 (PSEN2)

The locus is located on 1q42.13. PSEN2 is expressed in a variety of tissues including the brain, primarily in neurons. Their mutations are rare and only 14 variants have been described in six families.

#### 3.1.4 Apolipoprotein E epsilon (APOE-ε)

The role of variations in the gene APOE-ε on chromosome 19q13.2 as a risk factor for late onset AD has been demonstrated. Its variations are associated with both late-onset familial AD and 20% of sporadic AD.

This gene has multiple alleles: E2, E3 and E4. In both, normal subjects and AD patients the least common is E2 and the most common is E3, but in subjects with AD the E4 allele has a frequency almost equal to E3. In its heterozygous composition APOE-ε4 gene increases the risk four times, with onset between 5 and 10 years earlier.

In subjects homozygous for APOE-ε 4, the risk is increased fifteen times with onset between 10 and 20 years earlier. It is noteworthy that 42% of patients with LOAD have not alleles APOE-ε 4 as its absence does not rule out the disease.

Under normal conditions, APOE is produced predominantly in astrocytes, whereas under stress neurons are the main source. APOE participates in the distribution and metabolism of cholesterol and triglycerides. APOE-ε 4 is less efficient than E2 and E3 variants for the reuptake and efflux of cholesterol in neurons and astrocytes. On the other hand, APOE-ε4 is more efficient for the aggregation of beta-amyloid.

### 3.2 Sporadic AD

Sporadic forms have onset of symptoms later, over 60 years (LOAD). A large proportion of these cases have a family history of dementia suggesting a strong genetic component. On the other hand, the history of a first degree relative diagnosed with AD increase the risk of AD from two to seven times.

Attempts to demonstrate associations between genetic variations and sporadic AD others than APOE-ε4 has been inconsistent and rarely replicated. This scenario has been changing over the past three years with the results of studies of Genome Wide Association Studies (GWAS).

An article that reviews 15 GWAS (Bertram et al., 2010) confirms once again the relevance of the APOE gene variations as the most important risk factor in sporadic AD. At the same time new candidate genes have begun to emerge. Among the most notable are genes involved in beta-amyloid metabolism: Ataxin1 (ATX1), Siglec33 (CD33), Clusterin aka Apolipoprotein J (CLU-APOJ), Complement Component (3b/4b) receptor 1 (CR1); regulators of Tau phosphorylation: GRB2-Associated Binding Protein 2 (GAB2) and modulators of synaptic transmission as Protocadherin11 X linked (PCDH11X) and Inositol Phosphatydil Clathrin Assembly Binding Protein (PICALM).

However, it is appropriate to remember that these new variants increase the risk only from 0.10 to 0.15 times suggesting that, rather than the independent effect should be referred to the impact of gene networks. Overall, mutations in APOE and new variants described and confirmed could justify up to 50% of cases of sporadic AD.

Neuro Image Alzheimer's Disease Initiative (ADNI) extends the capacity of association between genetic variants and phenotypes of the AD because provides data from neuroimaging and other biomarkers. One of the most interesting findings of this study is the linear relationship between the number of alleles PICALM G and thinning of the entorhinal cortex, an effect that is independent of APOE variants (Saykin et al., 2010).

## 4. Pathogenesis

Traditionally attention has focused on the typical lesions and its primary components: the βA of the SP and tau protein in the NFT, examining the impact that the accumulation of these compounds in different parts of the brain tissue. Currently the research focus has shifted to the initial and solubles states of both metabolic pathways: amyloid cascade and tau phosphorylation, trying to unravel the relationship between them and their earlier effects.

### 4.1 Amyloid beta metabolism

The βA is a small peptide fragment of a transmembrane protein called amyloid precursor protein (APP). This protein is found in cytoplasmic membranes, endosomal and Golgi system of the nervous system and blood cells. Both the APP and its products, including the βA can also be located in mitochondria. Certain isoforms of APP have a domain protease inhibitor Kunitz regulating the coagulation cascade. In normal subjects the βA peptide is fragmented by a protein alpha-secretase which divides into two segments forming nexin II modulator action of coagulation and the βA of 16 amino acid peptide highly soluble.

This βA peptide binds to alpha 2 macroglobulin, which signals the proteins to be degraded and form a βA-A2M complex that binds to a protease. The product of these interactions is reintroduced into the nerve cell to adhere to them first through A2M for the membrane receptor that is common to LDL and APOE.

There is an alternative way that is the complete detachment of the peptide βA 40 to 42 amino acids. This occurs by the action of beta-secretase BACE (division 1) and gamma-secretase (split 40-42). The gamma secretase is composed of four segments: presenilin, nicastrin, APH-1 PEN2 and presenilin, the active site. βA 1-42 segments are more difficult to degrade and tend to aggregate to form oligomers (OM). Monomers do not produce damage, however, since dimers formed are capable of causing cell death mediated by microglia.

Although OM can be composed of aggregates of 2 to 100 peptides, the most frequents are the compounds for 3 to 7 segments. Unlike the SP, which are usually away from the regions of greatest damage, the OM has a wider distribution and can cause functional and structural changes in regions typically affected in AD, for example the entorhinal cortex and CA1, respecting initially CA3 and Cerebellum. Synapse loss and cognitive impairment correlates well with the concentration of OM, but not with SP. On the other hand, the OM may diminish or even abolish Long Term Potentiation (LTP), an effect that is selective because it does not affect Excitatory Post Synaptic Potential (EPSP) or Long Term Depression (LTD).

Apparently these changes in electrical activity are mediated by prion receptors PrPc, molecules with which the OM have a high affinity. Indeed, blocking these receptors with anti-PrPc antibodies can reverse the behavioral and learning disorders in experimental models of AD in mice (Chung et al., 2010). Larger aggregates called Proto fibrils (PF) are also able to induce toxicity and cell death, however, these molecules are less stable (Klein, 2002).

Apolipoprotein J (APOJ) secreted by astrocytes may prevent the formation of PF, but not of OM, in fact facilitates their aggregation by increasing the substrate and serve as a chaperone. Interestingly, Clum-APOJ mutations are well replicated as risk factors in GWAS studies.

Finally, the formation of insoluble fibrils, whose center is composed of 1-42 βA which is then added βA 1-40, accumulates in the interstice where suffers the loss of helical conformation (alpha helix) to adopt a beta sheet conformation, very difficult to degrade. These complexes achieve stability by association with several proteins, including SAP (Serum Amyloid Component) very stable and only degradable in the liver and accompanying amyloid deposits from any source (Figure 4A). The presence of these bodies cause the activation of the immune system, especially the microglia, which perpetuate the inflammation and injury by free radicals.

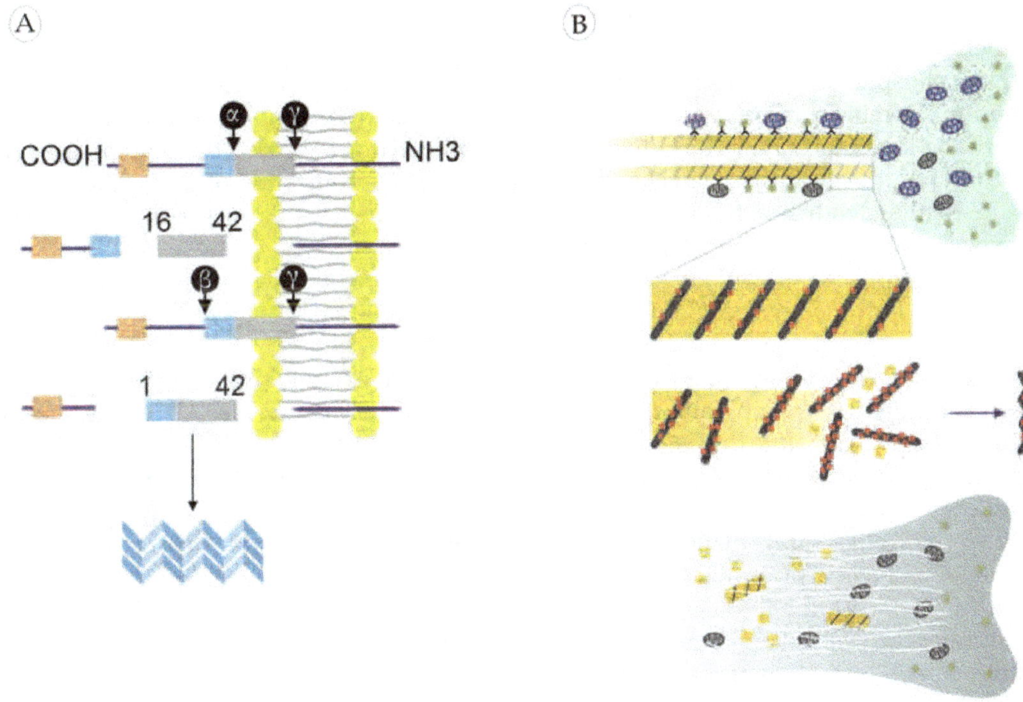


Fig. 4. A) The amyloid beta is part of a transmembrane protein whose end is intracellular NH3 and extracellular COOH. Cleavage by alpha and gamma secretases produces a peptide 16-42 very soluble and easily degradable. The alternative cleavage by beta and gamma secretases produces insoluble 1-42 peptide, then added in formation of folded sheets, very difficult to degrade.
B). Tau proteins are part of the microtubule-associated proteins. The hyperphosphorylation of these proteins causes a disruption of the cytoskeleton engaging features such as maintaining the structure and intracellular transport. Hyperphosphorylated tau proteins forming paired helices very difficult to degrade. This eventually leads to neuronal death and depopulation.

### 4.2 Neurofibrillary metabolism

The NFT are mainly composed of paired helical filaments formed by hyperphosphorylated tau protein. They are also formed by other proteins such as MAP2 (predominantly in dendrites), ubiquitin, and βA peptides, supporting the theory of amyloidogenesis as a primary lesion.
Tau proteins predominate in axons and form the group of MAP (Microtubule Associated Protein) interacting with microtubules during cell movement and transport assembling or disassembling the microtubules depending on whether there lengthening or shortening of the extensions, especially in axons. Recent research has found that tau proteins are also located in the dendrites, although in a much lower concentration. Here are involved in cytoskeletal functions and signal transduction by facilitating the activity of protein tyrosine kinase FYN (FYN), which phosphorylates the 2B subunit of N-Methyl-D-aspartate (NMDA)

receptors, mediating their interaction with Protein Posinaptic Density (PSD-95). This interaction is critical for the efficiency of the synapse and in its absence there is a decrease of experimental seizures (Ittner et al., 2010).

Tau hyperphosphorylation has several effects. First results in their haste and self-aggregation forming, in the case of AD paired helical filaments that impede axonal transport. On the other hand, Tau-p have a greater affinity for FYN and thereby increase its concentration in the dendrites. This leads to a shift in the concentration of Tau protein from the axon to the dendrites, finally occupying the soma and breaking the cell dynamics leading eventually apoptotic neurodegeneration (figure 4 B).

An interesting question is why does the progression and spread of Tau-p follows a route so stereotyped as proposed in the anatomical and pathological Braak´s stages?

In our view there are two possible answers:

1. This pattern shows a gradient of susceptibility to increasing exposure to an aggressor factor. In this case the obvious candidate would be the OM. However, as we have seen, after a first phase, the deposition rate of βA and PIB-PET load stabilizes, while the spread and damage induced by Tau-p continues at the same time that the neuronal loss and cognitive impairment
2. Tau-p molecules and their aggregates do not require external factors, but these formations have a prion-like behavior. Tau-p are seeds that can penetrate the cell and recruit Tau functional molecules making them hyper-phosphorylated forms. Thus continues the cycle of aggregation and spreading the damage to other areas.

The latter possibility seems to be reinforced by an experimental model that achieved with very small concentrations of Tau-p and in a short time, a degree of infection similar to that observed in tissues of patients with AD (prion-like dissemination). (Clavaguera et al., 2009;Guo and Lee, 2011).

### 4.3 Relationship between Tau and βA metabolism

A complex problem is determining which is the primary lesion and the relationship between them. There are some facts that suggest that the primary is the βA accumulation. For example, βA accumulation precedes the presence of NFT. Also been achieved KO mice that produce accumulation βA with all the features of these lesions without neurofibrillary tangles. These mice have cognitive deficits comparable to that human AD. Moreover, the demonstration of tau protein as a basis for degenerations with dementia that occur (Frontotemporal dementia and parkinsonism linked to chromosome 17; Progressive Supranuclear Palsy and Pick's dementia) in the absence of SP, support the protagonism of the NFT.

A very interesting hypothesis has been proposed by Ittner and Gotz, called "Tau Axis Hypothesis" (Ittner and Gotz, 2011). Here suggest that the presence of Tau protein in the dendrite is essential for OM mediated toxicity. In fact, in experimental models the absence of interaction Tau-FYN prevents the development of cognitive, behavioral disorders or neuronal degeneration induced by OM. On the other hand, increasing the concentration of OM increases the phosphorylation of Tau protein, which moves them to the dendrites and increases its affinity for FYN, closing a vicious circle.

### 4.4 Vascular factors

The frecuent presence of vascular lesions in patients with AD and the results of epidemiological studies suggest that vascular risk factors increase the likelihood of suffering from AD and once established, accelerate the progression of cognitive impairment. The most important are hypertension, advanced age, atherosclerosis, homocystinemia, hyperlipidemia, metabolic syndrome and obesity. Cerebral vascular lesions, especially lacunar infarcts increase to double the risk of AD (Ott et al., 1999).

It also showed that cerebral hypoperfusion precedes onset of clinical dementia and that the reduction in cerebral blood flow (CBF) occurs before cognitive impairment and hippocampal atrophy. This is consistent with results achieved by our group.

The Nun Study (Snowdon et al., 1997) relates the number of vascular lesions with the severity of Alzheimer's disease by showing that individuals with one or two lacunar infarctions had a greater cognitive deterioration than individuals who had no stroke, regardless of the number of neurofibrillary tangles in the cortex.

Experimental studies in rodents have shown that chronic cerebral hypo-perfusion and transient cerebral ischemia increases the production of amyloid peptide precursor, beta amyloid protein and the accumulation of hyperphosphorylated Tau protein, which simulates the changes of Alzheimer's disease. However, these conditions of intense ischemia are not present in normal subjects or patients with AD.

The beta amyloid peptide has a vasoconstrictor effect, which could be related to the early decrease in CBF and the narrowing of the average diameter capillary. In AD the mean diameter capillary is decreased, which is associated with cognitive impairment even before the accumulation of SP and NFT.

In the AD there is an increase of Advanced Glycation End products (AGE) that accumulate on the walls of blood vessels. In addition, the concentrations of AGE receptors (RAGE) are several times increased in vessels, microglia and neurons. The binding of βA to RAGE in the luminal membrane of the BBB leads to the peripheral βA input in to the brain followed by binding to neurons. Increased RAGE becomes a pro-inflammatory signal that activates microglia (Zlokovic, 2008).

Low density lipoprotein receptor related protein 1 (LRP) is a member of the family of LDL and a major clearance receptor for βA at the BBB. LRP concentrations decline with age and are particularly low in the elderly and patients with AD.

BBB dysfunction is early and confirmed by a series of morphological changes such as reducing the number of mitochondria, tight junctions, loss of pericytes and the presence of pinocytotic in cerebral microvessels.

In a clinical study showed the BBB impairement in 22% of patients with AD (Bowman et al., 2007). The rate of damage progression was measured by concentrations of albumin in Cerebrospinal Fluid (CSF) and correlated with worsening of cognitive performance.

Cholinergic nuclei, dramatically affected in AD, have a regulatory effect on CBF, particularly groups of the substantia innominata and the Nuclei basalis magnocellularis (SI / NBM). In healthy volunteers who were given Scopolamine, the CBF decreased from 20%.

The opposite effect was found in an experimental study where chronic deep electrical stimulation of the region SI / NBM produced a sustained increase in CBF in basal ganglion and Cortex, particularly in fronto parietal regions.

### 4.5 Cerebral insulin resistance

Insulin in the brain plays an important role in regulating metabolism, and alterations in activity are directly related to metabolic diseases such as obesity, diabetes or metabolic syndrome. In the mammalian brain, insulin induces anorexia, weight loss and regulates the hypothalamic control of food intake.

The insulin receptor (IR) is a glycoprotein of 300 to 400 kDa, formed by two identical alpha chains located in the extracellular region and two beta subunits that end within the cytosol, the beta chains have intrinsic tyrosine kinase activity. The IR is found in higher concentrations in neurons when compared with the glial cells. The IR is distribuited at the brain structures in different densities, they expression have proved at the olfactory bulb, hypothalamus, pituitary, choroid plexus, thalamus, piriform cortex, hippocampal formation, amygdaloid nuclei, prefrontal cortex and cerebellum. The IR largest concentrations are at the level of the olfactory bulb, hypothalamus, hippocampus and cerebellum. The IR is widely found in the synapses, especially in the dendritic tree where it regulates neurotransmitter release and the recruitment of receptors.

Within the brain, function of Insulin / Insulin like Growth Factor (IGF) include stimulation of neuronal and oligodendroglial survival, growth factor, regulation of mitochondrial function and energy metabolism, expression of Tau and acetylcholine transferase.

The IGF2 is abundantly expressed in the hippocampus. Recent research shows that IGF2 plays an essential role in the regulation of LTP and memory consolidation, one of the cognitive functions affected in early stages of AD (Chen et al., 2011).

The search for an association between insulin metabolism and AD brain has been extensively investigated in recent years. The starting point takes place in epidemiological studies wich strongly indicate that diabetes mellitus (DM) is a risk factor for AD. A closer look identifies insulin resistance as risk factor independent of changes in blood sugar levels. In people with insulin resistance and cognitive impairment without DM there is a reduction in the rate of cerebral glucose utilization. This pattern is also different in people with DM type 2 or pre DM during the execution of cognitive tasks, suggesting that insulin resistance could be taken as an early marker of AD (Baker et al., 2011).

Unlike the vascular brain disease that affects mainly CA1, a region highly susceptible to ischemia, insuline resistance selectively damaged the entorhinal cortex, one of the first areas involved in AD.

Biochemical and genetic data show that insulin degrading enzyme (IDE) is involved in insulin and Aβ homeostasis. The expression and activity of IDE is significantly decreased in AD brains compared with age-matched controls. In addition, IDE and Aβ are deposited in SP and vessels, indicating a gross conformational change by post-translational mechanisms. These changes in the distribution and activity of IDE may result in hormone resistance, insufficient degradation of insulin and Aβ, formation of Aβ oligomers and neurodegeneration.

The possibility that the AD is the result of a selective insulin resistance in the brain has been proposed by de la Monte et al. with solid clinical and experimental arguments that crystallize into a new concept: the DM type 3 (de la Monte and Wands, 2008).

In post mortem studies of brains affected by AD were significant decreases in concentrations of Insulin and Insulin like Growth Factor (IGF). By comparing the expression of IGF with Braak´s stages shows that the involvement is early and progressive decline increasingly as they progress Braak´s stages, what is more remarkable for IGF1.

Streptozocin experimental models in rats lead to a selective reduction of the expression of insulin / IGF in the brain without changing peripheral levels of glucose or insulin. In these animals are changes similar to the AD such as increased BA, Tau phosphorylation, neurodegeneration and gliosis and decreased genes associated with neurons,

oligodendroglia, and acetyl choline transferase, while increase genes related to microglia and inflammation (de la Monte and Wands, 2008).
Other factors that may have some weight in neuronal loss and progression of damage are: the development of inflammatory changes, damage to mitochondria, the energy imbalance, the increased production of free radicals, the problems of calcium metabolism, the toxicity of some elements such as aluminum, inefficient autophagy and suppression of neurogenesis.

## 5. Clinical expression

As we have seen, there are many factors which interact and are interwoven pathways, increasing the capacity of injury in different brain areas, which is expressed as a progressive cognitive deficit, which begins as a disorder of recent memory and then progresses to affect in advanced stages, the majority of brain functions. Each pathway described above can be added to the final damage but there are two main theories that justify the initial cognitive deficits of AD, these are: The "Theory of cortical disconnection" and "Cholinergic theory".

### 5.1 Theory of cortical disconnection

Neurofibrillary tangles in the entorhinal cortex, wich is the cortical portal of the hippocampus, are distributed in layers II, which together with the layer III form the perforant pathway to the hippocampus and the layer IV receiving eference from the hippocampus. In this way hippocampus is isolated from the neocortex. This adds to the deficit of glutamate and other neuropeptides such as neuropeptide Y, oxytocin, vasopressin and somatostatin in the association cortices adding a cortico-cortical disconnection that correlates with aphasia, apraxia and agnosia, as well as visuospatial and executives disorders. At first the degeneration is slight and apparently can be offset by the cognitive reserve, however, as neurodegeneration progresses, this mechanism is not sufficient. The techniques of functional magnetic resonance imaging at 7 Tesla can define in vivo the degree of atrophy of specific regions of the hippocampus (Kerchner et al., 2010)..

### 5.2 Cholinergic theory

In advanced stages there is a decrease of over 90% of the activity of acetylcholinesterase which identifies a dramatic impairment of the cholinergic system in this disease. This causes early and progressive memory affection. One study suggests that progression of cholinergic deficit is not linear but at an early stage levels rise, falling years later. This is similar to what occurs with serotonin (Dekosky et al., 2002).
The selective degeneration of the nucleus basalis of Meynert, principal cholinergic eference to neocortex and septal nuclei and diagonal band of Broca, subcortical cholinergic eference, especially to the hippocampus, cause a progressive anterograde memory. Some authors hypothesize that the clinical expresion of depression needs some indemnity of cholinergic pathways, close to normal levels, which occurs only in initial stages.
As mentioned before, there is evidence of early changes in regional CBF, which could be related to the degeneration of cholinergic population that has a regulatory effect. This is known as the cholinergic-vascular theory.
As part of a research project in our institution (International Center of Neurological Restauration-CIREN), and with the collaboration of other Cubans institutions, we compared the global cerebral blood flow (gCBF) in absolute units (ml/min/100 g) at resting state

between 38 controls and 40 amnestic MCI subjects, both groups with similar demographic and vascular risk factors (limited). We explored also a possible association between gCBF and cognitive function, after controlling for age, gender, level of education and global brain atrophy (quantified on 3D T1-weighted MRI images). gCBF was measured by spectral analysis of radionuclide angiography, which is a simple and non-invasive method for the quantification of gCBF (Murase et al., 1999;Van et al., 2001) and linearly correlated with gCBF measured by using PET (Takasawa et al., 2004). Our results show a significant decrease of gCBF in the MCI group as compared with controls ($p < 0.05$, Mann-Whitney U Test, figure 5).

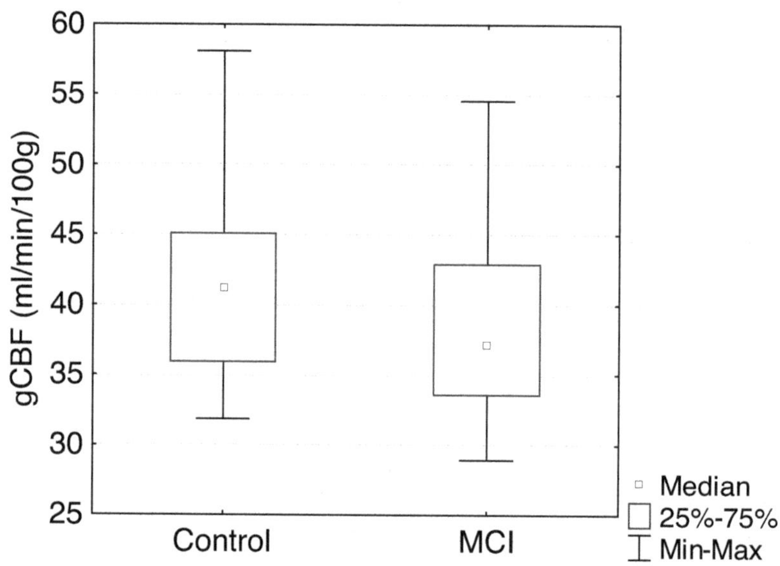


Fig. 5. MCI group show less gCBF than control group.

We also found in the MCI group a direct association between gCBF and semantically unrelated word-pairs learning (immediate recall) as measured by the hard-word pairs learning score of the Wechsler memory scale (Spearman $R = 0.46$, $p < 0.005$, figure 6), after removing the effects of age, gender, level of education and global brain atrophy (standardized z_scores). Control subjects show no association.

Interestingly, other domains of cognitive function (attention, episodic memory, working memory, verbal fluency, praxis and executive function) show no association with gCBF. Thus verbal learning is probably more sensitive than other cognitive functions in MCI patients, particularly semantically unrelated word-pairs learning. Many studies have reported very early deficits in associative memory in MCI patients, which is the ability to associate unrelated items presented together during the encoding phase, or to associate one item to its spatial or visual context (Belleville et al., 2008).

The decrease of gCBF observed in our MCI group cannot be explained by a clear vascular cause, related to demographic variables or brain atrophy. One possible explanation of our findings could be to assume a gradual reduction of cholinergic vasodilatory innervations of cerebral blood vessels as a result of a gradual cholinergic deficit originating in the basal forebrain, which also affect learning and memory (Schliebs and Arendt, 2006). This assumption is supported by previous studies (Claassen and Jansen, 2006;Farkas and Luiten, 2001).

A way to confirm a gradual reduction of regional vasodilatory innervations in the MCI state would be to study the cerebrovascular reserve and find out the connection with cognitive decline. This study will be the subject of further research. Perhaps a more complete evaluation of this topic could be the combined studies in the same MCI subjects (or equivalent animal model) of cerebral blood flow and direct measurements of cholinergic activity and plaque formation (for example, using PET imaging). Recent studies suggest an interaction between vascular, cholinergic and "amyloid β" hypotheses of AD.

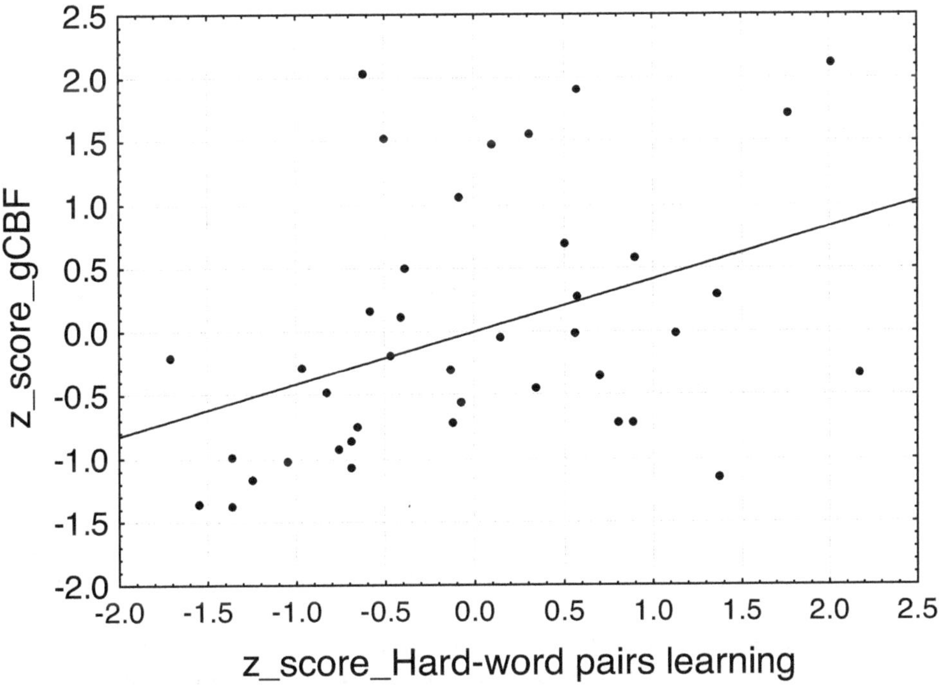


Fig. 6. There is a positive correlation between gCBF and semantically unrelated word-pairs learning in the MCI group.

### 5.3 Role of others neurotransmitters

Other neurotransmitter imbalances better explain the non-cognitive symptoms. As mentioned, there is a greater involvement of the raphe nuclei, the nucleus ceruleus and a relative sparing of the substantia nigra.

Serotonin deficit. It is related to depressive symptoms as well as obsession, compulsion and aggression. This is observed both in AD and in normal people. A study with Fluoro-benzamidoethylpiperazine-PET shows that in Mild Cognitive Impairment patients exists up-regulation of hippocampal serotonin, apparently as a compensatory mechanism. Once the AD is stablished, serotonin levels falls. (Truchot et al., 2007).

Noradrenaline deficit. It is also observed associated with depression and psychomotor agitation. With this neurotransmitter occurs something unique because although there is a depoblaction of nucleus ceruleus (where there are Lewy bodies), there is a cortical noradrenergic hyperactivity, which is attributed to an increased sensitivity and the production of cortical noradrenaline. The increased sensitivity is observed in the prefrontal

cortex and in the hippocampus. However, the increased concentration of noradrenaline is only found in the prefrontal cortex. In cases of depression there is noradrenaline decrease, while those with agitation there is an increase.
Relative dopamine preservation. This causes an imbalance choline / dopamine with the relative increase of the latter, a substrate of observed hallucinations, sleep disorders and psychosis. In 30% of AD patients there is a decrease of dopamine with the presence of a parkinsonian syndrome. However, the preservation of posture and gait to advanced stages is a characteristic of cortical dementia.

## 6. Conclusions

Currently there are notable advances in understanding the basic mechanisms of AD. This has allowed the design of biomarkers of the disease in vivo wich are able to define its presence, with a high degree of sensitivity and specificity, even before establishing the cognitive deficits characteristic of this entity. This has led to reconsider the diagnostic criteria and include diagnostic tools such as PIB-PET, Magnetic Resonance and Cerebrospinal Fluid (Dubois et al., 2007).
This extends the time for preventive or early intervention, using new treatments designed to block the damage in the early stages of the cascade of events. The prevention of risk factors and the use of new drugs such as fibrillar aggregation inhibitors, intranasal insulin and anti-PrPc antibodies promise to change the current scenario, dominated by discrete symptomatic treatment gains.

## 7. References


Alladi, S., J. Xuereb, T. Bak, P. Nestor, J. Knibb, K. Patterson, and J. R. Hodges, 2007, Focal cortical presentations of Alzheimer's disease: Brain, v. 130, no. Pt 10, p. 2636-2645.

Baker, L. D., D. J. Cross, S. Minoshima, D. Belongia, G. S. Watson, and S. Craft, 2011, Insulin resistance and Alzheimer-like reductions in regional cerebral glucose metabolism for cognitively normal adults with prediabetes or early type 2 diabetes: Arch.Neurol., v. 68, no. 1, p. 51-57.

Belleville, S., S. Sylvain-Roy, B. C. de, and M. C. Menard, 2008, Characterizing the memory changes in persons with mild cognitive impairment: Prog.Brain Res., v. 169, p. 365-375.

Bertram, L., C. M. Lill, and R. E. Tanzi, 2010, The genetics of Alzheimer disease: back to the future: Neuron, v. 68, no. 2, p. 270-281.

Bowman, G. L., J. A. Kaye, M. Moore, D. Waichunas, N. E. Carlson, and J. F. Quinn, 2007, Blood-brain barrier impairment in Alzheimer disease: stability and functional significance: Neurology, v. 68, no. 21, p. 1809-1814.

Chen, D. Y., S. A. Stern, A. Garcia-Osta, B. Saunier-Rebori, G. Pollonini, D. Bambah-Mukku, R. D. Blitzer, and C. M. Alberini, 2011, A critical role for IGF-II in memory consolidation and enhancement: Nature, v. 469, no. 7331, p. 491-497.

Chung, E., Y. Ji, Y. Sun, R. J. Kascsak, R. B. Kascsak, P. D. Mehta, S. M. Strittmatter, and T. Wisniewski, 2010, Anti-PrPC monoclonal antibody infusion as a novel treatment for cognitive deficits in an Alzheimer's disease model mouse: BMC.Neurosci., v. 11, p. 130.

Claassen, J. A., and R. W. Jansen, 2006, Cholinergically mediated augmentation of cerebral perfusion in Alzheimer's disease and related cognitive disorders: the cholinergic-vascular hypothesis: J.Gerontol.A Biol.Sci.Med.Sci., v. 61, no. 3, p. 267-271.

Clavaguera, F. et al., 2009, Transmission and spreading of tauopathy in transgenic mouse brain: Nat.Cell Biol., v. 11, no. 7, p. 909-913.

Cordonnier, C., and W. M. van der Flier, 2011, Brain microbleeds and Alzheimer's disease: innocent observation or key player?: Brain, v. 134, no. Pt 2, p. 335-344.

de la Monte, S. M., and J. R. Wands, 2008, Alzheimer's disease is type 3 diabetes-evidence reviewed: J.Diabetes Sci.Technol., v. 2, no. 6, p. 1101-1113.

Dekosky, S. T., M. D. Ikonomovic, S. D. Styren, L. Beckett, S. Wisniewski, D. A. Bennett, E. J. Cochran, J. H. Kordower, and E. J. Mufson, 2002, Upregulation of choline acetyltransferase activity in hippocampus and frontal cortex of elderly subjects with mild cognitive impairment: Ann.Neurol., v. 51, no. 2, p. 145-155.

Dubois, B. et al., 2007, Research criteria for the diagnosis of Alzheimer's disease: revising the NINCDS-ADRDA criteria: Lancet Neurol., v. 6, no. 8, p. 734-746.

Engler, H. et al., 2006, Two-year follow-up of amyloid deposition in patients with Alzheimer's disease: Brain, v. 129, no. Pt 11, p. 2856-2866.

Farkas, E., and P. G. Luiten, 2001, Cerebral microvascular pathology in aging and Alzheimer's disease: Prog.Neurobiol., v. 64, no. 6, p. 575-611.

Guo, J. L., and V. M. Lee, 2011, Seeding of normal tau by pathological tau conformers drives pathogenesis of Alzheimer-like tangles: J.Biol.Chem..

Ittner, L. M., and J. Gotz, 2011, Amyloid-beta and tau--a toxic pas de deux in Alzheimer's disease: Nat.Rev.Neurosci., v. 12, no. 2, p. 65-72.

Ittner, L. M. et al., 2010, Dendritic function of tau mediates amyloid-beta toxicity in Alzheimer's disease mouse models: Cell, v. 142, no. 3, p. 387-397.

Kerchner, G. A., C. P. Hess, K. E. Hammond-Rosenbluth, D. Xu, G. D. Rabinovici, D. A. Kelley, D. B. Vigneron, S. J. Nelson, and B. L. Miller, 2010, Hippocampal CA1 apical neuropil atrophy in mild Alzheimer disease visualized with 7-T MRI: Neurology, v. 75, no. 15, p. 1381-1387.

Klein, W. L., 2002, Abeta toxicity in Alzheimer's disease: globular oligomers (ADDLs) as new vaccine and drug targets: Neurochem.Int., v. 41, no. 5, p. 345-352.

Koivunen, J. et al., 2008, PET amyloid ligand [11C]PIB uptake shows predominantly striatal increase in variant Alzheimer's disease: Brain, v. 131, no. Pt 7, p. 1845-1853.

Murase, K., T. Inoue, H. Fujioka, Y. Ishimaru, A. Akamune, Y. Yamamoto, T. Mochizuki, and J. Ikezoe, 1999, An alternative approach to estimation of the brain perfusion index for measurement of cerebral blood flow using technetium-99m compounds: Eur.J.Nucl.Med., v. 26, no. 10, p. 1333-1339.

Ott, A., R. P. Stolk, H. F. van, H. A. Pols, A. Hofman, and M. M. Breteler, 1999, Diabetes mellitus and the risk of dementia: The Rotterdam Study: Neurology, v. 53, no. 9, p. 1937-1942.

Pimplikar, S. W., R. A. Nixon, N. K. Robakis, J. Shen, and L. H. Tsai, 2010, Amyloid-independent mechanisms in Alzheimer's disease pathogenesis: J.Neurosci., v. 30, no. 45, p. 14946-14954.

Saykin, A. J. et al., 2010, Alzheimer's Disease Neuroimaging Initiative biomarkers as quantitative phenotypes: Genetics core aims, progress, and plans: Alzheimers.Dement., v. 6, no. 3, p. 265-273.

Schliebs, R., and T. Arendt, 2006, The significance of the cholinergic system in the brain during aging and in Alzheimer's disease: J.Neural Transm., v. 113, no. 11, p. 1625-1644.

Schroeter, ML., Stein, T., Maslowski N. and Neumann J., 2009, Neural correlates of Alzheimer's disease and mild cognitive impairment: A systematic and quantitative meta-analysis involving 1351 patients. NeuroImage, v. 47, p. 1196–1206.

Snowdon, D. A., L. H. Greiner, J. A. Mortimer, K. P. Riley, P. A. Greiner, and W. R. Markesbery, 1997, Brain infarction and the clinical expression of Alzheimer disease. The Nun Study: JAMA, v. 277, no. 10, p. 813-817.

Takasawa, M. et al., 2004, Spectral analysis of 99mTc-HMPAO for estimating cerebral blood flow: a comparison with H2(15)O PET: Ann.Nucl.Med., v. 18, no. 3, p. 243-249.

Truchot, L. et al., 2007, Up-regulation of hippocampal serotonin metabolism in mild cognitive impairment: Neurology, v. 69, no. 10, p. 1012-1017.

Van, L. K., F. Dumont, M. Koole, and R. Dierckx, 2001, Non-invasive methods for absolute cerebral blood flow measurement using 99mTc-ECD: a study in healthy volunteers: Eur.J.Nucl.Med., v. 28, no. 7, p. 862-872.

Zlokovic, B. V., 2008, New therapeutic targets in the neurovascular pathway in Alzheimer's disease: Neurotherapeutics., v. 5, no. 3, p. 409-414.

# 8

# Selectivity of Cell Signaling in the Neuronal Response Based on NGF Mutations and Peptidomimetics in the Treatment of Alzheimer's Disease

Kenneth E. Neet[1], Sidharth Mahapatra[2], Hrishikesh M. Mehta[3]
[1]*Department of Biochemistry and Molecular Biology, The Chicago Medical School, Rosalind Franklin University of Medicine and Science, North Chicago*
[2]*Department of Pediatrics, School of Medicine, Stanford University, Palo Alto*
[3]*Department of Pediatrics, Division of Hematology/Oncology/Stem Cell Transplantation Children's Memorial Hospital, Northwestern Feinberg School of Medicine, Lurie Comprehensive Cancer Center, Chicago Northwestern University, Chicago USA*

## 1. Introduction

Neurotrophins are maintained at low concentrations by target tissues. They form highly selective interactions with their respective cognate receptors and maintain the viability of neurons in the central and peripheral nervous systems. Overlap in receptor specificities for neurotrophins, in the tissue distribution of the specific receptors, and in the expression of the high affinity receptors enable growth- and survival-enhancing signals to be transduced with great efficiency and specificity over a wide variety of neuronal cells. Early studies suggested that alterations in neurotrophin levels might underlie the pathogenesis of Alzheimer's disease (AD), Parkinson's disease (PD), Huntington's disease (HD) and other neurodegenerative disorders (Apfel et al., 1991; Emilien et al., 2000; Hefti, 1983) [reviewed in (Lad et al., 2003a)]. Today, a strong link between such a neurodegenerative condition and an imbalance in neurotrophin and/or receptor levels has been supported with nerve growth factor (NGF) and AD. A disruption or reduction in critical neurotrophin levels thus leads to widespread neurodegeneration. Conversely, administration of NGF and/or its related family of neurotrophins can potentially play a role in treatment of AD or other degenerative neurological disorders. NGF and its peptidomimetics have been proposed and tested in animal studies and clinical trials for AD with complex responses observed in some patients. Intracellular signaling from the NGF receptors is complex, giving rise to neuronal responses that include differentiation, survival, and apoptosis. This review will focus on novel approaches to eliciting selectivity of a cellular response, based on alterations in the NGF molecule or in the peptidomimetic, that may lead to more effective treatments of AD with NGF-related therapeutics. A conceptual comparison to selectivity in other growth factor receptor systems, such as epidermal growth factor (EGF) and insulin, will also be made.

## 2. Neurotrophins, their receptors, and neurodegenerative disease

### 2.1 Neurotrophin receptor interactions

Neurotrophins (NTs) are a family of closely related proteins that have diverse functions ranging from neuronal development, differentiation, and survival to regulation of axonal and dendritic outgrowth, activity-dependent synaptic formation and regulation, cell migration, and cellular proliferation (Diamond et al., 1992; Katz et al., 1990; Levi-Montalcini, 1987; Lindsay, 1988; Segal, 2003). The family of neurotrophins includes nerve growth factor (NGF), brain-derived neurotrophic factor (BDNF), neurotrophin 3 (NT-3), and neurotrophin 4 (NT-4) (Ibanez, 1994; Lad et al., 2003a) . They possess high sequence homology (ca. ~50%) and adopt similar tertiary structures (Fig. 1A) (Bibel & Barde, 2000; Korsching, 1993). The same neurotrophin can affect a variety of neuronal populations and, conversely, the same tissue is capable of receiving stimulatory inputs from multiple neurotrophins. For example, cholinergic basal forebrain (CBF) neurons are attuned to NGF for their maintenance but have been shown to respond to BDNF and NT-3 (Bibel & Barde, 2000; Korsching, 1993; Lad et al., 2003a). The viability of dopaminergic neurons of the substantia nigra has been linked to the actions of BDNF and NT-4 (Hyman et al., 1991; Lad et al., 2003a; Parain et al., 1999). Also, BDNF can act on the entorhinal cortex, the substantia nigra, and the striatum to affect AD, PD, and PD/HD, respectively (Nagahara & Tuszynski, 2011). Each of these neurotrophins binds selectively to a 140-kDa tropomyosin-receptor-kinase, i.e. NGF to TrkA, BDNF and NT-4 to TrkB, and NT-3 to TrkC (Cordon-Cardo et al., 1991; Kaplan et al., 1991; Soppet et al., 1991). Binding to Trk enables the transduction of positive signals, i.e. survival and differentiation through its intracellullar tyrosine kinase domain. In contrast, all neurotrophins can bind a 75-kDa common neurotrophin receptor, p75 (or $p75^{NTR}$), involved in the transduction of negative signals, i.e. growth arrest or apoptosis, when expressed exclusively, or positive signals when co-expressed with Trk receptors (Lad et al., 2003a). The central and peripheral nervous systems possess multiple neurotrophin-dependent cells and tissues that demonstrate co-expression of TrkA and p75.

### 2.2 Importance of neurotrophins in neurodegenerative disorders

Numerous studies have now demonstrated an imbalance between neurotrophins and their receptors in AD, appearing even in early cognitive defects (Mufson et al., 2007; 2008; Lad, et al., 2003a). In cholinergic basal forebrain (CBF) neurons in AD, TrkA and p75 are decreased at both the mRNA and proteins levels and NGF mRNA is not changed (Mufson et al., 1995; Salehi et al., 2000; S. A. Scott et al., 1995). NGF protein is down in CBF neurons with accumulation of NGF in the cortex, suggesting that retrograde transport to provide the neurotrophic factor to the basal forebrain is impaired (Schindowski et al., 2008). These changes begin to appear in early, pre-clinical stages of cognitive impairment (Ginsberg et al., 2006; Mufson et al., 1995; Mufson et al., 2000; Mufson et al., 2002; Schulte-Herbruggen et al., 2008). In addition, the pro-apoptotic proNGF is elevated, suggesting destruction of neurons containing p75 (Cuello et al., 2010; Fahnestock et al., 2001). A relationship of neurotrophins and their receptors to Aβ toxicity and/or deposition is also becoming apparent (Calissano et al., 2010a; Peng et al., 2004). Finally, BDNF, and possibly its precursor form, is implicated in neuronal survival imbalance in AD (Garzon & Fahnestock, 2007; Peng et al., 2005), particularly in the entorhinal cortex region of the brain (Nagahara & Tuszynski, 2011). Consequently, various treatment strategies have been suggested to slow or reverse cognitive symptoms, utilizing administration of neurotrophins (Mufson et al., 2008; Nagahara & Tuszynski, 2011; Nilsson et al., 2010; Schulte-Herbruggen et al., 2008).

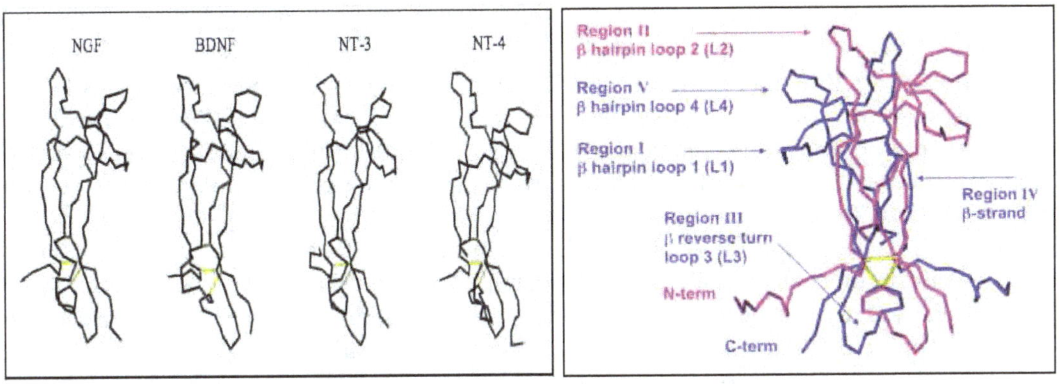


Fig. 1. A (left). Folding of the protomer of the four neurotrophins. B (right). Structure of dimeric NGF showing the loop regions that interact with the receptors. The yellow bonds represent the cystine knot motif. From PDB 1WWW. Note: the variable regions I, II and V defined by sequence homology (Ibanez et al., 1991; Ibanez et al., 1993; Ilag et al., 1994) are equivalent to loops 1, 2, and 4 (L1, L2, L4) defined in the structure (Wiesmann et al., 1999).

### 2.3 Alzheimer's disease – Treatment strategies

The pathogenesis of Alzheimer's disease is related to loss of NGF-mediated survival signals, receptor imbalances at the cell surface, and a shift to proprotein forms capable of inducing apoptosis. Without these positive signals, the progression of intracellular events that ultimately lead to deposition of tangles and plaques occurs uninterrupted. As a result, neurodegeneration in the cholinergic basal forebrain leads to cognitive and memory deficits demonstrable in AD patients. In the current treatment of Alzheimer's disease, the use of cholinesterase therapies to re-establish critical levels of acetylcholine in the inflicted areas are unable to deter the loss of neuronal populations from the CBF and hence to slow the progression of the disease (Bierer et al., 1995; Lad et al., 2003a). Based on these findings, an appropriate way to reduce or prevent neurodegeneration and maintain viability in Alzheimer's disease is to re-establish NGF signaling within the CBF. Additionally, the administered protein must be well-tolerated and stably released over a long period of time to achieve its trophic effects (Apfel, 2002). However, the direct administration of NGF to the CNS via the circulation is precluded by its inability to cross the blood brain barrier (BBB) (Lad et al., 2003a). Furthermore, subcutaneous delivery of NGF elicits acutely painful phenomena due to the presence of TrkA receptors at free nerve endings of pain fibers (Apfel et al., 1998; Lad et al., 2003a). Finally, gastric secretions would rapidly degrade the protein, making oral preparations ineffective.

Other methods have been considered for delivery of growth factors or protein drugs to the brain [for a broad review see references (Alam et al., 2010; Cattaneo et al., 2008)]. Intranasal inhalation has been demonstrated to be a promising mode of non-invasive, facile delivery of biologics to the brain (Benedict et al., 2011). Monocytes can be loaded to secrete NGF and, in proof of principle, shown to migrate across an *in vitro* BBB model consisting of a brain capillary endothelial cell system (Bottger et al., 2010). Encapsulated cell biodelivery is a modified gene therapy approach which encapsulates cells in a immunoprotective semi-permeable hollow fiber synthetic membrane to secrete the protein factor of interest into the desired region of the brain (Fjord-Larsen et al., 2010); NGF and glial derived neurotrophic factor (GDNF) are currently undergoing clinical trials with this method in Sweden. Transcranial focused ultrasound (FUS) has been shown to transiently-enhance the permeability of the BBB and permit antibodies, and probably other macromolecules into the intrathecal space (Jordão et al., 2010). Early interest in conjugation of NGF to transferrin or transferrin antibodies as a means of transport across the BBB (Friden et al., 1993; Liao et al., 2001) seems to have waned and shifted toward using this means of cellular uptake for anti-cancer or diabetic drugs.

Gene therapy presents the most-advanced, current means of delivering NGF in a cerebral region-specific manner (Lad et al., 2003a; Nagahara & Tuszynski, 2011). The two main forms of gene therapy that have been used in the delivery of NGF include an *in vivo* approach and an *ex vivo* approach. The former requires the injection of a viral vector containing the gene of interest directly into the region of interest. The latter can be done by transfecting cells with the gene of interest *in vitro* and subsequently transplanting the transfected cells into the region of interest. These techniques overcome the problems initially encountered with NGF delivery by circumventing the BBB, but require surgical manipulation. Additionally, by using viral vectors as the mode of NGF gene delivery into a specific target within the brain, these methods provide a stable, renewable system of NGF synthesis, which can help re-establish receptor levels and counter apoptosis driven by proNGF. However, these forms of therapy provide the greatest benefit during early stages of AD before cholinergic deficits set in.

Initial positive results in rat and primate animal models supported studies of NGF in clinical trials of AD (Bishop et al., 2008; Eriksdotter Jonhagen et al., 1998; Tuszynski et al., 2005). The early clinical trials met with a lack of success due to lack of efficacy, toxicity or both. Common problems in these clinical studies, as well as corresponding animal studies, include undesirable side effects (e.g. hyperinnervation, sprouting, sympathetic stimulation, cachexia, hyperalgesia) (Apfel, 2002; Thoenen & Sendtner, 2002; Winkler et al., 1997) [reviewed in (Nagahara & Tuszynski, 2011)]. Intriguingly, a phase I trial of *ex vivo* NGF gene delivery in mild Alzheimer's disease has shown some promise (Tuszynski et al., 2005). Briefly, eight individuals with early-stage, probable AD were administered primary autologous fibroblasts, which had been genetically modified to synthesize and secrete NGF, via stereotaxic injections to the CBF. This approach was shown to survive grafting into the brain and provided stable NGF secretion for up to 18 months in animal studies with improvement of cholinergic function and memory (Emerich et al., 1994; Tuszynski et al., 2002; Tuszynski et al., 2005). At 22 months of follow up, no adverse side effects were reported in the clinical trial. Mini-Mental State Exam scores demonstrated a reduction in the rate of cognitive decline and 18-fluorodeoxyglucose PET scans demonstrated significantly greater cortical glucose uptake (Tuszynski et al., 2005). Although these observations were encouraging, results must be considered with caution because of the small data set used and the absence of placebo groups. Additionally, NGF demonstrated a large trophic response in the CBF of some of these patients. While this response is necessary for target innervation during development of the nervous system, an adult brain where the axonal infrastructure is well-established might suffer from new and incomplete neuritogenesis in an area receiving dense axonal support. Hence, the generation of a more refined therapeutic molecule is desirable. Since this *ex vivo* trial, the focus of the scientific community has largely shifted to *in vivo* delivery with adeno-associated virus (AAV) (Table 1 and (Nagahara & Tuszynski, 2011; Nilsson et al., 2010).

Interestingly, monoclonal antibodies to NGF were so effective that a Phase III clinical trial for treatment of osteoarthritis of the knee was discontinued because of joint failure due to excessive wear and tear in the absence of the pain sensation (Lane et al., 2010; Wood, 2010).

| Disorder | Phase | # | Delivery* | Status | Sponsor |
|---|---|---|---|---|---|
| AD | I | 8 | ex vivo NGF | end 2005 some cognitive improvement (see text) | UCSD |
| AD | II | 50 | ICV AAV-NGF Cere-110 | Ongoing Recruiting | Ceregene |
| AD | Ib | 6 | Encapsulated cell biodelivery NGF | Ongoing | NsGene (Sweden) |
| HIV associated sensory neuropathy | II | 270 | SQ NGF | end 2005 | NIAID |
| Osteo-arthritis of knee | III | (a)697 (b)848 | IV mAb to NGF | Completed Discontinued (see text) | Pfizer |

Table 1. Selected clinical trials of NGF for AD or pain. From clinicaltrials.gov, April 2011. *Abbreviations: #, number of patients; ICV, intracerebroventricular; AAV, adeno-associated virus; SQ, subcutaneous; IV, intravenous.

## 3. Signal transduction by neurotrophins

### 3.1 TrkA signaling

Neurotrophin-mediated signal transduction via the Trk receptors leads to an activation of downstream signaling pathways for survival and differentiation (Bibel & Barde, 2000; Ibanez, 1994; Kaplan & Miller, 2000; Levi-Montalcini, 1987). NGF binding induces TrkA receptor dimerization, transautophosphorylation, and tyrosine kinase ICD activation (Bibel & Barde, 2000; Cunningham & Greene, 1998; Cunningham et al., 1997; Friedman & Greene, 1999). The three major signaling pathways are the phosphotidylinositol-3-kinase (PI3 kinase)/Akt pathway, the Ras/mitogen-activated protein kinase (MAPK) pathway, and the phospholipase C gamma (PLCγ) pathway (Bibel & Barde, 2000; Kaplan & Miller, 2000; Lad et al., 2003a) (See Fig. 2). The PI3 kinase pathway through Akt mediates survival via the suppression of apoptotic proteins and accounts for over 80% of neurotrophin-mediated survival in neurons (Bartlett et al., 1997; Crowder & Freeman, 1998; Kaplan & Miller, 2000). The MAPK pathway, has been implicated in both survival and differentiation, although it has also been implicated in such diverse functions as synaptic plasticity and long-term potentiation (Kaplan & Miller, 2000; Lad et al., 2003a). Depending on the upstream activators and downstream effectors of MAPK, survival, differentiation or both signals can be transduced. For the specific induction of differentiation, a sustained MAPK activation is necessary. The third signal transduction pathway is the PLCγ pathway, involved primarily in Ca2+ regulation of calcium regulated enzymes, neurotrophin secretion, and synaptic plasticity (Bibel & Barde, 2000; Canossa et al., 1997). These conclusions about distinct pathways have been reached by mutagenesis of the Tyr residues of the Trk-ICD and demonstrate that these signaling pathways can be individually dissected by manipulation of the intracellular initiation of each pathway. TrkB and TrkC have similar signaling pathways but with some individual differences because of the different neuronal environment of these receptors. The division of TrkA signaling into three discrete, but overlapping signal pathways, suggests that pharmaceutical approaches for design of signal selective neurotrophic therapeutics (see Section 5.2) may be able to discriminate among selected paths toward cellular outcomes.

| TrkA | Outcome |
|---|---|
| p-Y490→Ras→PI3K→Akt→ | *survival*[1] |
| p-Y490→Shc→MAPK→pMEK→Bcl2→ | *survival*[2] |
| p-Y490→FRS2→MAPK→p-Elk1, pCREB→ | *differentiation*[2] |
| p-Y785*→PLCγ→PI→DAG, IP3→$Ca^{++}$→ | *synaptic plasticity*[3] |

Fig. 2. Signaling pathways, PI3K, MAPK, PLCγ , from TrkA phospho-tyrosines to cell outcomes. *Phosphorylation of Y785 is dependent on phosphorylaton of Y670, Y674, Y675. [1]Bartlett et al., 1997; Crowder & Freeman, 1998; Rodriguez-Viciana et al., 1994; Holgado-Madruga et al., 1997. [2]Kao et al., 2001; Loeb et al., 1994; Gomez & Cohen, 1991; Qian et al., 1998; [3]Loeb et al., 1994; Canossa et al., 1997; Cunningham et al., 1997.

Phosphorylation of a specific set of tyrosines ensues within the activation loop of the kinase domain. These include two tyrosines located in the juxtamembrane domain (Y490) and C-terminus (Y785) of Trk that serve as docking sites for adaptor proteins and three tyrosines (Y670, Y674, and Y675) within the activation loop that interact with nearby basic residues to stabilize a fully functional, active catalytic core and potentiate transduction of downstream signals (Bibel & Barde, 2000; Cunningham & Greene, 1998; Friedman & Greene, 1999; Grewal et al., 1999; Huang & Reichardt, 2003; Kaplan & Miller, 2000; Lad et al., 2003a).

### 3.2 p75 signaling

Classically, p75 has been thought to be involved in the induction of negative signals like apoptosis and growth arrest in oligodendrocytes, Schwann cells, sympathetic neurons, motor neurons, and sensory neurons (Bamji et al., 1998; Barrett & Bartlett, 1994; Casaccia-Bonnefil et al., 1996; Kaplan & Miller, 2000) in a Trk-independent fashion, (Davey & Davies, 1998; Kaplan & Miller, 2000; Soilu-Hanninen et al., 1999). The co-presence of Trk on a neuron silences pro-apoptotic pathways by activation of the pro-survival transcription factor, NF-κB, which subsequently activates Akt (Bibel & Barde, 2000; Kaplan & Miller, 2000; Khursigara et al., 1999). Sympathetic neurons and basal forebrain neurons that were p75-deficient in p75-/- mice underwent robust axonal sprouting, hypertrophy, or target innervation with naturally-occurring developmental apoptosis being significantly delayed (Kaplan & Miller, 2000; Walsh et al., 1999; Yeo et al., 1997; Bamji et al., 1998). Without intrinsic catalytic activity, the p75 ICD appears to rely on docking of adaptor proteins. The complexities of the p75 signaling are outlined by representative examples shown in Fig. 3.

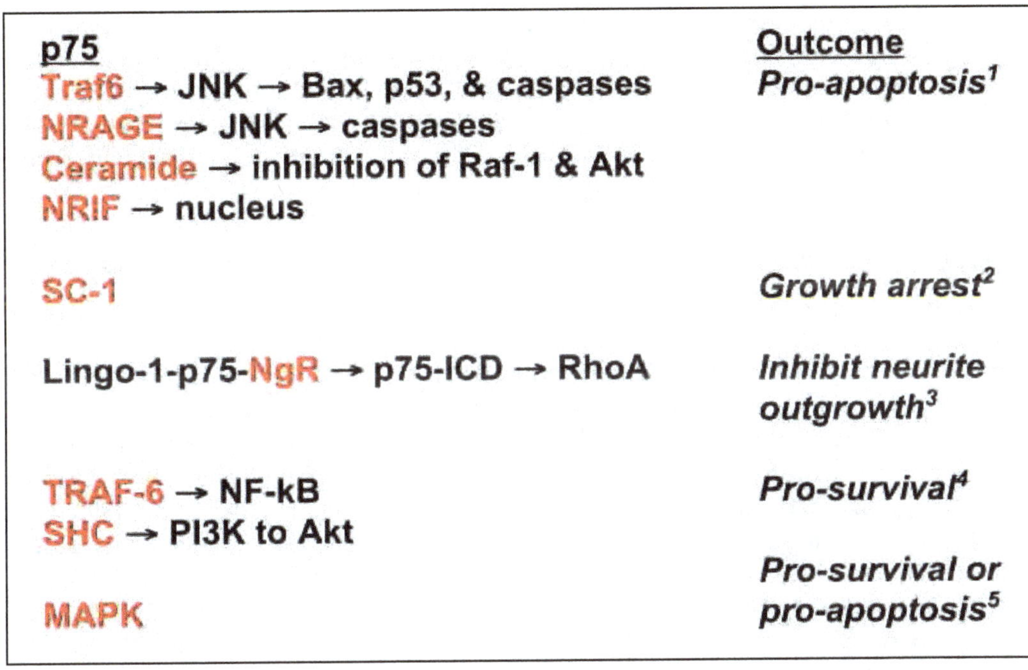


Fig. 3. Some signaling pathways from p75 to cell outcomes. Adaptor proteins interact with p75 to generate most cellular effects of a diverse nature. Uncommon abbrevations: NRAGE, Neurotrophin receptor-interacting MAGE homolog; NRIF, neurotrophin receptor interacting factor, Zn finger transcriptional factor; SC-1, Schwann cell factor 1; NgR, Nogo receptor. RhoA, Ras homolog A. (For reviews see Kaplan & Miller, 2000; Bibel & Barde, 2000; Schecterson & Bothwell, 2010). [1]Aloyz et al., 1998; Salehi, et al., 2002; Muller, et al., 1998; de Chaves et al., 1997; Casademunt, et al., 1999; [2]Chittka & Chao, 1999; [3]Domeniconi et al., 2005; [4]Khursigara et al., 1999; [5]Susen, et al., 1999; Lad & Neet, 2003.

The self-interaction of p75 also influences cellular outcome. Biophysical and biochemical methods have suggested that homomeric p75 plays a pro-apoptotic role while formation of oligomers abolishes this effect and may even serve an anti-apoptotic role (Kaplan & Miller, 2000; Lad et al., 2003a; Wang et al., 2000). Recently, evidence has been provided to support a model in which the formation of an inter-protomer disulfide bond in p75 allows a scissoring (or snail-tong) action upon NGF binding that promotes binding of intracellular adaptor proteins (Simi & Ibanez, 2010; Vilar et al., 2009).

As mentioned above (Section 2.2), proneurotrophins may play significant role in AD, due to their ability to stimulate p75 in the absence of positive Trk signals thereby promoting apoptosis and death of neurons or glia (Cuello et al., 2010; Fahnestock et al., 2001; Teng, et al. 2010). These effects are thought to be mediated by the same pathways (Fig. 3) as presented for mature NGF (or other neurotrophins). In addition, soluble oligomers of β-amyloid may also interact with p75 to cause apoptotic signals in neuronal tissue of AD or pre-AD patients (Dechant & Barde, 2002; Diarra et al. 2009; Coulson, et al., 2009; Calissano, et al. 2010a; 2010b; Peng, et al., 2004; Susen & Blochl, 2005).

These studies demonstrate that the interaction of neurotrophins or proneurotrophins with p75 can lead to diverse effects that are determined by the developmental state of the organism, the particular cell type within which it is expressed, the additional expression of co-receptors, receptor oligomerization states, and the binding of intracellular adaptors or effectors. The complexity of the p75 pathways suggests that developing signal selective muteins for this receptor would be much more difficult than those outlined for the Trk receptor (Section 5.2) with its more clearly initiated signaling. Since the response of cells is, basically, apoptosis or not, then there would be less advantage at this point in time in generating such reagents for p75.

## 4. Molecular analysis of neurotrophin structure and rationale of mutations

### 4.1 Conserved and variable regions defined from sequence and 3-D crystallographic structures

Functional data gathered from systematic mutagenesis studies and through the construction of inter-neurotrophin chimeras coupled with structural data from crystallographic studies have implicated several spatially distinct patches of residues in bestowing receptor specificity to each neurotrophin (Casademunt et al., 1999; de Chaves et al., 1997; Grimes et al., 1997; Ilag et al., 1994; Lad et al., 2003a; Ninkina et al., 1997; Rabizadeh et al., 1993; J. Scott et al., 1983; Walsh et al., 1999; Wiesmann et al., 1999; Yeo et al., 1997) . Sequence alignments of NGF, BDNF, and NT-3 (Ibanez et al., 1992; Ibanez et al., 1991; Ibanez et al., 1993; Ilag et al., 1994; Kullander & Ebendal, 1994; Kullander et al., 1997) demonstrate that each neurotrophin possesses seven variable regions that include the same residue positions. These are the N-terminus (residues 1-9), variable region I (β-hairpin loop 1, residues 23-35), variable region II (β-hairpin loop 2, residues 40-49), variable region III (β-reverse turn loop 3, residues 59-66), variable region IV (β-strand, residues 79-88), variable region V (β-hairpin loop 4, residues 95-99), and the C-terminus (residues 111-118) (Fig. 1B). This homology in clustering translates structurally to variable regions occupying complementary sites on each neurotrophin molecule, which are surface-exposed, enabling these regions to function as sites of receptor contacts (Fig. 4). These regions also define amino acid residues to target for redesign of molecules to alter signaling (see Section 5.2).

#### 4.1.1 The specificity patch

Chimeric molecules retaining the amino terminus, carboxyl terminus, and variable region II of NGF possessed the ability to differentiate sympathetic neurons and activate the TrkA receptor (Ibanez et al., 1991). However, a chimeric molecule that additionally replaced residues 3-9 of the N-terminus reduced TrkA binding, activation, and biological activity to <1% (Ibanez et al., 1993). Other substitution and deletion studies confirmed the importance of the N-terminus in specificity (Kullander et al., 1997; Woo et al., 1995; Kahle et al., 1992; Shih et al., 1994). Data from the crystal structure of human recombinant NGF complexed with the TrkA-d5 domains showed that the amino terminal residues 6-9, which were not well-defined in the original NGF crystal structure, adopted a helical conformation upon complex formation with their side chains almost completely buried in the interface (McDonald et al., 1991; Wiesmann et al., 1999) (Fig. 4). Within the same region, H4, I6, and E11 participated in strong interactions with residues in the ABED TrkA β-sheet. The authors labeled this region the specificity patch suggesting that the most important Trk receptor-binding determinants lie within the amino terminus (Wiesmann et al., 1999). Residues spanning the specificity patch, i.e. H4, P5, I6, F7, E11, and F12, are clearly important for neurotrophin-Trk interactions and activation.

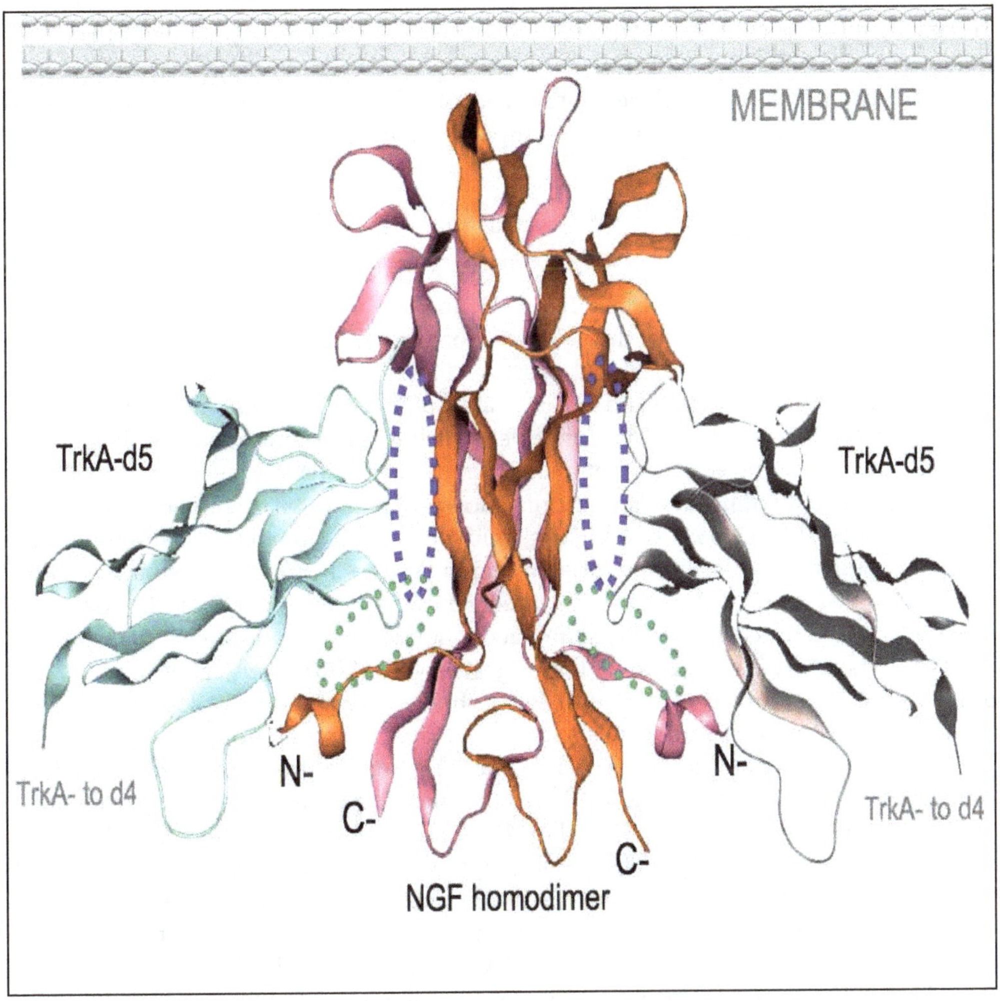


Fig. 4. Schematic representation of dimeric nerve growth factor complexed with two TrkA-d5 domains. NGF and TrkA (PDB 1WWW) form highly specific interactions at the specificity (green dotted oval) and the conserved patch (blue dotted oval). Additional contacts are provided by variable loops I, II, and V (loop 4) that form a continuous surface of binding. Each TrkA-d5 binding site is derived from contributions from loops in both protomers in the NGF dimer. NGF protomers, pink and orange. 1st TrkA-d5; cyan: 2nd TrkA-d5; grey.

#### 4.1.2 The variable regions

The variable regions (Fig. 1B), in general, correspond to loops and surface residues in NGF and the other neurotrophins. Generation of NGF-BDNF chimeras identified variable region II as holding important receptor binding determinants (Ibanez et al., 1991; Ibanez et al., 1993; Ilag et al., 1994; Kullander & Ebendal, 1994; Kullander et al., 1997). The variable region was further dissected into IIa (residues 40-44) and IIb (residues 45-49) (Ibanez et al., 1993). Region IIb was shown to play a more pivotal role than IIa when replacement of only the latter led to a dramatic reduction in receptor activation and biological activity (Ibanez et al., 1993). The variable region II, with help from variable region V (loop 4), was also shown to confer specificity between NT-3 and NGF (Ilag et al., 1994; Kullander & Ebendal, 1994; Kullander et al., 1997). The C-terminal linker region of TrkA could serve as a possible binding partner of this region (Wiesmann et al., 1999) (Fig. 4). Therefore, residues within variable regions IIa and IIb are considered important for neurotrophin activity, i.e. E41, N43, I44, N45, V48, and F49.

#### 4.1.3 The conserved patch

Crystallographic data of dimeric NGF complexed with TrkA-d5 demonstrated that 5 of 10 residues in variable region IV (Y79, T81, T83, H84, and F86) actually form part of the conserved patch that interacts intimately with the TrkA-d5 domains (Wiesmann & de Vos, 2001) (Fig. 4). This 'conserved' patch was so named because 14 of 23 NGF residues are occupied by homologous amino acids in BDNF and NT-3, while 8 of 15 TrkA residues are conserved in TrkB and TrkC (Wiesmann et al., 1999). The conserved patch forms a continuous binding surface for TrkA-d5 and retains high sequence homology across species (Wiesmann et al., 1999) (Fig. 4). Variable region IV, a β-strand, was specifically shown to retain ~90% homology across species. Within this region, T81 and H84 of NGF are replaced by non-homologous amino acids in the other neurotrophins, suggesting that variable region IV does form specific contacts with TrkA (Ibanez et al., 1993) (Fig. 4). Alanine point mutagenesis of H84 and H75 indicated that these residues participated in receptor binding and activation based on a decline in neuritogenesis in PC12 cells and the ability to compete for binding sites with radioactively-labeled wild-type NGF (Woo & Neet, 1996). Similarly, R100 and R103 showed trends akin to H84 with respect to sequence alignment analysis, mutagenesis studies, and crystallographic data. R100 and R103 are not only strictly conserved across species but also within the family of neurotrophins. Crystallographic data suggested that R103 was the most important binding determinant in the conserved patch (Wiesmann et al., 1999) (Fig. 4). [Also see Section 5.1.] Residues V22, I31, F53, and F54 within the conserved patch are also highly conserved across species and between neurotrophin family members. Alanine substitution of these four residues significantly affect TrkA binding by competition assays, intracellular receptor phosphorylation studies, and biological activity in PC12 cells (Ibanez et al., 1990; Ibanez et al., 1992; Ibanez et al., 1993; Guo et al., 1996). Hence, the conserved patch represents a binding epitope wherein residues help form critical interactions between neurotrophins and Trk receptors.

#### 4.1.4 Summary of important regions and residues of the neurotrophin family

Sixteen residues of NGF may be identified as most important for function (Table 2) and can be designated as the specificity patch (H4, P5, I6, F7, E11, and F12), the variable loops (I31, E41, N43, I44, N45, V48, and F49), or the conserved patch (I31, F54, H84, and R103). Additional residues, V22, F53, H75, and R100, may not occupy the conserved patch, *per se*, but are as highly conserved as residues residing within or near the patch. Similar considerations have been made for BDNF and NT-3 (Ibanez et al., 1992; Ibanez et al., 1991; Ibanez et al., 1993; Ilag et al., 1994; Kullander & Ebendal, 1994; Kullander et al., 1997; Suter et al., 1992; Urfer et al., 1997). These regions of the NGF molecule were targeted to obtain the signal selective muteins discussed in Section 5.2.

| | |
|---|---|
| **Specificity Patch** – induced N-terminal α-helix; mainly hydrophobic and some H-bond interactions to β-strands ABED of TrkA-d5. | **NGF:** H4, P5, I6, F7, E11, F12<br>**BDNF:** S4, D5, P6, A7, E11, L12 |
| **Conserved Patch** – part of hydrophobic core of NGF; interacts with loop EF and C-terminus of TrkA-d5 | **NGF:** V22, I31*, F53, F54, H75, H84*, R103<br>**BDNF:** V22, M31, F53, Y54, H75, Q84, R103 |
| Specificity for NGF vs NT-3: **Loop II-** | **NGF:** E41, N43, I44, N45, V48, F49<br>**BDNF:** K41, P43, V44, S45 - -<br>**NT-3:** E41, K43, T44, G45, P48, V49 |
| **N-terminus-** | **NGF:** P5, F7<br>**NT-3:** H5, S7 |

Table 2. Important regions of Trk receptor interaction in human NGF and BDNF. Based on crystal structure and mutagenesis analysis of NGF (Mahapatra, 2008; Ibanez et al., 1992; Ibanez et al., 1991; Ibanez et al., 1993; Ilag et al., 1994; Kullander & Ebendal, 1994; Kullander et al., 1997; Wiesmann & de Vos, 2001) and the corresponding regions in BDNF and NT-3. Note: I31 and H84 (with *) also participate in Loop 1 and Loop 4, respectively, as well as the conserved patch.

## 5. Development of neurotrophin muteins that have potentially improved therapeutic properties

### 5.1 Receptor selective muteins

Two interesting, complementary, and useful muteins have helped elucidate the role of the two receptors in neurotrophin action. The first discovery was that mutations in the 32-35, loop I area would greatly reduce or eliminate binding to the p75 receptor and leave TrkA binding unimpaired (Ibanez et al 1992; 1993). The triNGF (or KKE) mutein contained the three mutations, K32A/K34A/E35A, and was used to demonstrate the functional interaction between p75 and TrkA in the developing embryo (Ryden, et al., 1997). The mutations in the N-terminus of NGF were shown to be important for TrkA binding in several laboratories (Section 4.1.1). One noteable mutein was the Δ9/13 mutein that bound p75 but not TrkA (Woo et al., 1995), and helped distinguish between differentiation, cell cycle regulation, and apoptosis in PC12 cells (Hughes et al., 2001). Utilization of this Δ9/13 mutein also later indicated a unique role for the 'high affinity' binding complex of p75 and TrkA in PC12 cells (Lad, et al., 2003b). Indeed, the combination of these two receptor muteins, KKE/Δ9/13 has been studied, briefly, and shown to have no observable activity, as expected (Mahapatra, et al., 2009). Both muteins, KKE and Δ9/13, have been used in a rat glaucoma model to interpret the roles of TrkA (neuroprotective) and p75 (neurotoxic) in retinal degeneration (Bai, et al., 2010). KKE, but not wild type NGF, has recently been reported to partially improve learning in a transgenic APP mouse model (overexpression of Swedish and Indiana mutations) with a reduction of soluble cortical β-amyloid levels, but with no improvement in long-term memory (Aboulkassim, et al., 2011). These two receptor selective muteins have potential as an improved therapeutic for disorders in which either TrkA or p75 can be expected, with improved targeting in that case.

In the opposite direction, a neurotrophin mutein has been made that is less restrictive, rather than more restrictive, in binding to Trk receptors. The pan-neurotrophin, PNT, incorporated elements of variable and conserved regions to produce a mutein that binds to all three receptors, TrkA, TrkB, TrkC (Ibanez, et al., 1993; Ilag, et al., 1995). To the authors' knowledge, a pan-neurotrophin has not been made that was promiscuous for Trk receptors but restricted so as to not bind p75. Such pan-neurotrophins might have utility in the treatment of some neurodegenerative disorders in which multiple receptors indiscriminately needed extra support (Funakoshi, et al., 1998).

The observation of a mutation in NGF that affects the pain response suggests that changes in signaling from mutations in the ligand have already occurred in nature. A nociceptive response is mediated by NGF (Pezet & McMahon, 2006), partly through the TrkA receptor and partly through p75 (Einarsdottir et al., 2004; Indo, 2002; Nicol & Vasko, 2007). In a large family from northern Sweden, an R100W mutation was uncovered within the coding region of NGF. Individuals from this family suffered from insensitivity to both temperature and deep pain perception, while retaining normal mental abilities, a disorder termed hereditary sensory and autonomic neuropathy type V (HSANV) (Einarsdottir et al., 2004). The R100W mutation selectively disrupts binding of NGF to the p75 receptor, while the affinity for TrkA receptor is less affected (Covaceuszach et al., 2010). Also, the consequence of the R100W mutation on p75 receptor binding is greater for mature NGF rather than proNGF. Signaling pathways reflect this selectivity (Capsoni et al., 2011), suggesting that these findings might lead to a 'painless' NGF protein with therapeutic potential. This NGF mutation is an example of a naturally-occurring, receptor-selective change in the neurotrophin.

### 5.2 Development of signal selective muteins

To alleviate the potentially undesirable effects of inappropriate over extension of neurites during clinical trials (Section 2.3), designer neurotrophins have been developed (Mahapatra et al., 2009). Two survival-specific (or signal-selective, SS) recombinant NGF muteins with decreased differentiation potential were designed from a set of rationally selected mutations within the specificity, conserved, and variable regions of NGF that may play a discriminatory role in signal transduction. One of these muteins is the F7A/H84A/R103A NGF triple mutein, also called SS-1 or 7-84-103 for short. The other signal-selective hextuple mutein is the K32A/K34A/E35A/F7A/H84A/R103A NGF mutein, or called SS-2 or KKE/7-84-103 (Mahapatra et al., 2009). The main difference between the two SS muteins is that the KKE addition to the F7A/H84A/R103A mutation simply makes the hextuple mutein, SS2, incapable of binding p75 (see Section 5.1).

Survival in several cell lines and differentiation in PC12 cells were studied with these recombinant NGF triple and hextuple muteins and compared to wild type NGF. Each of these two muteins induced slightly lower levels of survival in MG139 and PC12 cells with greatly reduced neuritogenesis in PC12 cells. Neuritogenesis data indicated that residues Phe7, His84, and Arg103 played a critical role in biological activity, in agreement with earlier data in the literature (see Section 4). The observed neuritogenic potential of each recombinant triple mutein suggested that His84 (conserved patch) played a discriminatory role in neurite outgrowth. When His84 was mutated to alanine, to make 7-84-103 and KKE/7-84-103, the maximum neuritic response was almost 40% lower than when His84 was left unaltered. With 7-84-103 and KKE/7-84-103, a synergistic effect also occurred when combining mutations to these three residues. These data suggested that mutations within the specificity and conserved patches were more than additive and led to a reduction of neuritogenesis. In 7-84-103 and KKE/7-84-103, the two point mutations were made in close proximity within the same spatial region, *i.e.* His84 and Arg103, within the conserved patch. Combining mutations in close proximity may have a cumulative effect on ligand-receptor interactions and ultimately reduce the efficiency of some aspects of intracellular signaling. When independent single mutations were incorporated in close proximity within critical regions at the ligand-receptor interface, survival and differentiation were both affected, with a more pronounced effect on neuritogenesis. The greater decrease in differentiation suggests the possibility of multiple binding epitopes for the mediation of survival, while suggesting more limited patches needed for the induction of differentiation. Comparison with binding to immobilized TrkA by surface plasmon resonance suggested that differentiation more closely follows affinity than does survival. Furthermore, similarity in measurements between the recombinant NGF triple mutein and its KKE hextuple counterpart suggested that p75 binding was inconsequential to the induction of survival or differentiation in these cell lines. Studies with ectopically expressed receptors in fibroblast cell lines, MG139 (TrkA+, p75–) and PCNA (TrkA–, p75+), also supported the interpretation that the distinction in signaling properties was due to signaling from the TrkA tyrosine kinase receptor.

The 7-84-103 mutein supported better activation of the PI 3-kinase/Akt survival pathway than the Ras/MAPK pathway, from which differentiation results. These differences in signaling pathways (Akt vs MAPK, see Section 3) indicate that qualitative differences result from a different mode of binding to the receptor, or re-orientation of the receptor upon binding (see Section 6), and are not simply due to an affinity change that affects all signaling pathways equally. In other words, the level of TrkA phosphorylation with 7-84-103 is more efficiently transferred to MAPK and Akt activation for survival than it is for differentiation.

The discrimination ratio, or ratio of relative (to wtNGF) EC50 values, was 30-fold based on the relative EC50 values of 100 and 3.3 for differentiation and survival, respectively (Mahapatra et al., 2009). A 30-fold difference in effective EC50 values, in the pathophysiological context of an early cognitively diseased brain, might be sufficient to greatly reduce unwanted neuritic response while still maintaining neuronal viability. Whether the design of these two signal-selective muteins is optimal at this stage, or whether further improvement in discrimination between survival and differentiation pathways is possible, needs to be examined.

### 5.3 How can a transmembrane receptor be stimulated from the outside of a cell and initiate different kinds of intracellular signals?

The intricacies of intracellular signaling from tyrosine kinase ICDs are just now being elucidated and are more complicated than might be expected from the simple requirement of a receptor dimer to transautophosphorylate tyrosine residues on its ICD domain. Activation subsequent to ligand binding to the ECD typically requires phosphorylation of a tyrosine in a loop in the active site in order to auto-activate the ICD kinase by moving the loop out of its inhibitory position in the active site (Bae & Schlessinger, 2010; Lemmon & Schlessinger, 2010). Then the kinase continues to phosphorylate tyrosine residues in the C-terminal tail of the adjacent ICD of the receptor tyrosine kinase that provide a docking site for SH2 domain adaptor proteins or enzymes (Bae & Schlessinger, 2010; Jura et al., 2011; Lemmon & Schlessinger, 2010). Three distinct molecular mechanisms have been detected: (i) The activation loop interacts directly with the active site of the kinase and blocks access to substrates. (ii) The juxtamembrane region interacts with elements within the active site of the kinase to stabilize an inactive conformation. (iii) The C-terminal tail interacts with the active site of the tyrosine kinase domain to stabilize an inactive conformation. In each case, phosphorylation of the appropriate tyrosine relieves the kinase of its inactivation.

Evidence from crystallographic studies of the EGF receptor ICD has suggested an allosteric mechanism of initiating the signaling cascade (X. Zhang et al., 2006). Two distinct EGFR ICD interactions were described: one being a symmetric interaction and the other an asymmetric interaction that is capable of explaining how the EGF signal is transduced across the cell membrane (X. Zhang et al., 2006). Direct contacts occur between the C-lobe of one ICD, acting as an activator, and the N-lobe of another ICD, acting as a receiver. The activator kinase ICD destabilizes autoinhibitory interactions that involve the activation loop of the receiver ICD. Interactions between the docking proteins, Gab1 and Shc, and the EGFR-ICD generate kinetic discrimination between the unliganded and EGF-liganded states (Fan et al., 2004). The formation of the signal transduction 'signalosome' could well depend upon the intricate relationship of the ICDs with docking proteins and, thus, be susceptible to the manner in which the ligand (neurotrophin mutein or peptidomimetic) brought together two Trk ECDs and their connected ICDs with docking partners. In such a scenario, a larger protein ligand, such as EGF or NGF, would seem to be more capable of having multiple ways to force intracellular interactions in the signalosome than a much smaller peptidomimetic with limited 'hot spots' for interaction.

Thus, to explain the NGF mutein data discussed in Section 5.2 (Mahapatra et al., 2009), the wild-type NGF might orient the two ICDs in a signalosome that generates a "normal" ratio of MAPK to Akt activation. In the survival-selective muteins, 7-84-103 and KKE/7-84-103, the orientation of the ICDs or juxtamembrane regions would have been altered such that the output ratio has been shifted in favor of Akt over MAPK signaling and, hence, survival over neuritogenesis.

## 6. Neurotrophin peptidomimetics and cell signaling

The use of small molecules is often preferable over the use large proteins as pharmacological agents due to their stability, lower manufacturing costs, ability to pass tissue barriers and good pharmacokinetic profiles. The small molecules can be rationally designed to mimic a region of the ligand that is involved in binding to the receptor or involved in activation of the receptor, thus the term 'peptidomimetics'. Binding of a peptidomimetic to the target receptor may not necessarily result in activation and thus these mimetics may act as antagonists or agonists, depending on their ability to induce a functional response. An inability to induce a functional response would mean that a small molecule with good affinity would be a good inhibitor/antagonist. Two terms that are useful in the design of mimetics are pharmacophore and 'hot spots'. The term 'pharmacophore' relates to the steric and electronic interactions of the mimetic that are necessary to bind to the target receptor, either as an agonist or as an antagonist. The term 'hot spot' refers to the regions on the target protein that specifically interact with a ligand to induce a biological response. Hence, the rational design of mimetics utilizes the information from both the pharmacophore and the hot spots to create libraries of compounds that have subtle structural differences, but significant functional differences (Peleshok & Saragovi, 2006).

### 6.1 Early neurotrophomimetics

Early studies with cyclized monomeric peptides representing the four loop regions (see Fig. 1B) of NGF (LeSauteur et al., 1995) produced antagonists that competed with NGF for binding and inhibited its activity. The most potent antagonist was derived using amino acids from loop 4 (amino acids 92-97); the peptides designed around loop 2 (amino acids 43-48) or loop 1 (amino acids 30-35) were less effective. As expected, potency was also effected by length and amino acid substitution, with linear peptides showing no activity. Formation of the β-turn is not simply defined by the amino acid sequence and the activity requires mimicking of the 3-dimensional conformation (LeSauteur et al., 1995). Interestingly, in cells expressing both TrkA and p75, the addition of an anti-p75 monoclonal antibody (MC192) that synergizes with NGF caused the antagonistic loop 4 mimetics to behave as agonists with phosphorylation of TrkA and induction of neurites (Maliartchouk et al., 2000). Peptides that formed type I or type γL-αR turns showed greater activity in presence of MC192, suggesting that binding between TrkA and the loop 4 region may require an 'induced fit' mechanism (Beglova et al., 2000).

### 6.2 Small molecule Trk agonists and antagonists

Other studies, however, reported that cyclized monomeric loop 4 peptide mimetics had to be presented as dimers of cyclized peptides to show agonistic activity (Xie et al., 2000). Their dimeric cyclized peptide, involving amino acids 92-96, showed NGF like activity and induced neurite outgrowth and Akt activation in a TrkA- and ERK- dependent manner. Thus, the dimeric peptide was able to induce an NGF-like signal, by binding to and activating TrkA. Modifications in the peptide sequence abolished the agonistic activity, suggesting specificity conferred by the amino acid sequence (Xie et al., 2000). On the other hand, dimerization of a peptidomimetic does not always behave as expected. Conversion of a monovalent peptidomimetic into a divalent mimetic by chemical coupling resulted, surprisingly, in an antagonist (Brahimi et al., 2010).

Loop 1 peptidomimetics show very unique activity. The loop 1 region (amino acids 30-35) has not only been implicated in activation of TrkA, but amino acids K32, K34 and E35 are extremely important for p75 binding (Ibanez et al., 1992; Ibanez et al., 1993) (see Section 5.1). Therefore, this region influences both TrkA and p75 binding. Cyclized monomeric peptidomimetics designed using the β-turn of NT-3 are good TrkC agonists, however some of the peptides showed partial agonistic response towards TrkA. Interestingly, some of the mimetics were able to induce a neurite outgrowth response through TrkA or TrkC, but failed to induce a survival response on TrkA-only expressing cells (Zaccaro et al., 2005). Neurite outgrowth studies were done using PC12 cells which express both TrkA and p75, whereas survival studies were done using TrkA-only expressing 3T3 cells. The authors, therefore, argued that this peptidomimetic binds to a special 'hot spot' on TrkA that is accessible only when p75 is co-expressed. The co-expression of p75 with TrkA could result in formation of the TrkA-p75 heteroreceptor complex and binding of p75 to TrkA, perhaps, results in conformational changes in the receptor, making the 'hot spot' accessible (Zaccaro et al., 2005). The D3 mimetic in this series was also tested in cognitively impaired aged rats and showed rescue of the cholinergic phenotype in the cortex and nucleus basilis (Bruno, et al., 2004) and to improve learning and reduce β-amyloid in APP mice (Aboulkassim, et al., 2011).

### 6.3 Small molecule p75 agonists and antagonists

In contrast, Longo's group made loop 1 mimetics (LM11A-24 and LM11A-31) that targeted p75 and were able to induce a survival response through p75 in hippocampal neurons (Massa et al., 2006). Hippocampal neurons express TrkB and p75, but not TrkA; therefore, this survival induced by loop 1 mimetics was suggested to result via p75. They further showed that the survival response was lost in hippocampal neurons from p75-/- mice and that these peptides showed competitive binding to p75 but not TrkA, supporting the interpretation that the activity was through p75. The survival response observed was mediated by NF-κB and the PI3K-Akt pathway (Massa et al., 2006). They further demonstrated that the mimetics were able to rescue the neurons from proNGF-induced (Massa et al., 2006) or Aβ-induced (Yang et al., 2008) cell death, which have implications for Alzheimer's pathogenesis. NGF, even though it can bind p75, was not able to prevent the Aβ-induced neuritic dystrophy. Differences between the signaling by the mimetics vs NGF via p75 were also observed. Both NGF and the mimetics were able to inhibit the ability of Aβ to down regulate Akt signaling; in contrast, the peptidomimetics demonstrated p75-dependent inhibition of Aβ-induced GSK3b and Aβ-induced JNK activation, whereas NGF could not affect these latter two activities. Thus, these loop 1 peptidomimetics induced additional survival promoting cell signaling via p75 in presence of Aβ, not observed with NGF via p75 (Yang et al., 2008). Hence, the selectivity progressed from receptor to signaling pathway. From another laboratory, a different loop1-loop4 mimetic was shown to have some ability to reduce neuropathic pain in a rat model (Colangelo, et al., 2008).

### 6.4 The prognosis for signal selective mimetics

These studies with NGF peptidomimetics illustrate the advances that have been made as well as outlining the complexities involved. Whether a monovalent or a divalent (dimeric) NGF peptidomimetic is functional and most appropriate for clinical use is, as yet, unresolved. Good NGF mimetics at this stage appear to be D3 or its derivatives and LM11A-24 or LM11A-31, although each may potentially be useful for a distinct purpose. Also being developed are TrkB (O'Leary & Hughes, 2003; Fletcher, et al., 2008; Fletcher & Hughes, 2009) and TrkC (Brahimi, et al., 2009; Chen, et al., 2009; Liu, et al., 2010) antagonists/agonists. BDNF mimetics have made progress toward a useful therapeutic reagent with efficacy studies in rodents (Massa et al., 2010). Some of these neurotrophin reagents show receptor selectivity, as well as selective cellular response, i.e. survival vs differentiation (Saragovi et al., 2009). Whether a small peptidomimetic or a modified, full-length NGF protein will ultimately prove to be the most effective clinical reagent for treatment of AD is an open question at present. The pharmacokinetic advantages of a small molecule mimetic may eventually outweigh the limited information content, relative to the full length protein, provided by such a peptide. In other words, will the chemists be able to design sufficient specificity and selectivity into the peptidomimetics to compete with the potential specificity of a 26 kDa neurotrophin protein with its myriad interaction sites? The answer in some cases for selective signaling appears to be yes (Zaccaro et al., 2005; Longo, et al., 2007; Yang et al., 2008). Conversely, will the means of delivery (intracerebroventricular injection, intranasal inhalation, encapsulation) of a full-length neurotrophin mutein be developed sufficiently to make easy administration to the AD brain competitive with a, perhaps, less effective small molecule that is easily delivered? In either case, exquisite signal selectivity to allow ultra-focus may be most effective and/or desirable.

## 7. Other growth factors with cellular signaling selectivity

Neurotrophins are not the only ligand-receptor system in which molecular engineering approaches have been employed to improve the therapeutic potential. Mutants of both insulin and tumor necrosis factor (TNFα) have also been developed with enhancement of their therapeutic properties. TNFα was re-designed with the intent of improving its death-inducing targeting toward tumors and reducing its systemic side effects (Wajant, et al., 2005; Gerspach, et al., 2009). This attempt is a true challenge with a multifunctional, pleiotropic cytokine such as TNFα; nevertheless some progress has been made. Similarly, insulin has been engineered to improve its stability as a single chain (Hua, et al., 2008), its stability as a zinc 'stapled' hexamer with even longer lasting attributes (Phillips, et al., 2010), and its selectivity for the insulin receptor over the non-cognate IGF-1 receptor (Zhao, et al., 2009). A reported 3-fold improvement in receptor selectivity has the potential of reducing colorectal cancer risk for diabetic patients using insulin replacement therapy (Zhao, et al., 2009). How well these receptor and/or signal selective mutant cytokines/hormones may work in therapeutic trials is still uncertain.

## 8. Conclusions and the future

The importance of ligand-receptor interactions in AD and other neurodegenerative conditions is well appreciated. Protein levels and mRNA levels for both TrkA and p75 receptors are reduced in early AD even in the presence of stable NGF expression. A shift from mature NGF to proNGF, which binds p75 and induces apoptosis, has also been observed. Thus, the neurodegeneration in the basal forebrain in AD is aggravated by a reduction in signaling from TrkA receptors coupled with apoptotic signaling by proNGF binding to p75 (see Section 2.2). Animal studies and clinical trials of NGF gene delivery show promise in curtailing neuronal apoptosis in Alzheimer's disease or animal models. However, the CBF in some patients demonstrated a trophic response of immature neuritic processes, i.e. neurite outgrowth where it was not needed or useful. Adult brains with AD possessing an established axonal network may be adversely affected by this type of aberrant neuritogenesis. Survival support for existing neurons is preferable without inducing *de novo* connections that might be dysfunctional. A key goal for future intervention of this type is to promote viability of specific neurons without causing neuritic or axonal overgrowth.

The possibility and potential of designer growth factors has been highlighted in this review. Step-wise mutagenesis of NGF led to the generation of survival-selective muteins that are potentially therapeutic lead candidates for Alzheimer Disease or other neurodegenerative disorders. Two mechanism-selective recombinant NGF muteins show a marked difference in the ratio of survival to neuritogenesis in several assays, including signaling through the Akt survival pathway. Thus, in principle one can separate intracellular signaling pathways for a receptor via modifications to its ligand. Successful parallel studies with molecular engineering of insulin and TNFα support this viewpoint. Structural studies of other receptor systems, e.g., EGF, have provided a logical, molecular basis for understanding how these signals may be separately activated. Progress with small molecule mimetics of NGF that are agonists show some of the same receptor- and signaling- selectivity that receptor- or signal-selective muteins of the parent protein do. The future should provide major advances in this exciting area of improving upon nature and developing novel treatments for AD. Coupling of designer neurotrophins with improved delivery to the brain provides great promise.

## 9. Acknowledgements

We wish to acknowledge the generous support of the NINDS, NIH, USPHS, USA for nearly 20 years through the grant NS24380. We are grateful to many interesting and challenging discussions with other members of the Neet lab who indirectly contributed to this review. Finally, we would like to acknowledge the collegiality of the investigators in the neurotrophin field and all of their accomplishments that are summarized in this review.

## 10. Nomenclature

7-84-103, NGF mutein, F7A/H84A/R103A
Aβ, beta amyloid
AD, Alzheimer's disease
APP, amyloid precursor protein
Akt, a ser-thr kinase (also PKB)
BDNF, brain derived neurotrophic factor
BBB, blood brain barrier
CBF, cholinergic basal forebrain
ECD, extracellular domain
EGF, epidermal growth factor
EGFR, EGF receptor
GSK3b, glycogen synthase kinase 3b
ICD, intracellular domain
IGF-1, insulin like growth factor 1
JNK, c-Jun N-terminal kinase
KKE, K32A/K34A/E35A NGF mutein
KKE/7-84-103, hextuple mutein, K32A/K34A/E35A/F7A/H84A/R103A NGF mutein
MAPK, mitogen-activated protein kinase
NF-κB, Nuclear factor kappa-light-chain-enhancer of activated B cells
NGF, nerve growth factor (β-subunit)
NT-3, neurotrophin 3
NT-4, neurotrophin 4
p75, common neurotrophin receptor
PC12, pheochromocytoma 12 cell line
PI3K, phosphoinositide 3-kinase
PLCγ, phospholipase C gamma
proNGF, precursor form of NGF
TNFα, tumor necrosis factor alpha
Trk, tropomyosin related kinase
Δ9/13, NGF mutein with residues 9 through 13 deleted

## 11. References

Aboulkassim, T., Tong, X.-K., Tse, Y. C., Wong, T.-P., Woo, S. B., Neet, K. E., Brahimi, F., Hamel, E., & Saragovi, H. U. (2011). Ligand-dependent TrkA activity in brain impacts differently on spatial learning and long-term memory. *Molecular Pharmacology*, DOI 10.1124/mol.111.071332 in press.

Alam, M.I., Beg, S., Samad, A., Baboota, S., Kohli, K., Ali, J., Ahuja, A., & Akbar, M. (2010). Strategy for effective brain drug delivery. *European Journal of Pharmaceutical Sciences*, Vol. 40, No. 5, pp. 385-403.

Aloyz, R.S., Bamji, S.X., Pozniak, C.D., Toma, J.G., Atwal, J., Kaplan, D.R., & Miller, F.D. (1998). p53 is essential for developmental neuron death as regulated by the TrkA and p75 neurotrophin receptors. *Journal of Cell Biology*, Vol. 143, No. 6, pp. 1691-1703.

Apfel, S.C. (2002). Nerve growth factor for the treatment of diabetic neuropathy: what went wrong, what went right, and what does the future hold? *International Review of Neurobiology*, Vol. 50, pp. 393-413.

Apfel, S.C., Kessler, J.A., Adornato, B.T., Litchy, W.J., Sanders, C., & Rask, C.A. (1998). Recombinant human nerve growth factor in the treatment of diabetic polyneuropathy. NGF Study Group. *Neurology*, Vol. 51, No. 3, pp. 695-702.

Apfel, S.C., Lipton, R.B., Arezzo, J.C., & Kessler, J.A. (1991). Nerve growth factor prevents toxic neuropathy in mice. *Annals of Neurology*, Vol. 29, No. 1, pp. 87-90.

Bae, J., & Schlessinger, J. (2010). Asymmetric tyrosine kinase arrangements in activation or autophosphorylation of receptor tyrosine kinases. *Molecules and Cells*, Vol. 29, No. 5, pp. 443-448.

Bai, Y., Dergham, P., Nedev, H., Xu, J., Galan, A., Rivera, J. C., ZhiHua, S., Mehta, H. M., Woo, S. B., Sarunic, M. V., Neet, K. E., & Saragovi, H. U. (2010). Chronic and acute models of retinal neurodegeneration of TrkA activity are neuroprotective whereas p75NTR activity is neurotoxic through a paracrine mechanism. *Journal of Biological Chemistry*, Vol. 285, No. 50, pp. 39392-39400.

Bamji, S.X., Majdan, M., Pozniak, C.D., Belliveau, D.J., Aloyz, R., Kohn, J., Causing, C.G., & Miller, F.D. (1998). The p75 neurotrophin receptor mediates neuronal apoptosis and is essential for naturally occurring sympathetic neuron death. *J Cell Biol*, Vol. 140, No. 4, pp. 911-923.

Barrett, G.L., & Bartlett, P.F. (1994). The p75 nerve growth factor receptor mediates survival or death depending on the stage of sensory neuron development. *Proceedings of the National Academy of Sciences, U.S.A.*, Vol. 91, No. 14, pp. 6501-6505.

Bartlett, S.E., Reynolds, A.J., Weible, M., Heydon, K., & Hendry, I.A. (1997). In sympathetic but not sensory neurones, phosphoinositide-3 kinase is important for NGF-dependent survival and the retrograde transport of 125I-betaNGF. *Brain Research*, Vol. 761, No. 2, pp. 257-262.

Beglova, N., Maliartchouk, S., Ekiel, I., Zaccaro, M.C., Saragovi, H.U., & Gehring, K. (2000). Design and Solution Structure of Functional Peptide Mimetics of Nerve Growth Factor. *Journal of Medicinal Chemistry*, Vol. 43, No. 19, pp. 3530-3540.

Benedict, C., Frey, W.H., 2nd, Schioth, H.B., Schultes, B., Born, J., & Hallschmid, M. (2011). Intranasal insulin as a therapeutic option in the treatment of cognitive impairments. *Experimental Gerontology*, Vol. 46, No. 2-3, pp. 112-115.

Bibel, M., & Barde, Y.A. (2000). Neurotrophins: key regulators of cell fate and cell shape in the vertebrate nervous system. *Genes & Development*, Vol. 14, No. 23, pp. 2919-2937.

Bierer, L.M., Haroutunian, V., Gabriel, S., Knott, P.J., Carlin, L.S., Purohit, D.P., Perl, D.P., Schmeidler, J., Kanof, P., & Davis, K.L. (1995). Neurochemical correlates of dementia severity in Alzheimer's disease: relative importance of the cholinergic deficits. *Journal of Neurochemistry*, Vol. 64, No. 2, pp. 749-760.

Bishop, K.M., Hofer, E.K., Mehta, A., Ramirez, A., Sun, L., Tuszynski, M., & Bartus, R.T. (2008). Therapeutic potential of CERE-110 (AAV2-NGF): targeted, stable, and sustained NGF delivery and trophic activity on rodent basal forebrain cholinergic neurons. *Experimental Neurology*, Vol. 211, No. 2, pp. 574-584.

Bottger, D., Ullrich, C., & Humpel, C. (2010). Monocytes deliver bioactive nerve growth factor through a brain capillary endothelial cell-monolayer in vitro and counteract degeneration of cholinergic neurons. *Brain Research*, Vol. 1312, pp. 108-119.

Brahimi, F., Liu, J., Malakhov, A., Chowdhury, S., Purisima, E.O., Ivanisevic, L., Caron, A., Burgess, K., & Saragovi, H.U. (2010). A monovalent agonist of TrkA tyrosine kinase receptors can be converted into a bivalent antagonist. *Biochimica et Biophysica Acta (BBA) - General Subjects*, Vol. 1800, No. 9, pp. 1018-1026.

Brahimi, F., Malakhov, A., Lee, H. B., Pattarawarapan, M., Ivanisevic, L., Burgess, K., & Saragovi, H. U. (2009). A peptidomimetic of NT-3 acts as a TrkC antagonist. *Peptides*, Vol. 30, No. 10, pp. 1833-1839.

Bruno, M. A., Clarke, P. B., Seltzer, A., Quirion, R., Burgess, K., Cuello, A. C., & Saragovi, H. U. (2004). Long-lasting rescue of age-associated deficits in cognition and the CNS cholinergic phenotype by a partial agonist peptidomimetic ligand of TrkA. *Journal of Neuroscience*, Vol. 24, No. 37, pp. 8009-8018.

Calissano, P., Amadoro, G., Matrone, C., Ciafrè, S., Marolda, R., Corsetti, V., Ciotti, M. T., Mercanti, D., Di Luzio, A., Severini, C., Provenzano, C., & Canu, N. (2010a) Does the term trophic actually mean anti-amyloidogenic? The case of NGF. *Cell Death & Differentiation* Vol. 17, No. 7, pp. 1126-33.

Calissano, P., Matrone, C., & Amadoro, G. (2010b). Nerve growth factor as a paradigm of neurotrophins related to Alzheimer's disease. *Developmental Neurobiology*, Vol. 70, No. 5, pp. 372-383.

Canossa, M., Griesbeck, O., Berninger, B., Campana, G., Kolbeck, R., & Thoenen, H. (1997). Neurotrophin release by neurotrophins: implications for activity-dependent neuronal plasticity. *Proceedings of the National Academy of Sciences, U.S.A.*, Vol. 94, No. 24, pp. 13279-13286.

Capsoni, S., Covaceuszach, S., Marinelli, S., Ceci, M., Bernardo, A., Minghetti, L., Ugolini, G., Pavone, F., & Cattaneo, A. (2011). Taking Pain Out of NGF: A "Painless" NGF Mutant, Linked to Hereditary Sensory Autonomic Neuropathy Type V, with Full Neurotrophic Activity. *PLoS ONE*, Vol. 6, No. 2, pp. e17321.

Casaccia-Bonnefil, P., Carter, B.D., Dobrowsky, R.T., & Chao, M.V. (1996). Death of oligodendrocytes mediated by the interaction of nerve growth factor with its receptor p75. *Nature*, Vol. 383, No. 6602, pp. 716-719.

Casademunt, E., Carter, B.D., Benzel, I., Frade, J.M., Dechant, G., & Barde, Y.A. (1999). The zinc finger protein NRIF interacts with the neurotrophin receptor p75(NTR) and participates in programmed cell death. *EMBO Journal*, Vol. 18, No. 21, pp. 6050-6061.

Cattaneo, A., Capsoni, S., & Paoletti, F. (2008). Towards Non Invasive Nerve Growth Factor Therapies for Alzheimer's Disease. *Journal of Alzheimer's Disease*, Vol. 15, No. 2, pp. 255-283.

Chen, D., Brahimi, F., Angell, Y., Li, Y. C., Moscowicz, J., Saragovi, H. U., & Burgess, K. (2009). Bivalent peptidomimetic ligands of TrkC are biased agonists and selectively induce neuritogenesis or potentiate neurotrophin-3 trophic signals. *ACS Chemical Biology*, Vol. 4, No. 9, pp. 769-781.

Chittka, A., & Chao, M.V. (1999). Identification of a zinc finger protein whose subcellular distribution is regulated by serum and nerve growth factor. *Proceedings of the National Academy of Sciences, U.S.A.*, Vol. 96, No. 19, pp. 10705-10710.

Colangelo, A. M., Bianco, M. R., Vitagliano, L., Cavaliere, C., Cirillo, G., De Gioia, L., Diana, D., Colombo, D., Redaelli, C., Zaccaro, L., Morelli, G., Papa, M., Sarmientos, P., Alberghina, L., & Martegani, E. (2008). A new nerve growth factor-mimetic peptide active on neuropathic pain in rats. *Journal of Neuroscience*, Vol. 28, No. 11, pp. 2698-2709.

Cordon-Cardo, C., Tapley, P., Jing, S.Q., Nanduri, V., O'Rourke, E., Lamballe, F., Kovary, K., Klein, R., Jones, K.R., Reichardt, L.F., & Barbacid, M. (1991). The trk tyrosine protein kinase mediates the mitogenic properties of nerve growth factor and neurotrophin-3. *Cell*, Vol. 66, No. 1, pp. 173-183.

Coulson, J., May, L. M., Sykes, A. M., & Hamlin, A. S. (2009). The role of the p75 neurotrophin receptor in cholinergic dysfunction in Alzheimer's disease. *Neuroscientist*, Vol. 15, No. 4, pp. 317-23.

Covaceuszach, S., Capsoni, S., Marinelli, S., Pavone, F., Ceci, M., Ugolini, G., Vignone, D., Amato, G., Paoletti, F., Lamba, D., & Cattaneo, A. (2010). In vitro receptor binding properties of a "painless" NGF mutein, linked to hereditary sensory autonomic neuropathy type V. *Biochemical and Biophysical Research Communications*, Vol. 391, No. 1, pp. 824-829.

Crowder, R.J., & Freeman, R.S. (1998). Phosphatidylinositol 3-kinase and Akt protein kinase are necessary and sufficient for the survival of nerve growth factor-dependent sympathetic neurons. *Journal of Neuroscience*, Vol. 18, No. 8, pp. 2933-2943.

Cuello, A., Bruno, M., Allard, S., Leon, W., & Iulita, M. (2010). Cholinergic Involvement in Alzheimer's Disease. A Link with NGF Maturation and Degradation. *Journal of Molecular Neuroscience*, Vol. 40, No. 1, pp. 230-235.

Cunningham, M.E., & Greene, L.A. (1998). A function-structure model for NGF-activated TRK. *EMBO Journal*, Vol. 17, No. 24, pp. 7282-7293.

Cunningham, M.E., Stephens, R.M., Kaplan, D.R., & Greene, L.A. (1997). Autophosphorylation of activation loop tyrosines regulates signaling by the TRK nerve growth factor receptor. *Journal of Biological Chemistry*, Vol. 272, No. 16, pp. 10957-10967.

Davey, F., & Davies, A.M. (1998). TrkB signalling inhibits p75-mediated apoptosis induced by nerve growth factor in embryonic proprioceptive neurons. *Current Biology*, Vol. 8, No. 16, pp. 915-918.

de Chaves, E.I., Bussiere, M., Vance, D.E., Campenot, R.B., & Vance, J.E. (1997). Elevation of ceramide within distal neurites inhibits neurite growth in cultured rat sympathetic neurons. *Journal of Biological Chemistry*, Vol. 272, No. 5, pp. 3028-3035.

Dechant, G., Barde, Y. A. (2002). The neurotrophin receptor p75(NTR): novel functions and implications for diseases of the nervous system. *Nature Neuroscience*, Vol. 5, No. 11, pp. 1131-1136.

DeKosky, S.T., Ikonomovic, M.D., Styren, S.D., Beckett, L., Wisniewski, S., Bennett, D.A., Cochran, E.J., Kordower, J.H., & Mufson, E.J. (2002). Upregulation of choline acetyltransferase activity in hippocampus and frontal cortex of elderly subjects with mild cognitive impairment. *Annals of Neurology*, Vol. 51, No. 2, pp. 145-155.

Diamond, J., Foerster, A., Holmes, M., & Coughlin, M. (1992). Sensory nerves in adult rats regenerate and restore sensory function to the skin independently of endogenous NGF. *Journal of Neuroscience*, Vol. 12, No. 4, pp. 1467-1476.

Diarra, A., Geetha, T., Potter, P., & Babu, J. R. (2009). Signaling of the neurotrophin receptor p75 in relation to Alzheimer's disease. *Biochemical and Biophysical Research Communications*, Vol. 390, No. 3, pp. 352-356.

Domeniconi, M., Zampieri, N., Spencer, T., Hilaire, M., Mellado, W., Chao, M.V., & Filbin, M.T. (2005). MAG induces regulated intramembrane proteolysis of the p75 neurotrophin receptor to inhibit neurite outgrowth. *Neuron*, Vol. 46, No. 6, pp. 849-855.

Einarsdottir, E., Carlsson, A., Minde, J., Toolanen, G., Svensson, O., Solders, G., Holmgren, G., Holmberg, D., & Holmberg, M. (2004). A mutation in the nerve growth factor beta gene (NGFB) causes loss of pain perception. *Human Molecular Genetics*, Vol. 13, No. 8, pp. 799-805.

Emerich, D.F., Winn, S.R., Harper, J., Hammang, J.P., Baetge, E.E., & Kordower, J.H. (1994). Implants of polymer-encapsulated human NGF-secreting cells in the nonhuman primate: rescue and sprouting of degenerating cholinergic basal forebrain neurons. *Journal of Computational Neurology*, Vol. 349, No. 1, pp. 148-164.

Emilien, G., Maloteaux, J.M., Beyreuther, K., & Masters, C.L. (2000). Alzheimer disease: mouse models pave the way for therapeutic opportunities. *Archives of Neurology*, Vol. 57, No. 2, pp. 176-181.

Eriksdotter Jonhagen, M., Nordberg, A., Amberla, K., Backman, L., Ebendal, T., Meyerson, B., Olson, L., Seiger, Shigeta, M., Theodorsson, E., Viitanen, M., Winblad, B., & Wahlund, L. O. (1998). Intracerebroventricular infusion of nerve growth factor in three patients with Alzheimer's disease. *Dementia and Geriatric Cognitive Disorders*, Vol. 9, No. 5, pp. 246-257.

Fahnestock, M., Michalski, B., Xu, B., & Coughlin, M.D. (2001). The Precursor Pro-Nerve Growth Factor Is the Predominant Form of Nerve Growth Factor in Brain and Is Increased in Alzheimer's Disease. *Molecular and Cellular Neuroscience*, Vol. 18, No. 2, pp. 210-220.

Fan, Y.-X., Wong, L., Deb, T.B., & Johnson, G.R. (2004). Ligand Regulates Epidermal Growth Factor Receptor Kinase Specificity. *Journal of Biological Chemistry*, Vol. 279, No. 37, pp. 38143-38150.

Fjord-Larsen, L., Kusk, P., Tornoe, J., Juliusson, B., Torp, M., Bjarkam, C.R., Nielsen, M.S., Handberg, A., Sorensen, J.C.H., & Wahlberg, L.U. (2010). Long-term Delivery of Nerve Growth Factor by Encapsulated Cell Biodelivery in the Gottingen Minipig Basal Forebrain. *Molecular Therapy*, Vol. 18, No. 12, pp. 2164-2172.

Fletcher, J. M., Morton, C. J., Zwar, R. A., Murray, S. S., O'Leary, P. D., & Hughes, R. A. (2008). Design of a conformationally defined and proteolytically stable circular mimetic of brain-derived neurotrophic factor. *Journal of Biological Chemistry*, Vol. 283, No 48, pp. 33375-33383.

Fletcher, J. M. & Hughes, R. A. (2009). Modified low molecular weight cyclic peptides as mimetics of BDNF with improved potency, proteolytic stability and transmembrane passage in vitro. *Bioorganic Medicinal Chemistry*, Vol. 17, No. 7, pp. 2695-2702.

Friden, P., Walus, L., Watson, P., Doctrow, Kozarich, J., Backman, C., Bergman, H., Hoffer, B., Bloom, F., & Granholm, A. (1993). Blood-brain barrier penetration and in vivo activity of an NGF conjugate. *Science*, Vol. 259, No. 5093, pp. 373-377.

Friedman, W.J., & Greene, L.A. (1999). Neurotrophin signaling via Trks and p75. *Experimental Cell Research*, Vol. 253, No. 1, pp. 131-142.

Funakoshi, H., Risling, M., Carlstedt, T., Lendahl, U., Timmusk, T., Metsis, M., Yamamoto, Y., & Ibanez, C. F. (1998). Targeted expression of a multifunctional chimeric neurotrophin in the lesioned sciatic nerve accelerates regeneration of sensory and motor axons. *Proceedings of the National Academy of Sciences, U.S.A.*, Vol. 95, No. 9, pp. 5269-5274.

Garzon, D.J., & Fahnestock, M. (2007). Oligomeric Amyloid Decreases Basal Levels of Brain-Derived Neurotrophic factor (BDNF) mRNA via Specific Downregulation of BDNF Transcripts IV and V in Differentiated Human Neuroblastoma Cells. *The Journal of Neuroscience*, Vol. 27, No. 10, pp. 2628-2635.

Gerspach, J., Pfizenmaier, K., & Wajant, H. (2009). Improving TNF as a cancer therapeutic: tailor-made TNF fusion proteins with conserved antitumor activity and reduced systemic side effects. *Biofactors*. 35, No. 4, pp. 364-372.

Ginsberg, S.D., Che, S., Wuu, J., Counts, S.E., & Mufson, E.J. (2006). Down regulation of trk but not p75NTR gene expression in single cholinergic basal forebrain neurons mark the progression of Alzheimer's disease. *Journal of Neurochemistry*, Vol. 97, No. 2, pp. 475-487.

Gomez, N., & Cohen, P. (1991). Dissection of the protein kinase cascade by which nerve growth factor activates MAP kinases. *Nature*, Vol. 353, No. 6340, pp. 170-173.

Grewal, S.S., York, R.D., & Stork, P.J. (1999). Extracellular-signal-regulated kinase signalling in neurons. *Current Opinion in Neurobiology*, Vol. 9, No. 5, pp. 544-553.

Grimes, M.L., Beattie, E., & Mobley, W.C. (1997). A signaling organelle containing the nerve growth factor-activated receptor tyrosine kinase, TrkA. *Proceedings of the National Academy of Sciences, U.S.A.*, Vol. 94, No. 18, pp. 9909-9914.

Guo, M., Meyer, S.L., Kaur, H., Gao, J.J., & Neet, K.E. (1996). Mutational studies of conserved residues in the dimer interface of nerve growth factor. *Protein Science*, Vol. 5, No. 3, pp. 447-455.

Hefti, F. (1983). Is Alzheimer disease caused by lack of nerve growth factor? *Annals of Neurology*, Vol. 13, No. 1, pp. 109-110.

Holgado-Madruga, M., Moscatello, D.K., Emlet, D.R., Dieterich, R., & Wong, A.J. (1997). Grb2-associated binder-1 mediates phosphatidylinositol 3-kinase activation and the promotion of cell survival by nerve growth factor. *Proceedings of the National Academy of Sciences, U.S.A.*, Vol. 94, No. 23, pp. 12419-12424.

Hua, Q. X., Nakagawa, S. H., Jia, W., Huang, K., Phillips, N. B., Hu, S. Q., & Weiss, M. A. (2008). Design of an active ultrastable single-chain insulin analog: synthesis, structure, and therapeutic implications. *Journal of Biological Chemistry*, Vol. 283, No. 21, pp. 14703-14716.

Huang, E.J., & Reichardt, L.F. (2003). Trk receptors: roles in neuronal signal transduction. *Annual Review of Biochemistry*, Vol. 72, pp. 609-642.

Hubbard, S.R., Wei, L., Ellis, L., & Hendrickson, W.A. (1994). Crystal structure of the tyrosine kinase domain of the human insulin receptor. *Nature*, Vol. 372, No. 6508, pp. 746-754.

Hughes, A. L., Messineo-Jones, D., Lad, S. P., & Neet, K. E. (2001). Distinction between differentiation, cell cycle, and apoptosis signals in PC12 cells by the nerve growth factor mutant delta9/13, which is selective for the p75 neurotrophin receptor. *Journal of Neuroscience Research*, Vol. 63, No. 1, pp. 10-19.

Hyman, C., Hofer, M., Barde, Y.-A., Juhasz, M., Yancopoulos, G.D., Squinto, S.P., & Lindsay, R.M. (1991). BDNF is a neurotrophic factor for dopaminergic neurons of the substantia nigra. *Nature*, Vol. 350, No. 6315, pp. 230-232.

Ibanez, C.F., Hallbook, F., Ebendal, T., & Persson, H. (1990). Structure-function studies of nerve growth factor: functional importance of highly conserved amino acid residues. *EMBO Journal*, Vol. 9, No. 5, pp. 1477-1483.

Ibanez, C.F., Ebendal, T., & Persson, H. (1991). Chimeric molecules with multiple neurotrophic activities reveal structural elements determining the specificities of NGF and BDNF. *EMBO Journal*, Vol. 10, No. 8, pp. 2105-2110.

Ibanez, C.F., Ebendal, T., Barbany, G., Murray-Rust, J., Blundell, T.L., & Persson, H. (1992). Disruption of the low affinity receptor-binding site in NGF allows neuronal survival and differentiation by binding to the trk gene product. *Cell*, Vol. 69, No. 2, pp. 329-341.

Ibanez, C.F., Ilag, L.L., Murray-Rust, J., & Persson, H. (1993). An extended surface of binding to Trk tyrosine kinase receptors in NGF and BDNF allows the engineering of a multifunctional pan-neurotrophin. *EMBO Journal*, Vol. 12, No. 6, pp. 2281-2293.

Ibanez, C.F. (1994). Structure-function relationships in the neurotrophin family. *Journal of Neurobiolgy*, Vol. 25, No. 11, pp. 1349-1361.

Ilag, L.L., Lonnerberg, P., Persson, H., & Ibanez, C.F. (1994). Role of variable beta-hairpin loop in determining biological specificities in neurotrophin family. *Journal of Biological Chemistry*, Vol. 269, No. 31, pp. 19941-19946.

Ilag, L. L., Curtis, R., Glass, D., Funakoshi, H., Tobkes, N. J., Ryan, T. E., Acheson, A., Lindsay, R. M., Persson, H., Yancopoulos, G. D., DiStefano, P. S. & Ibanez, C. F. (1995). Pan-neurotrophin 1: a genetically engineered neurotrophic factor displaying multiple specificities in peripheral neurons in vitro and in vivo. *Proceedings of the National Academy of Sciences, U.S.A.*, Vol. 92, No. 2, pp. 607-611.

Indo, Y. (2002). Genetics of congenital insensitivity to pain with anhidrosis (CIPA) or hereditary sensory and autonomic neuropathy type IV. Clinical, biological and molecular aspects of mutations in TRKA(NTRK1) gene encoding the receptor tyrosine kinase for nerve growth factor. *Clinical Autonomic Research*, Vol. 12, Suppl 1, pp. I20-32.

Jordão, J.F., Ayala-Grosso, C.A., Markham, K., Huang, Y., Chopra, R., McLaurin, J., Hynynen, K., & Aubert, I. (2010). Antibodies Targeted to the Brain with Image-Guided Focused Ultrasound Reduces Amyloid-β Plaque Load in the TgCRND8 Mouse Model of Alzheimer's Disease. *PLoS ONE*, Vol. 5, No. 5, pp. e10549.

Jura, N., Zhang, X., Endres, Nicholas F., Seeliger, Markus A., Schindler, T., & Kuriyan, J. (2011). Catalytic Control in the EGF Receptor and Its Connection to General Kinase Regulatory Mechanisms. *Molecular Cell*, Vol. 42, No. 1, pp. 9-22.

Kahle, P., Burton, L.E., Schmelzer, C.H., & Hertel, C. (1992). The amino terminus of nerve growth factor is involved in the interaction with the receptor tyrosine kinase p140trkA. *Journal of Biological Chemistry*, Vol. 267, No. 32, pp. 22707-22710.

Kao, S., Jaiswal, R.K., Kolch, W., & Landreth, G.E. (2001). Identification of the mechanisms regulating the differential activation of the mapk cascade by epidermal growth factor and nerve growth factor in PC12 cells. *Journal of Biological Chemistry*, Vol. 276, No. 21, pp. 18169-18177.

Kaplan, D.R., Hempstead, B.L., Martin-Zanca, D., Chao, M.V., & Parada, L.F. (1991). The trk proto-oncogene product: a signal transducing receptor for nerve growth factor. *Science*, Vol. 252, No. 5005, pp. 554-558.

Kaplan, D.R., & Miller, F.D. (2000). Neurotrophin signal transduction in the nervous system. *Current Opinion in Neurobiology*, Vol. 10, No. 3, pp. 381-391.

Katz, D.M., Erb, M., Lillis, R., & Neet, K. (1990). Trophic regulation of nodose ganglion cell development: evidence for an expanded role of nerve growth factor during embryogenesis in the rat. *Experimental Neurology*, Vol. 110, No. 1, pp. 1-10.

Khursigara, G., Orlinick, J.R., & Chao, M.V. (1999). Association of the p75 neurotrophin receptor with TRAF6. *Journal of Biological Chemistry*, Vol. 274, No. 5, pp. 2597-2600.

Korsching, S. (1993). The neurotrophic factor concept: a reexamination. *Journal of Neuroscience*, Vol. 13, No. 7, pp. 2739-2748.

Kullander, K., & Ebendal, T. (1994). Neurotrophin-3 acquires NGF-like activity after exchange to five NGF amino acid residues: molecular analysis of the sites in NGF mediating the specific interaction with the NGF high affinity receptor. *Journal of Neuroscience Research*, Vol. 39, No. 2, pp. 195-210.

Kullander, K., Kaplan, D., & Ebendal, T. (1997). Two restricted sites on the surface of the nerve growth factor molecule independently determine specific TrkA receptor binding and activation. *Journal of Biological Chemistry*, Vol. 272, No. 14, pp. 9300-9307.

Lad, S. P. & Neet, K. E. (2003). Activation of the mitogen-activated protein kinase pathway through p75NTR: a common mechanism for the neurotrophin family. *Journal of Neuroscience Research*, Vol. 73, No. 5, pp. 614-626.

Lad, S.P., Neet, K.E., & Mufson, E.J. (2003a). Nerve growth factor: structure, function and therapeutic implications for Alzheimer's disease. *Current Drug Targets- CNS and Neurological Disorders*, Vol. 2, No. 5, pp. 315-334.

Lad, S.P., Peterson, D.A., Bradshaw, R.A., & Neet, K.E. (2003b). Individual and combined effects of TrkA and p75NTR nerve growth factor receptors. A role for the high affinity receptor site. *Journal of Biological Chemistry*, Vol. 278, No. 27, pp. 24808-24817.

Lane, N.E., Schnitzer, T.J., Birbara, C.A., Mokhtarani, M., Shelton, D.L., Smith, M.D., & Brown, M.T. (2010). Tanezumab for the Treatment of Pain from Osteoarthritis of the Knee. *New England Journal of Medicine*, Vol. 363, No. 16, pp. 1521-1531.

Lemmon, M.A., & Schlessinger, J. (2010). Cell Signaling by Receptor Tyrosine Kinases. *Cell*, Vol. 141, No. 7, pp. 1117-1134.

LeSauteur, L., Wei, L., Gibbs, B.F., & Saragovi, H.U. (1995). Small Peptide Mimics of Nerve Growth Factor Bind TrkA Receptors and Affect Biological Responses. *Journal of Biological Chemistry*, Vol. 270, No. 12, pp. 6564-6569.

Levi-Montalcini, R. (1987). The nerve growth factor 35 years later. *Science*, Vol. 237, No. 4819, pp. 1154-1162.

Liao, G.S., Li, X.B., Zhang, C.Y., Shu, Y.Y., & Tang, S.X. (2001). Pharmacological actions of nerve growth factor-transferrin conjugate on the central nervous system. *Journal of Natural Toxins*, Vol. 10, No. 4, pp. 291-297.

Lindsay, R.M. (1988). Nerve growth factors (NGF, BDNF) enhance axonal regeneration but are not required for survival of adult sensory neurons. *Journal of Neuroscience,* Vol. 8, No. 7, pp. 2394-2405.

Liu, J., Brahimi, F., Saragovi, H. U., & Burgess K. (2010) Bivalent diketopiperazine-based tropomysin receptor kinase C (TrkC) antagonists. *Journal of Medicinal Chemistry,* Vol. 53, No. 13, pp. 5044-5048.

Loeb, D.M., Stephens, R.M., Copeland, T., Kaplan, D.R., & Greene, L.A. (1994). A Trk nerve growth factor (NGF) receptor point mutation affecting interaction with phospholipase C-gamma 1 abolishes NGF-promoted peripherin induction but not neurite outgrowth. *Journal of Biological Chemistry,* Vol. 269, No. 12, pp. 8901-8910.

Longo, F. M., Yang, T., Knowles, J. K., Xie, Y., Moore, L. A., & Massa, S. M. (2007). Small molecule neurotrophin receptor ligands: novel strategies for targeting Alzheimer's disease mechanisms. *Currents in Alzheimer Research,* Vol 4, No. 5, pp. 503-506.

Mahapatra, S. (2008). *Identification of Critical Residues within the Conserved and Specificity Patches of Nerve Growth Factor Leading to Survival or Differentiation.* Ph.D. Thesis, Rosalind Franklin University of Medicine and Science, North Chicago.

Mahapatra, S., Mehta, H., Woo, S.B., & Neet, K.E. (2009). Identification of Critical Residues within the Conserved and Specificity Patches of Nerve Growth Factor Leading to Survival or Differentiation. *Journal of Biological Chemistry,* Vol. 284, No. 48, pp. 33600-33613.

Maliartchouk, S., Debeir, T., Beglova, N., Cuello, A.C., Gehring, K., & Saragovi, H.U. (2000). Genuine Monovalent Ligands of TrkA Nerve Growth Factor Receptors Reveal a Novel Pharmacological Mechanism of Action. *Journal of Biological Chemistry,* Vol. 275, No. 14, pp. 9946-9956.

Massa, S.M., Xie, Y., Yang, T., Harrington, A.W., Kim, M.L., Yoon, S.O., Kraemer, R., Moore, L.A., Hempstead, B.L., & Longo, F.M. (2006). Small, Nonpeptide p75NTR Ligands Induce Survival Signaling and Inhibit proNGF-Induced Death. *The Journal of Neuroscience,* Vol. 26, No. 20, pp. 5288-5300.

Massa, S.M., Yang, T., Xie, Y., Shi, J., Bilgen, M., Joyce, J.N., Nehama, D., Rajadas, J., & Longo, F.M. (2010). Small molecule BDNF mimetics activate TrkB signaling and prevent neuronal degeneration in rodents. *The Journal of Clinical Investigation,* Vol. 120, No. 5, pp. 1774-1785.

McDonald, N.Q., Lapatto, R., Murray-Rust, J., Gunning, J., Wlodawer, A., & Blundell, T.L. (1991). New protein fold revealed by a 2.3-A resolution crystal structure of nerve growth factor. *Nature,* Vol. 354, No. 6352, pp. 411-414.

Mufson, E.J., Conner, J.M., & Kordower, J.H. (1995). Nerve growth factor in Alzheimer's disease: defective retrograde transport to nucleus basalis. *Neuroreport,* Vol. 6, No. 7, pp. 1063-1066.

Mufson, E.J., Counts, S.E., Fahnestock, M., & Ginsberg, S.D. (2007). Cholinotrophic molecular substrates of mild cognitive impairment in the elderly. *Current Alzheimer Research,* Vol. 4, No. 4, pp. 340-350.

Mufson, E.J., Counts, S.E., Perez, S.E., & Ginsberg, S.D. (2008). Cholinergic system during the progression of Alzheimer's disease: therapeutic implications. *Expert Review of Neurotherapeutics,* Vol. 8, No. 11, pp. 1703-1718.

Mufson, E.J., Ma, S.Y., Cochran, E.J., Bennett, D.A., Beckett, L.A., Jaffar, S., Saragovi, H.U., & Kordower, J.H. (2000). Loss of nucleus basalis neurons containing trkA immunoreactivity in individuals with mild cognitive impairment and early Alzheimer's disease. *Journal of Computational Neurology*, Vol. 427, No. 1, pp. 19-30.

Mufson, E.J., Ma, S.Y., Dills, J., Cochran, E.J., Leurgans, S., Wuu, J., Bennett, D.A., Jaffar, S., Gilmor, M.L., Levey, A.I., & Kordower, J.H. (2002). Loss of basal forebrain p75NTR immunoreactivity in subjects with mild cognitive impairment and Alzheimer's disease. *The Journal of Comparative Neurology*, Vol. 443, No. 2, pp. 136-153.

Muller, G., Storz, P., Bourteele, S., Doppler, H., Pfizenmaier, K., Mischak, H., Philipp, A., Kaiser, C., & Kolch, W. (1998). Regulation of Raf-1 kinase by TNF via its second messenger ceramide and cross-talk with mitogenic signalling. *EMBO Journal*, Vol. 17, No. 3, pp. 732-742.

Nagahara, A.H., & Tuszynski, M.H. (2011). Potential therapeutic uses of BDNF in neurological and psychiatric disorders. *Nature Reviews Drug Discovery*, Vol. 10, No. 3, pp. 209-219.

Nicol, G.D., & Vasko, M.R. (2007). Unraveling the Story of NGF-mediated Sensitization of Nociceptive Sensory Neurons: ON or OFF the Trks? *Molecular Interventions*, Vol. 7, No. 1, pp. 26-41.

Nilsson, P., Iwata, N., Muramatsu, S.-i., Tjernberg, L.O., Winblad, B., & Saido, T.C. (2010). Gene therapy in Alzheimer's disease - potential for disease modification. *Journal of Cellular and Molecular Medicine*, Vol. 14, No. 4, pp. 741-757.

Ninkina, N., Grashchuck, M., Buchman, V.L., & Davies, A.M. (1997). TrkB variants with deletions in the leucine-rich motifs of the extracellular domain. *Journal of Biological Chemistry*, Vol. 272, No. 20, pp. 13019-13025.

O'Leary, P. D. & Hughes, R. A. (2003). Design of Potent Peptide Mimetics of Brain-derived Neurotrophic Factor. *Journal of Biological Chemistry*, Vol. 278, No. 28, pp. 25738–25744.

Parain, K., Murer, M.G., Yan, Q., Faucheux, B., Agid, Y., Hirsch, E., & Raisman-Vozari, R. (1999). Reduced expression of brain-derived neurotrophic factor protein in Parkinson's disease substantia nigra. *Neuroreport*, Vol. 10, No. 3, pp. 557-561.

Peleshok, J., & Saragovi, H.U. (2006). Functional mimetics of neurotrophins and their receptors. *Biochemical Society Transactions*, Vol. 34, No. Pt 4, pp. 612-617.

Peng, S., Wuu, J., Mufson, E.J., & Fahnestock, M. (2004). Increased proNGF Levels in Subjects with Mild Cognitive Impairment and Mild Alzheimer Disease. *Journal of Neuropathology & Experimental Neurology*, Vol. 63, No. 6, pp. 641-649.

Peng, S., Wuu, J., Mufson, E.J., & Fahnestock, M. (2005). Precursor form of brain-derived neurotrophic factor and mature brain-derived neurotrophic factor are decreased in the pre-clinical stages of Alzheimer's disease. *Journal of Neurochemistry*, Vol. 93, No. 6, pp. 1412-1421.

Pezet, S., & McMahon, S.B. (2006). Neurotrophins: Mediators and Modulators of Pain. *Annual Review of Neuroscience*, Vol. 29, pp. 507-538.

Phillips, N. B., Wan, Z. L., Whittaker, L., Hu, S. Q., Huang, K., Hua, Q. X , Whittaker, J., Ismail-Beigi, F., & Weiss, M. A. (2010). Supramolecular protein engineering: design of zinc-stapled insulin hexamers as a long acting depot. *Journal of Biological Chemistry*, Vol. 285, No. 16, pp. 11755-11759.

Qian, X., Riccio, A., Zhang, Y., & Ginty, D.D. (1998). Identification and characterization of novel substrates of Trk receptors in developing neurons. *Neuron*, Vol. 21, No. 5, pp. 1017-1029.

Rabizadeh, S., Oh, J., Zhong, L.T., Yang, J., Bitler, C.M., Butcher, L.L., & Bredesen, D.E. (1993). Induction of apoptosis by the low-affinity NGF receptor. *Science*, Vol. 261, No. 5119, pp. 345-348.

Rodriguez-Viciana, P., Warne, P.H., Dhand, R., Vanhaesebroeck, B., Gout, I., Fry, M.J., Waterfield, M.D., & Downward, J. (1994). Phosphatidylinositol-3-OH kinase as a direct target of Ras. *Nature*, Vol. 370, No. 6490, pp. 527-532.

Rydén, M., Hempstead, B., & Ibáñez, C. F. (1997). Differential modulation of neuron survival during development by nerve growth factor binding to the p75 neurotrophin receptor. *Journal of Biological Chemistry*, Vol. 272, No. 26, 16322-16328.

Salehi, A., Ocampo, M., Verhaagen, J., & Swaab, D.F. (2000). P75 neurotrophin receptor in the nucleus basalis of meynert in relation to age, sex, and Alzheimer's disease. *Experimental Neurology*, Vol. 161, No. 1, pp. 245-258.

Salehi, A. H., Xanthoudakis. S., & Barker, P. A. (2002). NRAGE, a p75 neurotrophin receptor-interacting protein, induces caspase activation and cell death through a JNK-dependent mitochondrial pathway. *Journal of Biological Chemistry*, Vol. 277, No. 50, pp. 48043-48050.

Saragovi, H.U., Hamel, E., & Di Polo, A. (2009). A neurotrophic rationale for the therapy of neurodegenerative disorders. *Current Alzheimer Research*, Vol. 6, No. 5, pp. 419-423.

Schecterson, L. C. & Bothwell, M. (2010). Neurotrophin receptors: Old friends with new partners. *Developmental Neurobiology*, Vol. 70, No. 5, pp. 332-338.

Schindowski, K., Belarbi, K., & Buée, L. (2008). Neurotrophic factors in Alzheimer's disease: role of axonal transport. *Genes, Brain and Behavior*, Vol. 7, pp. 43-56.

Schulte-Herbruggen, O., Jockers-Scherubl, M.C., & Hellweg, R. (2008). Neurotrophins: from pathophysiology to treatment in Alzheimer's disease. *Current Alzheimer Research*, Vol. 5, No. 1, pp. 38-44.

Scott, J., Selby, M., Urdea, M., Quiroga, M., Bell, G.I., & Rutter, W.J. (1983). Isolation and nucleotide sequence of a cDNA encoding the precursor of mouse nerve growth factor. *Nature*, Vol. 302, No. 5908, pp. 538-540.

Scott, S.A., Mufson, E.J., Weingartner, J.A., Skau, K.A., & Crutcher, K.A. (1995). Nerve growth factor in Alzheimer's disease: increased levels throughout the brain coupled with declines in nucleus basalis. *Journal of Neuroscience*, Vol. 15, No. 9, pp. 6213-6221.

Segal, R.A. (2003). Selectivity in neurotrophin signaling: theme and variations. *Annual Review of Neuroscience*, Vol. 26, pp. 299-330.

Shih, A., Laramee, G.R., Schmelzer, C.H., Burton, L.E., & Winslow, J.W. (1994). Mutagenesis identifies amino-terminal residues of nerve growth factor necessary for Trk receptor binding and biological activity. *Journal of Biological Chemistry*, Vol. 269, No. 44, pp. 27679-27686.

Simi, A., & Ibanez, C.F. (2010). Assembly and activation of neurotrophic factor receptor complexes. *Developmental Neurobiology*, Vol. 70, No. 5, pp. 323-331.

Soilu-Hanninen, M., Ekert, P., Bucci, T., Syroid, D., Bartlett, P.F., & Kilpatrick, T.J. (1999). Nerve growth factor signaling through p75 induces apoptosis in Schwann cells via a Bcl-2-independent pathway. *Journal of Neuroscience*, Vol. 19, No. 12, pp. 4828-4838.

Soppet, D., Escandon, E., Maragos, J., Middlemas, D.S., Reid, S.W., Blair, J., Burton, L.E., Stanton, B.R., Kaplan, D.R., Hunter, T., Nikolics, K., & Parada L.F. (1991). The neurotrophic factors brain-derived neurotrophic factor and neurotrophin-3 are ligands for the trkB tyrosine kinase receptor. *Cell*, Vol. 65, No. 5, pp. 895-903.

Susen K., Heumann, R., & Blöchl, A. (1999). Nerve growth factor stimulates MAPK via the low affinity receptor p75(LNTR). *FEBS Letters*. Vol. 463, No. 3, pp. 231-234.

Susen, K. & Blöchl, A. (2005). Low concentrations of aggregated beta-amyloid induce neurite formation via the neurotrophin receptor p75. *Journal of Molecular Medicine*, Vol. 83, No. 9, pp. 720-735.

Suter, U., Angst, C., Tien, C., Drinkwater, C., Lindsay, R., & Shooter, E. (1992). NGF/BDNF chimeric proteins: analysis of neurotrophin specificity by homolog-scanning mutagenesis. *The Journal of Neuroscience*, Vol. 12, No. 1, pp. 306-318.

Teng, K. K., Felice, S., Kim, T., & Hempstead, B. L. (2010). Understanding proneurotrophin actions: Recent advances and challenges. *Developmental Neurobiology*, Vol. 70, No. 5, pp. 350-359.

Thoenen, H., & Sendtner, M. (2002). Neurotrophins: from enthusiastic expectations through sobering experiences to rational therapeutic approaches. *Nature Neuroscience*, Vol. 5, No. 11s, pp. 1046-1050.

Tuszynski, M.H., Conner, J., Blesch, A., Smith, D., Merrill, D.A., & Vahlsing, H.L. (2002). New strategies in neural repair. *Progress in Brain Research*, Vol. 138, pp. 401-409.

Tuszynski, M.H., Thal, L., Pay, M., Salmon, D.P., U, H.S., Bakay, R., Patel, P., Blesch, A., Vahlsing, H.L., Ho, G., Tong, G., Potkin, S. G., Fallon, J., Hansen, L., Mufson, E. J., Kordower J. H., Gall, C., & Conner, J. (2005). A phase 1 clinical trial of nerve growth factor gene therapy for Alzheimer disease. *Nature Medicine*, Vol. 11, No. 5, pp. 551-5.

Urfer, R., Tsoulfas, P., O'Connell, L., & Presta, L.G. (1997). Specificity Determinants in Neurotrophin-3 and Design of Nerve Growth Factor-Based trkC Agonists by Changing Central β-Strand Bundle Residues to Their Neurotrophin-3 Analogs. *Biochemistry*, Vol. 36, No. 16, pp. 4775-4781.

Vilar, M., Charalampopoulos, I., Kenchappa, R.S., Reversi, A., Klos-Applequist, J.M., Karaca, E., Simi, A., Spuch, C., Choi, S., Friedman, W.J., Ericson, J., Schiavo, G., Carter, B. D., & Ibáñez, C. F. (2009). Ligand-independent signaling by disulfide-crosslinked dimers of the p75 neurotrophin receptor. *Journal of Cell Science*, Vol. 122, No. 18, pp. 3351-3357.

Wajant, H., Gerspach, J., & Pfizenmaier, K. (2005). Tumor therapeutics by design: targeting and activation of death receptors. *Cytokine Growth Factor Reviews*. Vol. 16, No. 1, pp. 55-76.

Walsh, G.S., Krol, K.M., Crutcher, K.A., & Kawaja, M.D. (1999). Enhanced neurotrophin-induced axon growth in myelinated portions of the CNS in mice lacking the p75 neurotrophin receptor. *Journal of Neuroscience*, Vol. 19, No. 10, pp. 4155-4168.

Wang, J.J., Rabizadeh, S., Tasinato, A., Sperandio, S., Ye, X., Green, M., Assa-Munt, N., Spencer, D., & Bredesen, D.E. (2000). Dimerization-dependent block of the proapoptotic effect of p75(NTR). *Journal of Neuroscience Research*, Vol. 60, No. 5, pp. 587-593.

Wiesmann, C., Ultsch, M.H., Bass, S.H., & de Vos, A.M. (1999). Crystal structure of nerve growth factor in complex with the ligand-binding domain of the TrkA receptor. *Nature*, Vol. 401, No. 6749, pp. 184-188.

Wiesmann, C., & de Vos, A.M. (2001). Nerve growth factor: structure and function. *Cellular and Molecular Life Sciences*, Vol. 58, No. 5-6, pp. 748-759.

Winkler, J., Ramirez, G.A., Kuhn, H.G., Peterson, D.A., Day-Lollini, P.A., Stewart, G.R., Tuszynski, M.H., Gage, F.H., & Thal, L.J. (1997). Reversible Schwann cell hyperplasia and sprouting of sensory and sympathetic neurites after intraventricular administration of nerve growth factor. *Annals of Neurology*, Vol. 41, No. 1, pp. 82-93.

Woo, S.B., Timm, D.E., & Neet, K.E. (1995). Alteration of NH2-terminal residues of nerve growth factor affects activity and Trk binding without affecting stability or conformation. *Journal of Biological Chemistry*, Vol. 270, No. 11, pp. 6278-6285.

Woo, S.B., & Neet, K.E. (1996). Characterization of histidine residues essential for receptor binding and activity of nerve growth factor. *Journal of Biological Chemistry*, Vol. 271, No. 40, pp. 24433-24441.

Wood, J.N. (2010). Nerve Growth Factor and Pain. *New England Journal of Medicine*, Vol. 363, No. 16, pp. 1572-1573.

Xie, Y., Tisi, M.A., Yeo, T.T., & Longo, F.M. (2000). Nerve Growth Factor (NGF) Loop 4 Dimeric Mimetics Activate ERK and AKT and Promote NGF-like Neurotrophic Effects. *Journal of Biological Chemistry*, Vol. 275, No. 38, pp. 29868-29874.

Yang, T., Knowles, J.K., Lu, Q., Zhang, H., Arancio, O., Moore, L.A., Chang, T., Wang, Q., Andreasson, K., Rajadas, J., Fuller, G.G., Xie, Y., Massa, S.M., & Longo, F.M. (2008). Small Molecule, Non-Peptide $p75^{NTR}$ Ligands Inhibit Aβ-Induced Neurodegeneration and Synaptic Impairment. *PLoS ONE*, Vol. 3, No. 11, pp. e3604.

Yeo, T.T., Chua-Couzens, J., Butcher, L.L., Bredesen, D.E., Cooper, J.D., Valletta, J.S., Mobley, W.C., & Longo, F.M. (1997). Absence of p75NTR causes increased basal forebrain cholinergic neuron size, choline acetyltransferase activity, and target innervation. *Journal of Neuroscience*, Vol. 17, No. 20, pp. 7594-7605.

Yoon, S.O., Soltoff, S.P., & Chao, M.V. (1997). A dominant role of the juxtamembrane region of the TrkA nerve growth factor receptor during neuronal cell differentiation. *Journal of Biological Chemistry*, Vol. 272, No. 37, pp. 23231-23238.

Zaccaro, M.C., Lee, H.B., Pattarawarapan, M., Xia, Z., Caron, A., L'Heureux, P.-J., Bengio, Y., Burgess, K., & Saragovi, H.U. (2005). Selective Small Molecule Peptidomimetic Ligands of TrkC and TrkA Receptors Afford Discrete or Complete Neurotrophic Activities. *Chemistry & Biology*, Vol. 12, No. 9, pp. 1015-1028.

Zhang, X., Gureasko, J., Shen, K., Cole, P.A., & Kuriyan, J. (2006). An Allosteric Mechanism for Activation of the Kinase Domain of Epidermal Growth Factor Receptor. *Cell*, Vol. 125, No. 6, pp. 1137-1149.

Zhang, Y., Moheban, D.B., Conway, B.R., Bhattacharyya, A., & Segal, R.A. (2000). Cell surface Trk receptors mediate NGF-induced survival while internalized receptors regulate NGF-induced differentiation. *Journal of Neuroscience*, Vol. 20, No. 15, pp. 5671-5678.

Zhao, M., Wan, Z. L., Whittaker, L., Xu, B., Phillips, N. B., Katsoyannis, P, G., Ismail-Beigi, F., Whittaker, J., & Weiss, M. A. (2009). Design of an insulin analog with enhanced receptor binding selectivity: rationale, structure, and therapeutic implications. *Journal of Biological Chemistry*, Vol. 284, No. 46, pp. 32178-32187.

9

# Oxidative Stress in Alzheimer's Disease: Pathogenesis, Biomarkers and Therapy

Alejandro Gella and Irene Bolea
*Universitat Internacional de Catalunya*
*Universitat Autònoma de Barcelona*
*Spain*

## 1. Introduction

Alzheimer's disease (AD) is the most common cause of dementia in the elderly with profound medical and social consequences. The pathogenesis of AD is a complex and heterogeneous process which classical neuropathological hallmarks found in the brain are extracellular deposits of beta-amyloid (Aβ)-containing plaques and intracellular neurofibrillary tangles (NFTs) composed of hyperphosphorylated tau protein. Mutation of *presenilin-1* (PS-1), *presenilin-2* (PS-2), and altered *amyloid precursor protein* (APP) genes has been reported to cause inherited AD. In addition, other genes such as apolipoprotein E-4 (APOE), endothelial nitric oxide synthase-3, and alpha-2-macroglubulin have also been associated with AD. A further number of hypothesis have been proposed for AD mechanism, which include: the amyloid cascade, vascular damage, excitotoxicity, deficiency of neurotrophic factors, mitochondrial dysfunction, trace element neurotoxicity, inflammation and oxidative stress hypothesis.

The oxidative stress (OS) hypothesis of aging postulated by Dr. Denham Harman in 1956 proposed that brain aging is associated to a progressive imbalance between the anti-oxidant defenses and the pro-oxidant species that can occur as a result of either an increase in free radical production or a decrease in antioxidant defence. The fact that age is the main risk factor for AD development provides considerable support to the OS hypothesis since the effects produced by reactive oxygen species (ROS) can accumulate over the years (Nunomura et al., 2001). The link between AD and OS is additionally supported by the finding of decreased levels of antioxidant enzymes, increased protein, lipid and DNA oxidation and advanced glycation end products (AGEs) and ROS formation in neurons of AD patients (Perry et al., 2000; Barnham et al., 2004). It has been reported that the accumulation of the oligomeric form of Aβ, the most toxic form of the peptide, induces OS in neurons (Butterfield, 2002), supporting the hypothesis and suggesting that OS plays a causative role in the development of AD. Then, a large amount of literature has demonstrated that OS is an important feature in AD pathogenesis that deserves to be deeply studied (Perry et al, 2002: Markesbery et al, 1999). In this Chapter, we address the main factors involved in the generation of oxidative stress and provide an overview of the oxidative stress biomarkers status in Alzheimer's disease. The Chapter concludes with a revision of the controversial efficacy of antioxidants as potential treatment in AD therapy as well as an update of the main antioxidant compounds found to have a beneficial effect in AD.

## 2. Mitochondria as a source of reactive oxygen species

Several years after the postulation of the OS hypothesis, Dr. Harman proposed that life span is determined by the rate of ROS damage to the mitochondria (Harman, 1972) giving for the first time an important role to this organelle in the ageing process and establishing the basis for "mitochondrial theory of ageing". It is important to note that the central nervous system (CNS) is especially vulnerable to oxidative damage as a result of the high oxygen consumption rate (20% of the total oxygen consumption), the abundant content of easily peroxidizable fatty acids, and the relative paucity of antioxidant enzymes compared to other tissues. In aerobic organisms, mitochondria produce semireduced oxygen species during respiration. The initial step of the respiratory chain reaction yields the superoxide radical ($^{\bullet}O_2^-$), which produces hydrogen peroxide ($H_2O_2$) by addition of an electron. The reduction of $H_2O_2$ through the Fenton reaction produces the highly reactive hydroxyl radical ($OH^{\bullet}$), which is the chief instigator of oxidative stress damage and reacts indiscriminately with all biomacromolecules (Figure 1). Under normal conditions, damage by ROS is prevented by an efficient antioxidant cascade, including both enzymatic and non-enzymatic entities. The enzymes responsible of the detoxification machinery are the cytosolic copper-zinc superoxide dismutase (CuZnSOD) and the mitochondrial manganese superoxide dismutase (MnSOD), which convert superoxide to $O_2$ and $H_2O_2$. Moreover, monoamine oxidases (MAOs) and L-amino acid oxidase can also produce $H_2O_2$ during its metabolism which is effectively removed by catalase (CAT) and peroxidases (e.g. glutathione peroxidase, GPx). Since CAT is compartmentalized into peroxisomes the detoxification of cytosolic and mitochondrial peroxides depends predominantly on GPx.

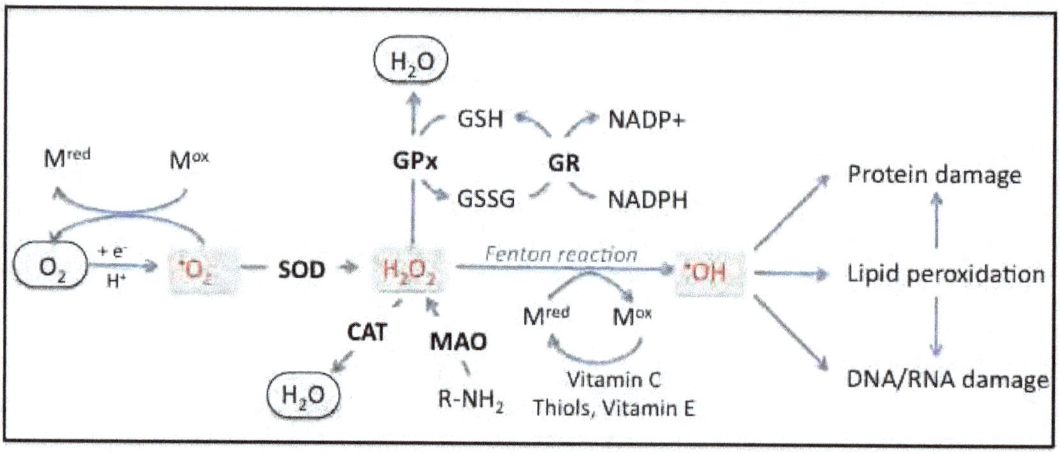


Fig. 1. Schematic illustration of the mechanism involved in reactive oxygen species (ROS) formation and elimination. Glutathione peroxidase (GPx), glutathione reductase (GR), superoxide dismutase (SOD), catalase (CAT), monoamine oxidase (MAO), glutathione (GSH), glutathione disulfide (GSSG).

The non-enzymatic antioxidant defenses include the reduction of the resulting oxidized transition metal ions (usually $Fe^{3+}$ and $Cu^{2+}$) by cellular reductants such as vitamin C, thiols and perhaps even vitamin E. In this context, SOD can also serve as the reductant of oxidized metal ions for the production of hydroxyl radical from $H_2O_2$, which coupled with the Fenton reaction, is known as the Haber-Weiss reaction. In AD, this situation is further exacerbated by the fact that redox active transition metals are aberrantly accumulated in cytoplasm of neurons. Moreover, Aβ peptide is considered a strong redox active agent capable of reducing transition metals and allowing for conversion of $O_2$ to $H_2O_2$ (Bondy et al, 1998).

## 3. Biomarkers of oxidative stress in Alzheimer's disease

Biomarkers, as indicators of signalling events in biological systems or samples, can be used as intermediate endpoints or early-outcome predictors of disease development for preventive purposes. Most effort is nowadays focused on the search of reliable and robust biomarkers which would be useful for an earlier AD diagnosis. The emphasis is being placed on the incorporation of oxidative stress biomarkers to study the increased oxidative damage (Lovell & Markesbery, 2007a). It has recently been a significant improvement in assay methods and measurement accuracy for oxidative biomarkers. Nevertheless, it appears imperative that biomarkers of oxidative damage must be validated (Dalle-Donne et al., 2006a) in order to incorporate them into epidemiological studies and provide a better understanding regarding the role of ROS in the pathogenesis and progression of AD, as well as to assess the possible effectiveness of an antioxidant therapy (Griffiths et al., 2002). Strong evidence show that oxidative markers are more prevalent in initial rather than in later stages of the disease, and thus suggesting that targeting the earlier events of the disease may be more successful that targeting the later events (e.g. beta-amyloid (Aβ) plaque deposition and/or intracellular neurofibrillary tangles formation). On the other hand, many studies provided evidence for the deleterious consequences of oxidative stress products on certain cellular targets in AD. Therefore, most highly reactive oxidants react with virtually all biomolecules, including, lipids, DNA/RNA, carbohydrates and proteins. Table 1 summarizes the main OS biomarker candidates for MCI and AD diagnosis.

| Biomarker | Specimen | Diagnosis | Reference |
|---|---|---|---|
| **Lipid Peroxidation** | | | |
| 4-HNE | Plasma | AD | Mc Grath et al., 2001 |
| | Ventricular fluid | AD | Lovell et al., 1997 |
| F2-Isoprostanes | Urine | AD | Kim et al., 2004 |
| | CSF | AD | Montine et al., 2011 |
| | CSF, plasma and urine | MCI | Pratico et al., 2002 |
| **DNA oxidation** | | | |
| 8-OHdG | Peripheral lymphocytes | MCI | Migliore et al., 2005 |
| | | AD | Mecocci et al., 2002 |
| **AGEs** | | | |
| CML | CSF | AD | Ahmed et al., 2005 |
| **Oxidized Protein** | | | |
| α-1-antitrypsin | CSF | AD | Puchades et al., 2003 |
| Ig λ light chain | CSF | MCI | Korolainen et al., 2007 |
| α-1-antitrypsin | Plasma | AD | Yu et al., 2003; Choi et al., 2002 |

Table 1. Potential OS biomarkers under validation for Alzheimer's disease. MCI, mild cognitive impairment; AD, Alzheimer's disease; CSF, cerebrospinal fluid; Ig, immunoglobulin; 4-HNE, 4-hydroxy-2-nonenal; 8-OHdG, 8-oxo-7,8-dihydro-2'-deoxyguanosine; AGEs, Advanced Glycation end products; CML, N-carboxymethyl-lysine.

### 3.1 Biomarkers of lipid peroxidation

Lipid oxidation (also called lipid peroxidation) has drammatic consequences in ageing and age-related disorders. Phospholipids present in brain membranes are mainly polyunsaturated fatty acids (PUFAs: arachidonic acid, linoleic acid, linolenic acid, docosahexaenoic acid, etc...), which are especially vulnerable to a free radical attack since their double bonds allow an easy removal of hydrogen ions. Oxidation of PUFAs produces a variety of reactive α,β-unsaturated aldehydes such as, acrolein, 4-hydroxy-2-nonenal (4-HNE), 4-oxo-2-nonenal (4-ONE), 4-hydroxy-2-hexanal (4-HHE), 2-hexenal, crotonaldehyde as well as the dialdehydes glyoxal and malondialdehyde (MDA). These species are highly reactive cytotoxic substances than can form stable covalent adducts with free amino groups of proteins (Lys, His and Cys residues) through Michael addition (Calingasan et al., 1999; Carini et al., 2004; Esterbauer et al., 1991; Montine et al., 1997) whick are known as advanced lipoxidation end products (ALEs). 4-HNE is a major and toxic aldehyde generated by free radical attack on PUFAs and is considered a second toxic messenger of oxygen free radicals. Therefore, it has a high biological activity and exhibits numerous cytotoxic, mutagenic, genotoxic, and signalling effects in neurons (Eckl et al., 1993; Williams et al., 2006). In addition, 4-HNE may be an important mediator of OS-induced apoptosis, cellular proliferation and signalling pathways (Uchida, 2003). HNE is permanently formed at basal concentrations under physiologic conditions, but its production is greatly enhanced in the AD brain where increased lipid peroxidation occurs (Butterfield et al., 2010; McGrath et al., 2001). Increased concentrations of 4-HNE, 4-HHE and acrolein have been found in cerebrospinal fluid (CSF) and in multiple brain regions from individuals with mild cognitive impairment and early AD compared with age-matched controls (Bradley et al., 2010a and 2010b; Lovell et al., 1997; Williams et al, 2006). In addition, a positive feedback in the pathogenesis of AD is provoked by HNE that increases Aβ production (Tamagno et al., 2008) which, in turns, induces lipid peroxidation (Butterfield et al., 2002). Furthermore, HNE-adducts have been identified in amyloid plaques and neurofibrillary tangles, the two hallmarks of AD pathogenesis (Sayre et al., 1997; Ando et al., 1998; Wataya et al., 2002).

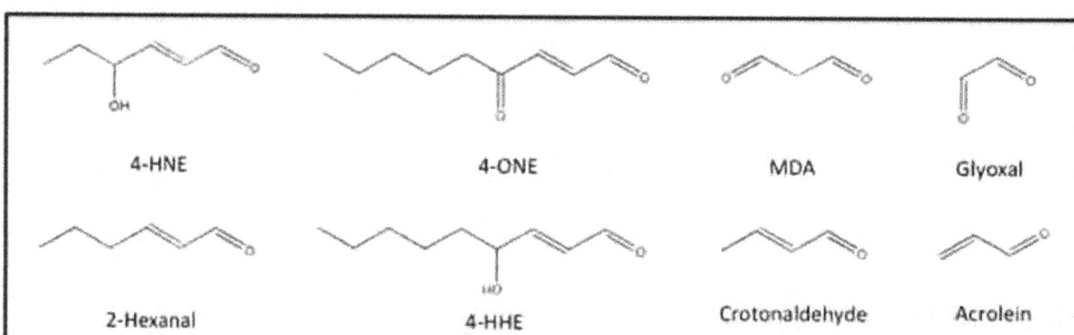


Fig. 2. Lipid peroxidation products. ROS stimulate peroxidation of polyunsaturated fatty acids (PUFA) to generate α-β-unsaturated aldehydes and dialdehydes.

F2-Isoprostanes (F2-IsoPs), which contain an F-type prostane ring, are a group of bioactive prostaglandin-like compounds generated via a non-enzymatic mechanism involving the free radical-initiated peroxidation of esterified arachidonic acid (AA). Then, they are cleaved and released into the circulation by phospholipases before excretion in the urine as free isoprostanes (Basu, 1998). The most studied class of isoprostanes, due to their urine stability, is 8-iso-Prostaglandin $F_{2a}$ (8-iso-PGF$_{2a}$; Figure 3). Urinary F2-IsoPs determination has been proposed as specific, reliable, and non-invasive marker to assess lipid peroxidation in vivo (Cracowski et al., 2002; Montushchi et al., 2004) since an increase in 8-iso-PGF$_{2a}$ levels in CSF and urine have been found in subjects with AD (Montine et al., 1998 and 2011; Kim et al., 2004). On the other hand, oxidation of docosahexanoic acid (DHA) produces F4-neuroprostanes (F4-NeuroPs; Figure 3) (Morrow et al., 1999; Roberts et al., 1998) which levels are elevated in postmortem ventricular CSF of AD patients and are more abundant in the brain that F2-isoprostanes. Nevertheless, plasma F2-IsoPs and F4-NeuroPs do not accurately reflect central nervous system levels and are not reproducibly elevated in body fluids outside of central nervous system in Alzheimer's disease patients (Montine et al., 2002).

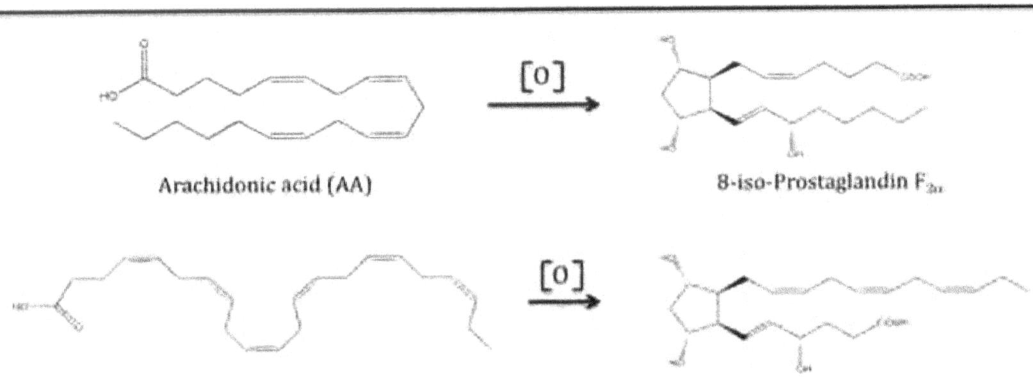


Fig. 3. Chemical structures of F4-neuroprostane and 8-iso-Prostaglandin $F_{2a}$ arising from direct oxidation of docosahexanoic and arachidonic acids, respectively.

### 3.2 Biomarkers of oxidative DNA damage

Among over 30 nucleobase modifications that have been described, the most extensively studied that reflect oxidative DNA damage is 8-oxo-7,8-dihydro-2′-deoxyguanosine (8-oxodG; also known as 8-OHdG), a product of oxidatively modified DNA base guanine (Figure 4). The detection of this oxidation is important not only due to its abundance but also to its mutagenic potential through GC-to-TA transversion mutations upon replication of DNA (Cheng et al., 1992). Nevertheless, oxidatively damaged DNA can be repaired and released into the bloodstream and consequently appear without further metabolism in the urine (Fraga et al., 1990; Shigenaga et al., 1989). In addition, urinary levels of 8-OHdG have been found to be independent of dietary influence in humans. The modified base 8-oxo-7,8-dihydroguanine (8-oxoGua; Figure 4) and modified nucleoside (8-oxodG; Figure 4), which are found in urine, represent the major repair products of oxidatively damaged DNA in vivo and have been considered to reflect the whole-body oxidative DNA damage (Hamilton et al., 2001; Olinnski et al., 2007). There is considerable evidence supporting that oxidative stress occurs in AD, and increased 8-oxodG levels have been found in DNA isolated from brain tissues, leukocytes and ventricular CSF of AD patients. In contrast, free 8-OHdG was found dramatically decreased in AD samples as compared to the controls (Lovell & Markesbery, 2001; Markesbery & Carney, 1999; Mecocci et al., 2002; Migliore et al., 2005).

Taken together, these data indicate a double insult in AD patients by increasing oxidative damage and decreasing DNA repair mechanisms efficiency. More recent studies showed an elevated 8-OHdG in both nuclear and mitochondrial DNA (mtDNA) isolated from vulnerable brain regions in amnestic mild cognitive impairment (MCI), the earliest clinical manifestation of AD, and thus suggesting that oxidative DNA damage is an early event in AD and is not merely a secondary phenomenon (Lovell & Markesbery, 2007b).
Many methods such as HPLC-ECD, GC-MS, LC-MS, and immunoassay have been established to measure 8-OHdG in biological specimens. In this concern, the European Standards Committee of Urinary (DNA) Lesions Analysis (ESCULA) was formed in 2006 in order to validate the measurement methods of oxidatively damaged DNA and to establish reference urine values (Cooke et al., 2008; Evans et al., 2010). Finally, it is important to mention that DNA can also be modified by products of lipid peroxidation (ALEs). These α-β-unsaturated aldehydes can react with deoxyguanosine through an initial Michael addition of the exocyclic amino group followed by ring closure of N-1 onto the aldehydic group to generate a bulky exocyclic 1-$N^2$-propanodeoxyguanosine adduct (Liu et al., 2006; Kozekov et al., 2003) and therefore participate in the propagation of the oxidative DNA damage.

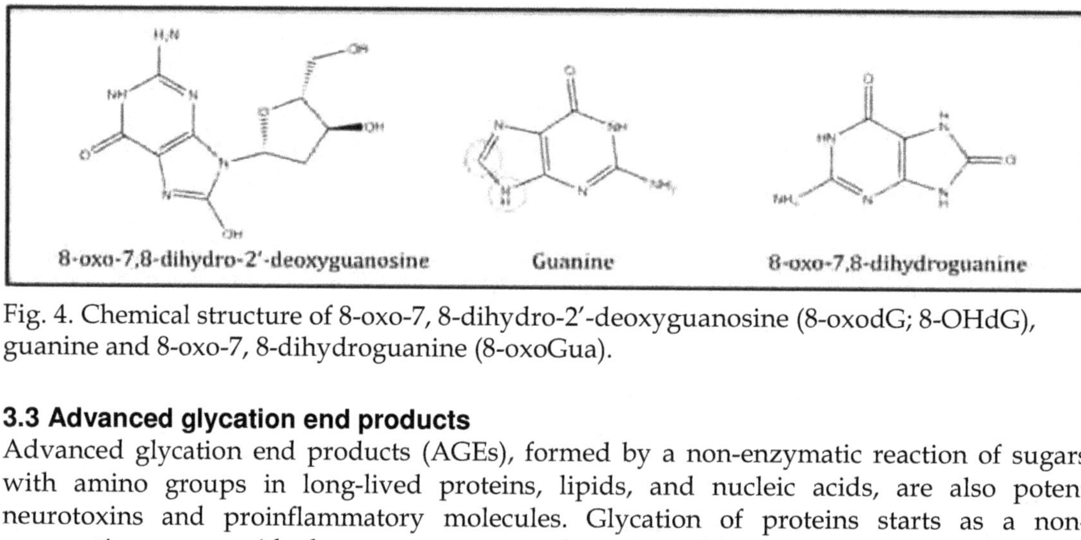


Fig. 4. Chemical structure of 8-oxo-7, 8-dihydro-2'-deoxyguanosine (8-oxodG; 8-OHdG), guanine and 8-oxo-7, 8-dihydroguanine (8-oxoGua).

### 3.3 Advanced glycation end products

Advanced glycation end products (AGEs), formed by a non-enzymatic reaction of sugars with amino groups in long-lived proteins, lipids, and nucleic acids, are also potent neurotoxins and proinflammatory molecules. Glycation of proteins starts as a non-enzymatic process with the spontaneous condensation of ketone or aldehyde groups of sugars with a free aminoacid group of proteins to form a labile Schiff base, consistent with the classical reaction described by Louis Camille Maillard in 1912 (Figure 5).

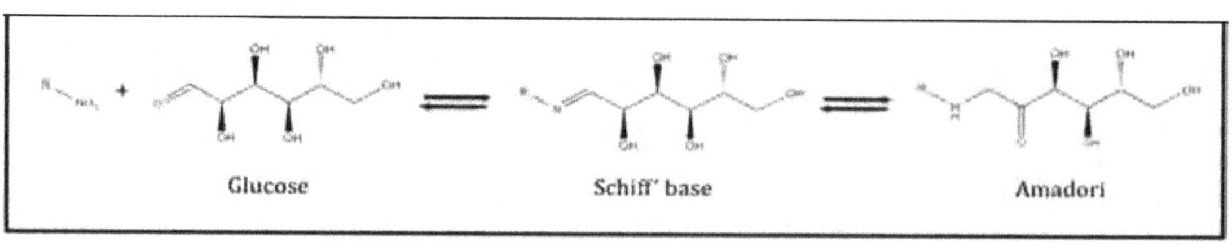


Fig. 5. Non-enzymatic reaction of the carbonyl groups of reducing sugars with primary amino groups produce corresponding Schiff bases, which undergo Amadori rearrangement to give ketoamines.

Glycation is the first step in the cascade of a complex series of very slow reactions in the body known as Amadori reactions, Schiff base reactions and Maillard reactions, all leading to the formation of irreversibly cross-linked heterogeneous aggregates. AGEs are continuously formed in the human body and progressively accumulate with age in plasma and tissues. In diabetes mellitus and AD the rate of AGEs formation is accelerated and consequently, they have been considered potentially useful biomarkers for monitoring the treatment of these disorders. Chemical structures of representative markers of AGEs are summarized in Figure 6. Supporting the argument that AGEs are involved in the pathogenesis of AD, some studies have shown the presence of AGEs in association with two major proteins of AD, Aβ and MAP-tau (Smith et al., 1995; Vitek et al., 1994; Yan et al., 1994). Extracellular AGEs accumulation has been demonstrated in senile plaques in different cortical areas. Intracellular proteins deposits including NFTs, Lewy bodies of patients with Parkinson's disease and Hirano bodies are also crosslinked by AGEs, which may explain their insolubility in detergents and resistance to proteases (Loske et al., 2000). The major component of the NFTs, the microtubuli-associated protein tau (MAP-tau) has been shown to be subject to intracellular AGEs formation. MAP-tau

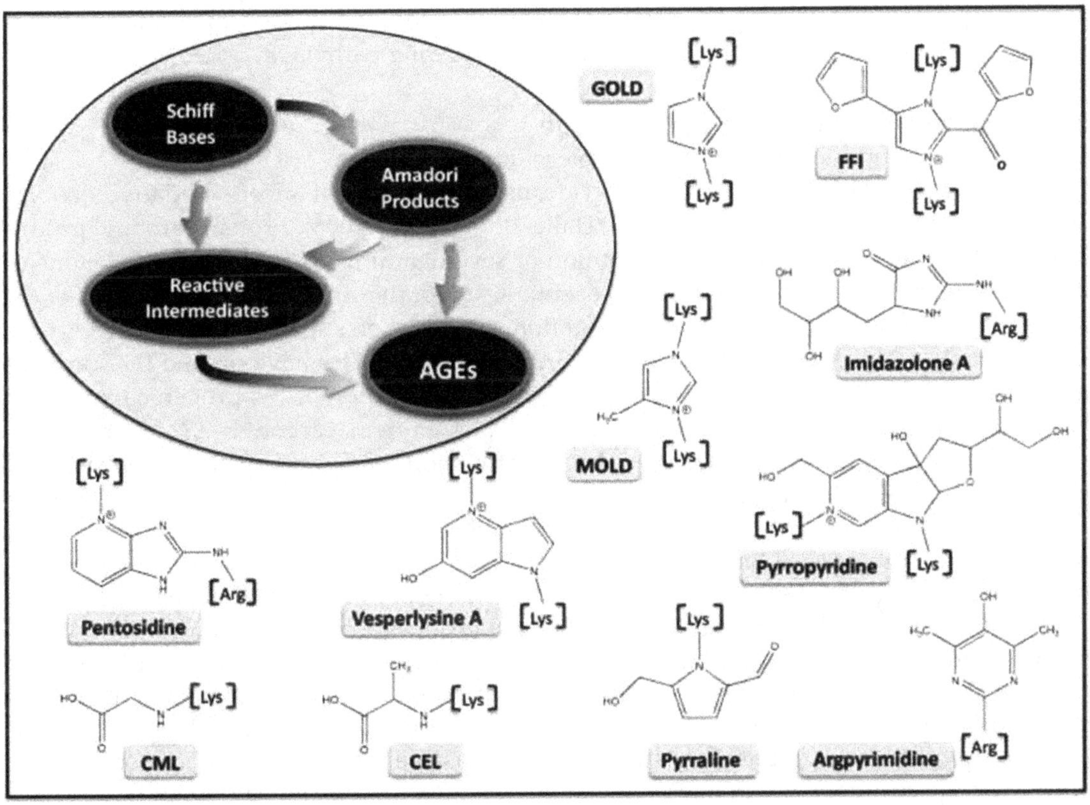


Fig. 6. A variety of highly reactive carbonyl intermediates such as 3-deoxy-glucosone, glyoxal and methyl-glyoxal can be formed by glucose or Schiff's base or Amadori product auto-oxidation which, in turn, can react with free amino groups to form AGE products. N-carboxymethyl-lysine (CML), N- carboxyethyl-lysine (CEL), glyoxal-derived lysine dimer (GOLD), methylglyoxal-derived lysine dimer (MOLD), furoyl-furanyl-imidazole (FFI), Lysine (Lys) and arginine (Arg).

can be glycated in vitro, inhibiting its ability to bind to microtubules. In addition, MAP-tau isolated from brains of AD patients is glycated in the tubulin-binding region, giving rise to the formation of β-sheet fibrils (Ledesma et al., 1998). AGEs accumulate in the human brain during aging (Kimura et al., 1996) and are present in neurofibrillary tangles and senile plaques in patients with AD (Castellani et al., 2001). Furthermore; AGE-modified Aβ peptides accelerate aggregation of soluble nonfibrillar Aβ peptides. In older adults with cerebrovascular disease, elevated N-carboxymethyl-lysine (CML) has been found in cortical neurons and cerebral vessels and has been related to the severity of cognitive impairment (Southern et al., 2007). Brain tissue AGEs can therefore be considered tissue biomarkers for AD, and increased brain AGEs concentrations are reflected in CSF (Ahmed et al., 2005) but no necessarily in plasma (Thome et al., 1996).

A positive feedback loop in the pathogenesis of AD is provoked by AGEs which increase OS and inflammation through binding with AGEs receptor (RAGE). The RAGE signalling pathway, found upregulated in AD brains, can be initiated by a diverse repertoire of pro-inflammatory ligands that include AGEs, S100/calgranulins, amphoterin, and amyloid-β peptide. Ligand binding with RAGE triggers the induction of increased reactive oxygen species, activates NADH oxidase, increases the expression of adhesion molecules, and up-regulates inflammation through NF-kB and other signalling pathways.

### 3.4 Biomarkers of oxidative protein damage

Carbonylation of proteins is an irreversible oxidative process, often leading to a loss of protein function, which is considered a widespread indicator of severe oxidative damage and disease-derived protein dysfunction (Dalle-Donne et al., 2006). Protein carbonyl groups are introduced to proteins by direct oxidation of several amino acid residues into ketone or aldehyde derivates (particularly lysine, arginine, threonine and proline; Figure 7) or by secondary reaction with the primary oxidation products of sugars (forming AGEs) and lipids (forming ALEs) (Berlett & Stadtman, 1997). Several studies have proved that proteins are major initial cell targets of ROS, leading to earlier formation of the protein carbonyls in biological systems. Detection of increased levels of protein carbonyls in AD has been proposed as a sign of disease-associated dysfunction, suggesting the potentiality as biomarkers for early AD diagnosis.

Recent studies show an increase in protein carbonyls together with NFTs in multiple brain regions of AD subjects (Sultana & Butterfield, 2011). Oxidative modifications of proteins can cause cross-linking of covalent bonds of proteins leading to fibril formation and insolubility. NFTs are characterized by the aggregation and hyperphosphorilation of tau proteins which is linked to oxidation through the microtubule-associated protein kinase pathway and through the activation of the transcription factor NF-kB. A wide number of studies have reported differences in specific carbonated proteins in brain, plasma and CSF of AD patients compared with control group by using 2-dimensional gel electrophoresis in combination with mass spectroscopy techniques (Castegna et al., 2002a, 2002b; Davidsson et al., 2001; Puchades et al., 2003). Some of these studies reveal the presence of specific targets of protein oxidation in AD brain: creatine kinase BB, glutamine synthase, ubiquitin carboxy-terminal hydrolase L-1, dihydropyrimidinase-related protein 2, alpha-enolase and heat shock cognate 71. Glutamine synthase and creatine kinase, both markedly decreased in AD brains, are especially sensitive to oxidative modifications since they may cause alteration of glutamate concentrations (glutamine sinthase), and therefore enhance excitotoxicity, and decrease energy metabolism (creatine kinase). Recently, several oxidized carbonylated proteins have been characterized in frontal cortex (Korolainen et al., 2006), plasma (Yu et al., 2003; Choi et al., 2002) and CSF (Korolainen et al., 2007) of patients suffering from AD by two-dimensional oxyblotting technique.

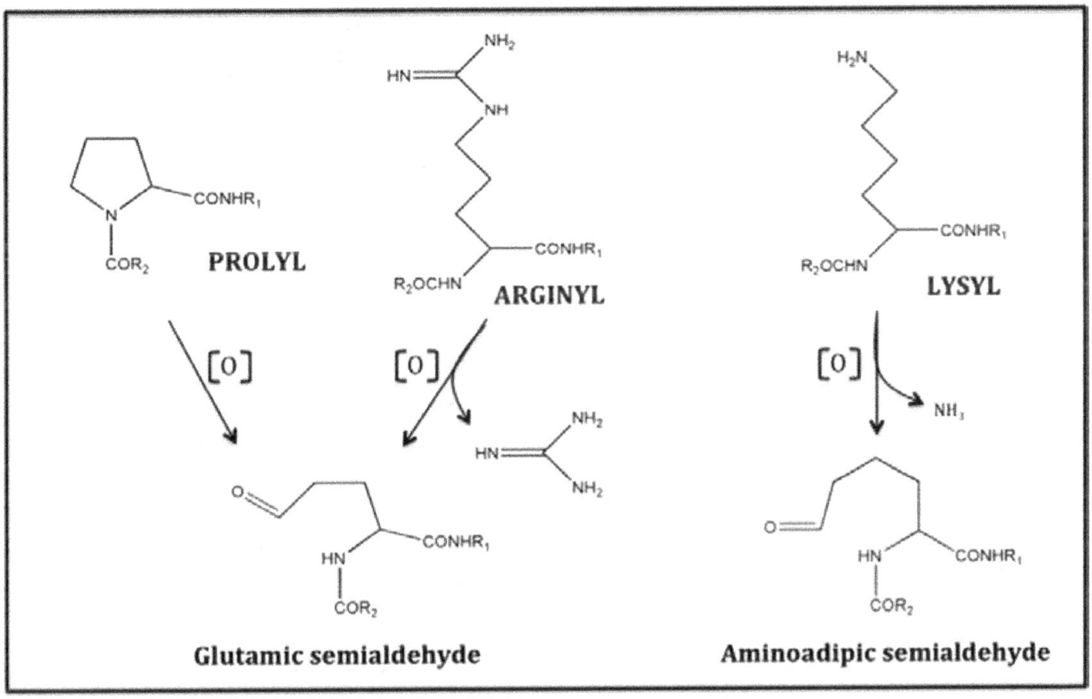


Fig. 7. Chemical structures of protein carbonyls arising from direct oxidation of aminoacid side chains. Glutamic semialdehyde (resulting from direct oxidation of arginyl and prolyl residues) and aminoadipic semialdehyde (resulting from direct oxidation of lysyl residue).

## 4. Antioxidant therapies in Alzheimer's disease

Currently, the only Food and Drug Administration (FDA) approved treatment for AD is the administration of the cholinesterase inhibitors (AChEI) donepezil, galantamine and rivastigmine and the N-methyl-D-aspartate (NMDA) receptor antagonist, memantine (Birks et al., 2000, 2006; Loy et al., 2004; Areosa et al., 2005). Nevertheless, to date, these drugs have demonstrated to produce only modest symptomatic improvements in some of the patients, but not to cure or stop the disease progression. Moreover, AChEI are expensive and may have side effects resulting from activation of peripheral cholinergic systems (Green et al., 2005). Then, effective treatments are greatly needed. The current therapeutic strategies being investigated for AD include targeting neurotransmission with multifunctional compounds, anti-amyloid and anti-tau therapies, drugs targeting mitochondrial dysfunction, neurotrophins, statins and also other approaches such us PUFAs and antioxidants (for review see Mangialasche et al., 2010). Among them, antioxidant therapies and PUFAs are particularly attractive due to their low toxicity, low cost and their ability to target earlier changes of the disease (e.g oxidative stress) which are linked to cognitive and functional decline. However, there is still much skepticism regarding the likelihood of success with an antioxidant therapy since to date these compounds tested in randomised controlled trials (RCTs) have given controversial results.

### 4.1 Vitamins

A large amount of literature exists in relation to the potential benefits of vitamins, which act as natural free radical scavengers, in the prevention of AD (Figure 8). Vitamin A has been traditionally considered as antioxidant and it seems essential for learning, memory and cognition. Retinoic acid, a metabolic product of vitamin A, is known to slow cell death and protect from Aβ (Sahin et al., 2005). Thus, since levels of vitamin A decline with age and are found lower in AD individuals (Goodman et al., 2006) vitamin A supplementation might be useful for the treatment of some features in the ageing process. B-vitamins ($B_6$, $B_{12}$ and folic acid) are lipid soluble antioxidants involved in the methylation of homocysteine (Hcy) which is highly cytotoxic. Cellular catabolism and cellular export mechanisms are the responsible for keeping low intracellular Hcy concentration. AD patients tipically present high levels of Hcy (McIlroy et al., 2002) and low levels of vitamin $B_{12}$ and folate which appear to be associated with an increased rate of cognitive decline (Tucker et al., 2006; Morris et al., 2007). Nevertheless, in a recent study, a combination of vitamins $B_{12}$, $B_6$ and folate in mild to moderate AD individuals, although lowering Hcy, did not produce any effect on cognition compared to controls. Vitamin C (ascorbic acid), found in many fruits and vegetables, is the major water-soluble antioxidant and acts as first defence against free radicals in blood and plasma. Bagi et al, 2003, have shown that chronic vitamin C treatment is able to decrease high levels of isoprostanes in animal models. In contrast, other studies have shown that it can also act as pro-oxidant inducing neuronal oxidative stress via its

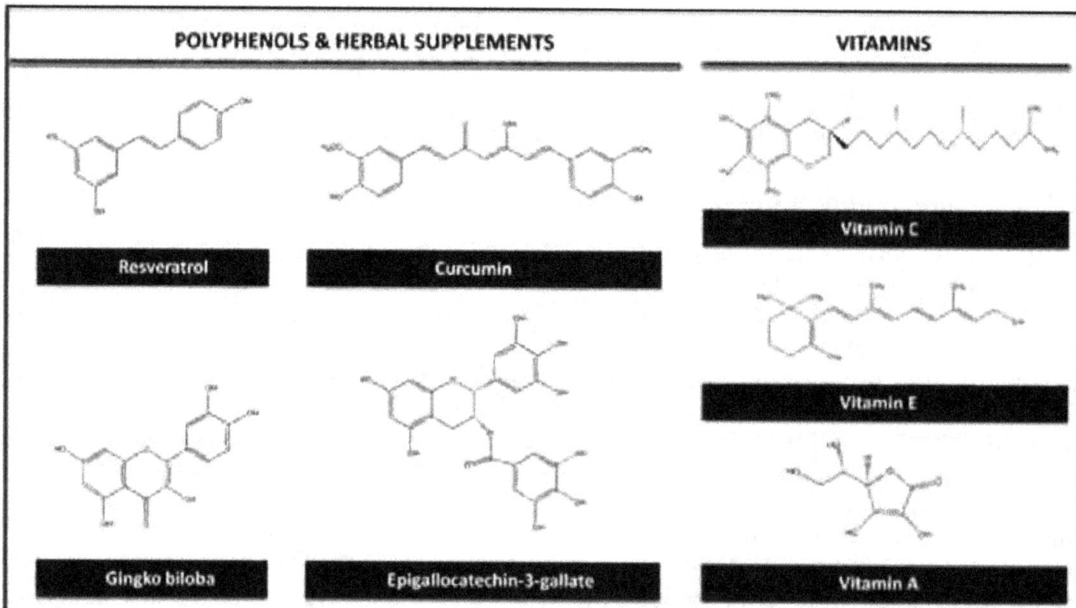


Fig. 8. Chemical structures of the principal polyphenols, herbal suplements and vitamins investigated as promising agents for the treatment of AD.

interaction with metal ions (White et al., 2004). Vitamin E (α-tocopherol), present in whole grains, cereals and vegetable oils, is a lipid-soluble vitamin found in cell membranes and circulating lipoproteins. Its antioxidant capacity acts directly to a variety of ROS. It is found low in AD patients (Jiménez-Jiménez et al., 1997) and although in vitro and animal studies have been encouraging, human trials have produced conflicting results (Berman et al., 2004). A Cochrane study shows that tocopherol is not effective in a prevention trial in mild cognitive impairment (MCI) to reduce progression to AD nor clearly effective in AD patients (Tabet et al., 2000; Luchsinger et al., 2003). Besides, a harmfull effect of tocopherol at high doses has also been suggested (Tucker et al., 2005). However, several studies correlate a reduced risk to AD in elderly persons treated with vitamin E and C alone or in combination (Grundman et al., 2004; Morris et al., 1998; 2002; 2005). On the other hand, brain bioavailability of vitamin E in humans is very low and, as suggested elsewhere may not be enough to quickly inhibit AD neuropathology unless administered as a prophylactic at very early ages. The large amount of contradictory data found in literature about the use of vitamins as antioxidants indicates intricate physiological and pharmacological features of AD and remain questionable its use in human.

### 4.2 Polyphenols and herbal supplements

Polyphenols are a group of plant-derived chemical substances which protect plants from the stress induced by physical damage, disease, radiation and pests (Figure 8). It has been suggested that curcumin, the yellow pigment extracted from the plant *curcuma longa* (turmeric), may be a promising therapy for AD due to its extended neuroprotective actions (Mishra et al., 2008; Cole et al., 2007), including antioxidant, anti-inflammatory, inhibition of Aβ formation and removal of existing Aβ, as well as cooper and iron chelation. Epigallocathechin-3-gallate (EGCg) is found in green tea and it has been described that prevents Aβ aggregation by directly binding to the unfolded peptide. It also modulates signal transduction pathways, expression of genes regulating cell survival and apoptosis and its actions in mitochondrial function make it a potent antioxidant (Mandel et al., 2008). Resveratrol is present in red wine, peanuts and other plants and it has been found that it reduces OS, inflammation and Aβ deposition, decreases cell death and protects DNA (Mishra et al., 2008; Karuppagounder et al., 2009). A recent study suggests that moderate consumption of red wine reduces the risk of developing AD. Nevertheless, the translation to humans is still somewhat problematic and has some caveats since although polyphenols easily penetrate blood-brain barrier, they show bioavailabity problems such us low absorption, rapid metabolism and quick elimination. Efforts to increase bioavailability have been reviewed (Anand et al., 2007) and the adjuvant use widely extended (Shoba et al., 1998). Indeed, there is currently a clinical trial underway addressing curcumin bioavailability (http://clinicaltrials.gov/NCT01001637). Furthermore, the anti-AD effects of polyphenols may not be mediated solely through their direct antioxidant action but rather indirectly through any other functions. Then, it is still to be clarified whether polyphenols are able to slow the progression of AD. Herbal supplements such us *gingko biloba* have been suggested to possess beneficial properties against AD (Luo et al, 2002). Numerous animal and in vitro studies report that *gingko biloba* extract EGb761 possess neuroprotective benefits (Defeudis et al., 2002) including antioxidant, anti-inflammatory, and regulator of Aβ processing. It has also been described that *gingko* improves cognitive function in mild to moderate AD patients (Oken et al., 1998; Le Bars et al., 2003) and reduces deterioration in subjects with more severe dementia via inhibition of the Aβ induced free radical generation (Napryeyenko et al., 2009; Yao et al., 2001). Nevertheless, a double-blind placebo controlled study found no beneficial effect of *gingko* on dementia in AD patients (Schneider et al, 2005) and DeKosky et al, 2008 showed that gingko was not better than placebo at preventing the onset of dementia. Additionally, there are two more studies finding no correlation between cognitive decline and the use of *gingko biloba* (Snitz et al., 2009; Dodge et al., 2008). Although data is controversial, it then appears that *gingko* may be useful delaying cognition impairment but not preventing the onset of AD. The ongoing clinical trial will help to elucidate this question (http://clinicaltrials.gov/NCT00814346).

### 4.3 Mitochondrial-related antioxidants

Since mitochondria are the major sources of ROS in the central nervous system, therapeutic strategies have largely focused in targeting mitochondria and mitochondrial-related pathways. There are several compounds showing an in vitro and in vivo antioxidant and neuroprotective action but only a few have been tested in human clinical trials with mixed results.

#### 4.3.1 Quinone family

Ubiquinone (Coenzyme Q, CoQ) and idebenone, a synthetic analog of CoQ, (Figure 9) are the major mitochondrial targets used as therapeutics against ROS-mediated damage. They have demonstrated antioxidant properties in vitro and in animal models (Wadsworth et al., 2008). CoQ has not been yet tested in humans but idebenone has been investigated in clinical trials for its capacity to inhibit lipid peroxidation. Several studies report a significant effect in memory and attention improvements (Gutzmann et al., 2002; Senin et al., 1992; Weyer et al., 1997) but a larger study reported no effect in slowing the disease progression (Thal et al., 2003).

#### 4.3.2 Other mitochondrial antioxidants

Alpha-lipoic acid (LA) is an organosulfur compound derived from octanoic acid and primarily a cofactor in aerobic metabolism for pyruvate dehydrogenase complex. Its reduced bioactive form produced into cells provides its antioxidant properties (Haenen et al., 1991). Acetyl L-carnitine (ALCAR) is formed within mitochondria by carnitine-*O*-acetyltransferase. Both LA and ALCAR (Figure 9) are good candidates for being used therapeutically as mitochondrial antioxidants since it was found that a combination of both decreased mitochondrial dysfunction and its consequent ROS-mediated damage in aged rats, improving cognitive functions (Aliev et al., 2009). Additional neuroprotective functions, including binding to targets involved in Aβ production have been reported (Epis et al., 2008). However, several clinical trials with ALCAR have been conducted with contradictory results: one showed no effectiveness in early onset AD (Thal et al., 2000) whereas another showed a slower deterioration in cognition (Pettergrew et al., 1995). A recent meta-analysis of ALCAR treatment trials showed an improvement in clinical scales in patients with MCI and AD (Montgomery et al., 2003). Dimebon (Figure 9), a non selective antihistamine, possesses several mechanisms of action including the inhibition of Aβ toxicity and the prevention of ROS-mediated damage (Doody et al., 2009; Okun et al., 2010). Several clinical trials have been performed in AD patients with contradictory results: in a phase 2 clinical trial, dimebon improved cognition and behaviour, overall function in MCI and AD (Doody et al., 2008) whereas more recently, a phase 3 CONNECTION trial with AD patients showed no improvement in any parameter (http://clinicaltrials.gov/NCT00675623).

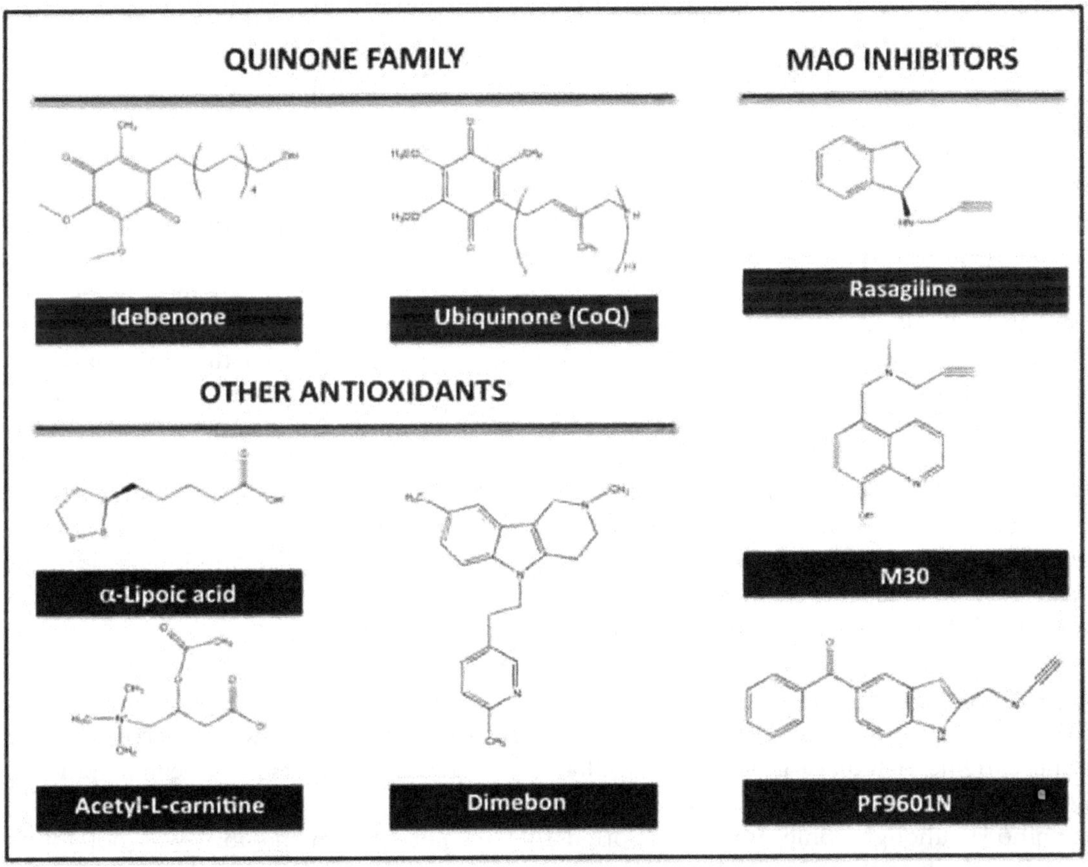


Fig. 9. Chemical structures of mitochondrial-related antioxidants investigated as promising agents for the treatment of AD.

### 4.3.3 Monoamine oxidase inhibitors

The therapeutic potential of monoamine oxidase inhibitors (MAOIs) for the treatment of AD has been largely reported (Thomas, 2000; Riederer et al., 2004; Youdim et al., 2005) due to their capacity to reduce the formation of toxic metabolites or oxygen radicals by blocking the catalytic activity of monoamine oxidase (MAO), enzyme located in the mitochondrial membrane and responsible of amine metabolism. It has been extensively reported that MAO-B activity besides increasing with age is found in high levels in AD patients. Selegiline, the classic MAO-B inhibitor, and also other propargylamines (Figure 9) possess potent antioxidant properties (Kitani et al., 2000; Sanz et al., 2004). Moreover, it has also been described that propargylamine-derived MAOIs exert neuroprotective effects by acting in very diverse type of targets, including metal chelation (e.g M30), reduction of Aβ aggregation and toxicity (Bar-Am et al., 2009; Youdim et al., 2005) as well as direct actions on diverse mitochondrial-related components. Among this direct functions, propargylamines increase the expression of anti-apoptotic proteins (Akao et al., 2002), prevent citocrom c release and preserve the mitochondrial membrane potential (Mayurama et al., 2000). The great amount of beneficial functions found for MAOIs make them promising molecules for the treatment of AD. Indeed, current pharmacological challenges in AD involve the design and development of multifunctional compounds able to bind to a very diverse type of targets and among them MAO inhibition is strongly recommended.

### 4.4 PUFAs

The beneficial effects of omega-3 polyunsaturated fatty acids (PUFAs) have been widely reported which make them good candidates for AD therapy (Cole et al., 2005) since they act directly on intracellular pathways and regulate oxidative stress mechanisms. DHA is the major omega-3 fatty acid in the brain. A recent study although showing no effect of DHA on subjects with mild-to-moderate AD it found a slower rate of cognitive decline among those patients without de APO ε4 allele (Quinn et al., 2009). As reviewed by Mangialasche et al, 2010, some studies have reported a beneficial effect of DHA on cognitive function in patients with AD (Yurko-Mauro et al., 2009; Chiu et al., 2008) whereas others did not found a correlation (Quinn et al., 2009). In effect, a recent study showed that treatment of patients with PUFAs did not modify the neuropathology of this disorder in CSF or plasma, nor the biomarkers of inflammation (Freund-Levi et al., 2009) and a randomised control trial in patients with mild to moderate AD did not delay the rate of cognitive decline (Freund-Levi et al., 2006). Some authors suggest that benefits of omega-3 fatty acids are limited to those with very mild cognitive impairment. A phase 2 randomised clinical trial is currently ongoing (http://clinicaltrials.gov/NCT01058941).

### 4.5 Multiple nutrients

Dietary supplementation with a plethora of nutrients such us apple juice concentrate, red wine, caffeine, fish oil or green tea as well as calorie restriction diets have been conducted. Diverse human studies have shown that multiple formulations improve all measures of cognition, although some authors reported that the increase in memory was not found significant (Chan et al., 2008). A recent study correlates frequent consumption of fruits and vegetables, fish, and omega-3 rich oils with a decreased risk of dementia in AD (Barberger-Gateau et al., 2007). In contrast, interventional trials with antioxidants, B-vitamines and DHA did not give the promising expectations from the epidemiological data. As reported by Von Arnim et al., 2010, although some trials are encouraging, larger randomised clinical trials with combined supplements are needed to draw any conclusion. Supplement composition is still a matter of debate, because high doses of a single antioxidant have been associated with no beneficial effects for AD patients and even with an increase in mortality risk (e.g vitamin E). Many interventional studies are started very late in the disease state, when AD pathology is already at a fulminant level which severely reduces therapeutic effectiveness of tested agents. The multifactorial nature of AD and the necessity to target the earlier production of OS makes important the combination of multiple supplements. Therefore, studies combining nutrients are of particular interest and at present in progress (e.g. T-diet, NKO™, and Memory XL; http://clinicaltrials.gov/NCT01192529, NCT00867828, NCT00903695).

| Exposure | Assessment | Design | Case source | Major findings | Reference |
|---|---|---|---|---|---|
| EGb 761 (intravenous) | NA | RCT | AD VaD | ADL improvement. Clinical impression of change | Haase et al, 1996 |
| EGb 761 (oral) | NA | RCT | AD VaD | Cognitive improvement | Le Bars et al, 2000 |
| PUFAs | Plasma assay | Cross-sectional | Normal, CI, dementia | Low n-3 and high n-6 associated with CI and AD | Conquer et al, 2000 |
| PUFAs | Plasma assay | Cross-sectional | Normal, CI, dementia | High n-3 associated with CI and AD. Strengthened in ApoEe4 non-carriers | Laurin et al, 2003 |
| PUFAs | Plasma assay | Prospective | Normal | No association between PUFAs and reduced risk of dementia | Kroger et al, 2009 |
| Fish intake | FFQ | Prospective | Normal | Reduced risk of incident dementia | Barberger-Gateau et al, 2002 |
| DHA | Serum assay | Case-control | Normal AD | MMSE and CDR improvement | Tully et al, 2003 |
| Fish oil | FFQ | Prospective | Elderly | Slow rate of decline but not on overall cognitive status | Morris et al, 2005 |
| PUFA | FFQ | Prospective | Elderly | Reduced MMSE decline over 5 years | Van Gelder et al, 2007 |
| β-carotene | NA | Prospective | Elderly | Less cognitive decline only in ApoE4 carriers | Hu et al, 2006 |
| Vitamin E | NA | RCT | MCI | No significant differences compared to placebo or donepezil | Petersen, 2005 |
| α-tocopherol and/or selegiline | NA | RCT | Moderate AD | Longer time to institutionalization in all cases | Sano et al, 1997 |

Table 2. Studies on antioxidants. EGb 761, Gingko biloba special extract 761; NA, not applicable; VaD, Vascular Disease; ADL, Activities of Daily Living; RCT, Randomised Controlled Trial; ApoE, apolipoprotein E; n-3, omega-3 fatty acids; n-6, omega-6 fatty acids; FFQ, food frequency questionnaire; AD, Alzheimer's Disease; CI, cognitive impairment; MCI, Mild cognitive impairment; DHA, docohexanoic acid; PUFAs, polyunsaturated fatty acids; MMSE, Folstein Mini- Mental State examination; CDR, Clinical Dementia Rating Scale.

## 5. Conclusions

Oxidative stress increases with ageing and seems to be a consequence of an imbalance between ROS production and antioxidant defences. The accumulation of endogenous oxygen radicals generated in mitochondria and the consequent oxidative modifications of biological molecules have been indicated as responsible for the ageing process. There is therefore an urgent need to identify biomarkers that would help to diagnose and monitor the early AD or "preclinical AD". Indeed, a few CSF proteins (e.g. amyloid-$\beta_{1-42}$, total tau and phospho-tau) have already shown promise as diagnostic biomarkers for AD. Nevertheless, these biomarkers are not yet optimal diagnostic tools to identify those MCI patients at higher risk of conversion to AD. Thus, a key objective in the research of OS biomarkers is to identify prodromal stages of the disorder, prior to cognitive decline, for gauging the long-term therapeutic effects of drugs. The contradictory results obtained with diverse antioxidants in clinical trials may be explained by other related differences in health problems as well as due to the fact that most studies are very short and conducted with very few subjects. Methodological problems and poorly matched epidemiological studies have also been pointed as reasons for mixed findings. In fact, very few trials are adequately addressing the effect of antioxidants in AD. Although at this time there is no rationale for recommending antioxidant use for prevention or treatment of AD, the current epidemiologic evidence points toward an important role of nutrition in this pathology. The optimal time for prevention seems to be important and still to be determined. Nevertheless, it seems clear that therapies acting in the beginning of the pathological cascade may be more effective than treatments that act after the fact (e.g., removal of amyloid plaques). Then, therapy should begin as early as possible while reversal of cellular pathologies is still achievable. In conclusion, properly addressed studies with antioxidants are greatly needed to obtain convincing data about its beneficial effects as anti-AD. There is also an urgent need for better formulations with increased bioavailability. Due to the multifactorial nature of AD, it seems imperative that future trials may use drug combinations or even multifunctional molecules, rather than a single compound, able to bind to a very diverse type of target and that an antioxidant capacity may be contemplated.

## 6. Acknowledgment

The authors gratefully acknowledge Professors Nuria Durany (Universitat Internacional de Catalunya) and Peter Riederer (University of Würzburg).

## 7. References

Ahmed N, Ahmed U, Thornalley PJ, Hager K, Fleischer G, Münch G. (2005). Protein glycation, oxidation and nitration adduct residues and free adducts of cerebrospinal fluid in Alzheimer's disease and link to cognitive impairment. *J Neurochem,* 92:255-63.

Aliev G, Liu J, Schenk JC et al. (2009). Neuronal mitochondrial amelioration of alpha-lipoic acid and acetyl-L-carnitine. *J Cell Mol Med,* 13:320-333.

Akao I. (2002). Mitochondrial permeability transition mediates apoptosis induced by N-methyl(R)salsolinol, an endogenous neurotoxin, and is inhibited by Bcl-s and rasagiline. *J Neurochem,* 82:913-923.

Anand P, Kunnumakkara AB, Newman RA et al. (2007). Bioavailability of curcumin: problems and promises. *Mol Pharm,* 4:807-818.

Ando Y, Brännström T, Uchida K, Nyhlin N, Näsman B, Suhr O, Yamashita T, Olsson T, El Salhy M, Uchino M, Ando M. (1998). Histochemical detection of 4-hydroxynonenal protein in Alzheimer amyloid. *J Neurol Sci,* Apr 1;156(2):172-6.

Areosa SA, Sheriff F, Mc Shane R. (2005). Memantine for dementia. *Cochrane Database Syst Rev* (2) CD003154 .

Bagi Z, CSeko C, Toth E et al. (2003). Oxidative stress-induced dysregulation of arteriosal wall shear stress and blood pressure in hyperhomocysteinemia is prevented by chronic vitamin C treatment. *Am J Physiol Heart Circ Physiol,* 285:H2277-H2283.

Bar-Am O, Weinreb O, Amit T et al. (2009). The novel cholinesterase-monoamine oxidase inhibitor and antioxidant, ladostigil, confers neuroprotection in neuroblastoma cells and aged rats. *J Mol Neurosci,* 37:135-145.

Barberger-Gateau P, Letenneur L, Deschamps V et al. (2002). Fish, meat, and risk of dementia: cohort study. *BMJ,* 325(7370):932-933.

Barberger-Gateau P, Raffaitin C, Letenneur L et al. (2007). Dietary patterns and risk of dementia : The Three-city chort study. *Neurology,* 69(20):1921-1930.

Barnham KJ, Masters CL, Bush AI. (2004). Neurodegenerative diseases and oxidative stress. *Nat Rev Drug Discov,* Mar;3(3):205-14.

Basu S. Metabolism of 8-iso-prostaglandin F2alpha. (1998). *FEBS Lett.* May 22;428(1-2):32-6.

Berman K & Brodaty H. (2004). Tocopherol (vitamin E) in Alzheimer's disease and other neurodegenerative disorders. *Drugs,* 18:807-825.

Berlett BS, Stadtman ER. (1997). Protein oxidation in aging, disease, and oxidative stress. *J Biol Chem.* Aug 15;272(33):20313-6.

Birks J & Harvey R. (2006). Donepezil for dementia due to Alzheimer's disease. *Cochrane Database Syst Rev* (1) CD001190.

Birks J, Grimley EJ, Iakovidou V et al. (2000). Rivastigmine for Alzheimer's disease. *Cochrane Database Syst Rev* (4) CD001191.

Bondy SC, Guo-Ross SX, Truong AT. (1998). Promotion of transition metal-induced reactive oxygen species formation by beta-amyloid. *Brain Res,* 799:91-96.

Bradley MA, Markesbery WR, Lovell MA. (2010a). Increased levels of 4-hydroxynonenal and acrolein in the brain in preclinical Alzheimer disease. *Free Radic Biol Med,* Jun 15;48(12):1570-6.

Bradley MA, Xiong-Fister S, Markesbery WR, Lovell MA. (2010b). Elevated 4-hydroxyhexenal in Alzheimer's disease (AD) progression. *Neurobiol Aging,* Oct 19.

Butterfield DA, Bader Lange ML, Sultana R. (2010). Involvements of the lipid peroxidation product, HNE, in the pathogenesis and progression of Alzheimer's disease. *Biochim Biophys Acta,* Aug;1801(8):924-9.

Butterfield DA, Castegna A, Lauderback CM, Drake J. (2002). Evidence that amyloid beta-peptide-induced lipid peroxidation and its sequelae in Alzheimer's disease brain contribute to neuronal death. *Neurobiol Aging,* Sep-Oct;23(5):655-64.

Butterfield DA, Griffin S, Munch G, Pasinetti GM. (2002). Amyloid beta-peptide and amyloid pathology are central to the oxidative stress and inflammatory cascades under which Alzheimer's disease brain exists. *J Alzheimers Dis,* Jun;4(3):193-201.

Calingasan NY, Uchida K, Gibson GE. (1999). Protein-bound acrolein: a novel marker of oxidative stress in Alzheimer's disease. *J Neurochem,* Feb;72(2):751-6.

Carini M, Aldini G, Facino RM. (2004). Mass spectrometry for detection of 4-hydroxy-trans-2-nonenal (HNE) adducts with peptides and proteins. *Mass Spectrom Rev*, Jul-Aug;23(4):281-305.

Castegna A, Aksenov M, Aksenova M, Thongboonkerd V, Klein JB, Pierce WM, Booze R, Markesbery WR, Butterfield DA. (2002a). Proteomic identification of oxidatively modified proteins in Alzheimer's disease brain. Part I: creatine kinase BB, glutamine synthase, and ubiquitin carboxy-terminal hydrolase L-1. *Free Radic Biol Med,*. Aug 15;33(4):562-71.

Castegna A, Aksenov M, Thongboonkerd V, Klein JB, Pierce WM, Booze R, Markesbery WR, Butterfield DA. (2002b). Proteomic identification of oxidatively modified proteins in Alzheimer's disease brain. Part II: dihydropyrimidinase-related protein 2, alpha-enolase and heat shock cognate 71. *J Neurochem*, 2002 Sep;82(6):1524-32.

Castellani RJ, Harris PL, Sayre LM, Fujii J, Taniguchi N, Vitek MP, Founds H, Atwood CS, Perry G, Smith MA. (2001). Active glycation in neurofibrillary pathology of Alzheimer disease: N(epsilon)-(carboxymethyl) lysine and hexitol-lysine. Free Radic Biol Med, Jul 15;31(2):175-80.

Chan A, Paskavitz J, Remington R et al. (2008). Efficacy of a vitamin/nutraceutical formulation for early stage Alzheimer's disease: a 1 year, open-label pilot study with a 16-month caregiver extension. *Am J Alzheimer Dis Other Demen*, 23:571-585.

Chen X, Walker DG, Schmidt AM, Arancio O, Lue LF, Yan SD. (2007). RAGE: a potential target for Abeta-mediated cellular perturbation in Alzheimer's disease. Curr Mol Med, Dec;7(8):735-42.

Chiu CC, Su KP, Cheng TC et al. (2008). The effects of omega-3 fatty acids monotherapy in Alzheimer's disease and mild cognitive impairment: a preliminary randomised double-blind placebo controlled study. *Prog Neuropsychopharmacol Biol Psychiatry*, 32:1538-1544.

Cheng KC, Cahill DS, Kasai H, Nishimura S, Loeb LA. (1992). 8-Hydroxyguanine, an abundant form of oxidative DNA damage, causes G----T and A----C substitutions. *J Biol Chem*, Jan 5;267(1):166-72.

Choi J, Malakowsky CA, Talent JM, Conrad CC, Gracy RW. (2002). Identification of oxidized plasma proteins in Alzheimer's disease. *Biochem Biophys Res Commun*, May 24;293(5):1566-70.

Cole GM, Teter B, Frautschy SA. (2007). Neuroprotective effects of curcumin. *Adv Exp Med Biol*, 595:197-212.

Conquer JA, Tierney MC, Zecevic J et al. (2000). Fatty acid analyisis of blood plasma of patients with Alzheimer's disease, other types of dementia, and cognitive impairment. *Lipids*, 35(12):1305-1312.

Cooke MS, Olinski R, Loft S. (2008). European Standards Committee on Urinary (DNA) Lesion Analysis. Measurement and meaning of oxidatively modified DNA lesions in urine. *Cancer Epidemiol Biomarkers Prev*, Jan;17(1):3-14.

Cracowski JL, Durand T, Bessard G. (2002). Isoprostanes as a biomarker of lipid peroxidation in humans: physiology, pharmacology and clinical implications. *Trends Pharmacol Sci*, Aug;23(8):360-6.

CTdotgovdimebon ClinicalTrials.gov study NCT00675623, a safety and efficacy study of oral dimebon in patients with mild-to-moderate Alzheimer's disease (CONNECTION)

Dalle-Donne I, Rossi R, Colombo R, Giustarini D, Milzani A. (2006a). Biomarkers of oxidative damage in human disease. Clin Chem, Apr;52(4):601-23.

Dalle-Donne I, Aldini G, Carini M, Colombo R, Rossi R, Milzani A. (2006b). Protein carbonylation, cellular dysfunction, and disease progression. J Cell Mol Med, Apr-Jun;10(2):389-406.

Davidsson P, Paulson L, Hesse C, Blennow K, Nilsson CL. (2001). Proteome studies of human cerebrospinal fluid and brain tissue using a preparative two-dimensional electrophoresis approach prior to mass spectrometry. *Proteomics*, Mar;1(3):444-52.

Defeudis FV (2002). Bilobalide and neuroprotection. *Pharmacol Res* 46: 565-568.

DeKosky ST, Williamson JD, Fitzpatrick AL et al (2008) Gingko biloba for prevention of dementia: a randomised controlled trial. *JAMA,* 300:2253-2262.

Dodge HH, Zitzelberger T, Oken BS et al. (2008). A randomised placebo-controlled trial of Gingko biloba for the prevention of cognitive decline. *Neurology,* 70:1809-1817.

Doody RS. (2009). Dimebon as a potential therapy for Alzheimer's disease. *CNS Spectrosc,* 14:14-16;discussion 16-18

Doody RS, Gavrilova SI, Sano M et al. (2008). Effect of dimebon on cognition, activities of daily living, behaviour, and global function in patients with mild-to-moderate Alzheimer's disease: a randomised, double-blind, placebo-controlled study. *Lancet* 372:207-215

Epis R, Marcello E, Gardoni F et al. (2008). Modulatory effect of acetyl-L-carnitine on amyloid precursor protein metabolism in hippocampal neurons. *Eur J Pharmacol* 597:51-56

Eckl PM, Ortner A, Esterbauer H. (1993). Genotoxic properties of 4-hydroxyalkenals and analogous aldehydes. *Mutat Res.* Dec;290(2):183-92.

Esterbauer H, Schaur RJ, Zollner H. (1991). Chemistry and biochemistry of 4-hydroxynonenal, malonaldehyde and related aldehydes. *Free Radic Biol* Med. 11(1):81-128.

Evans MD, Olinski R, Loft S, Cooke MS. (2010). Toward consensus in the analysis of urinary 8-oxo-7,8-dihydro-2'-deoxyguanosine as a noninvasive biomarker of oxidative stress. European Standards Committee on Urinary (DNA) Lesion Analysis, *FASEB J.* Apr;24(4):1249-60.

Freund-Levi Y, Eriksdotter-Jönhagen M, Cederholm T et al. (2006). Omega-3 fatty acids treatment in 174 patients with mild to moderate Alzheimer disease: OmegAD study: a randomised, double-blind trial. *Arch Neurol,* 63(10):1402-1408.

Freund-Levi Y, Hjorth E, Lindberg C et al. (2009). Effects of omega-3 fatty acids on inflammatory markers in cerebrospinal fluid and plasma in Alzheimer's disease: the OmegAD Study. *Dement Geriatr Cogn Disord,* 27:481-490.

Fraga CG, Shigenaga MK, Park JW, Degan P, Ames BN. Oxidative damage to DNA during aging: 8-hydroxy-2'-deoxyguanosine in rat organ DNA and urine. *Proc Natl Acad Sci USA,* 1990 Jun;87(12):4533-7.

Goodman AB. (2006). Retinoid receptors, transporters, and metabolizers as therapeutic targets in late onset Alzheimer disease. *J Cell Physiol,* 209:598-60.

Green C, Picot J, Loveman E et al. (2005). Modelling the cost effectiveness of cholinesterase inhibitors in the management of mild to moderately severe Alzheimer's disease. *Pharmacoeconomics,* 23:1271-1282.

Griffiths HR, Møller L, Bartosz G, Bast A, Bertoni-Freddari C, Collins A, Cooke M, Coolen S, Haenen G, Hoberg AM, Loft S, Lunec J, Olinski R, Parry J, Pompella A, Poulsen H, Verhagen H, Astley SB. (2002). Biomarkers. *Mol Aspects Med,* Feb-Jun;23(1-3):101-208.

Grundman M, Petersen RC, Ferris SH et al. (2004). Mild cognitive impairment can be distinguished from Alzheimer disease and normal aging for clinical trials. *Arch Neurol,* 61:59-66.

Gutzmann H, Khul KP, Hadler D et al. (2002). Safety and efficacy of idebenone versus tacrine in patients with Alzheimer's disease:results of a randomised, double-blind, parallel group multicenter study. *Pharmacopsychiatry,* 35:12-18.

Haase J, Halama P and Horr R. (1996). Effectiveness of brief infusions with Gingko biloba Special Extract EGb 761 in dementia of the vascular and Alzheimer type. *Z Gerontol Geriatr,*29:302-309.

Haenen GR & Bast A. (1991). Scavenging of hypochlorus acid by lipoic acid. *Biochem Pharmacol,* 42:2244-2246.

Hamilton ML, Van Remmen H, Drake JA, Yang H, Guo ZM, Kewitt K, Walter CA, Richardson A. (2001). Does oxidative damage to DNA increase with age? *Proc Natl Acad Sci USA,* Aug 28;98(18):10469-74.

Harman D. (1956). Aging: a theory based on free radical and radiation chemistry. *J Gerontol,* Jul;11(3):298-300.

Harman D. (1972). The biologic clock: the mitochondria?. *J Am Geriatr Soc,* Apr;20(4):145-7.

Hu P, Brestky P, Crimmins EM. (2006). Association between serum beta-carotene levels and decline of cognitive function in high functioning older persons with or without apolipoprotein E 4 alleles: MacArthur studies of successful aging. *J Gerontol A Biol Sci Med Sci,* 61:616-620.

Jiménez-Jiménez FJ, de Bustos F, Molina JA et al. (1997). Cerebrospinal fluid levels of alpha-tocopherol (vitamin E) in Alzheimer's disease. *J Neural Transm,* 104:703-710.

Karuppagounder SS, Pinto JT, Xu H et al. (2009). Dietary supplementation with resveratrol reduces plaque pathology in a transgenic model of Alzheimer's disease. *Neurochem Int,* 54:111-118.

Kim KM, Jung BH, Paeng KJ, Kim I, Chung BC. (2004). Increased urinary F(2)-isoprostanes levels in the patients with Alzheimer's disease. *Brain Res Bull,* Jul 30;64(1):47-51.

Kimura T, Takamatsu J, Ikeda K, Kondo A, Miyakawa T, Horiuchi S. (1996). Accumulation of advanced glycation end products of the Maillard reaction with age in human hippocampal neurons. *Neurosci Lett,* Apr 12;208(1):53-6.

Kitani KA et al. (2000). Common properties for propargylamines of enhancing superoxide dismutase and catalase acivities in the dopaminergic system in the rat: implications for the life prolonging effect of (-)deprenyl. *J Neural Transm,* 60 (Suppl) 139-156.

Korolainen MA, Nyman TA, Nyyssönen P, Hartikainen ES, Pirttilä T. (2007). Multiplexed proteomic analysis of oxidation and concentrations of cerebrospinal fluid proteins in Alzheimer disease. *Clin Chem,* Apr;53(4):657-65.

Korolainen MA, Goldsteins G, Nyman TA, Alafuzoff I, Koistinaho J, Pirttilä T. (2006). Oxidative modification of proteins in the frontal cortex of Alzheimer's disease brain. *Neurobiol Aging,* Jan;27(1):42-53.

Kozekov ID, Nechev LV, Moseley MS, Harris CM, Rizzo CJ, Stone MP, Harris TM. (2003). DNA interchain cross-links formed by acrolein and crotonaldehyde. *J Am Chem Soc*, Jan 8;125(1):50-61.

Kroger E, Verreault R, Carmicael PH et al. (2009). Omega-3 fatty acids and risk of dementia: the Canadian Study of Health and Aging. *Am J Clin Nutr*, 90(1):184-192.

Laurin D, Verreault R, Lindsay J et al. (2003). Omega-3 fatty acids and risk of cognitive impairment and dementia. *J Alzheimers Dis* 5(4):315-322.

Ledesma MD, Pérez M, Colaco C et al (1998) Tau glycation is involved in aggregation of the protein but not in the formation of filaments. *Cell Moll Biol* Nov 44(7):1111-1116.

Liu X, Lovell MA, Lynn BC. (2006). Detection and quantification of endogenous cyclic DNA adducts derived from trans-4-hydroxy-2-nonenal in human brain tissue by isotope dilution capillary liquid chromatography nanoelectrospray tandem mass spectrometry. *Chem Res Toxicol*, May;19(5):710-8.

Le Bars PL, Kieser M and Itil KZ. (2000). A 26-week analysis of a double-blind, placebo-controlled trial of the gingko biloba extract EGb 761 in dementia. *Dement Geriatr Cogn Disord*, 11:230-237.

Le Bars PL. (2003). Response patterns of EGb 761 in Alzhemier's disease: influence of neuropsychological profiles. *Pharmacopsychiatry*, 36 (Suppl 1) S50-S55.

Loske C, Gerdemann A, Schepl W, Wycislo M, Schinzel R, Palm D, Riederer P, Münch G. (2000). Transition metal-mediated glycoxidation accelerates cross-linking of beta-amyloid peptide. Eur J Biochem, Jul;267(13):4171-8.

Lovell MA, Ehmann WD, Mattson MP, Markesbery WR. (1997). Elevated 4-hydroxynonenal in ventricular fluid in Alzheimer's disease. *Neurobiol Aging*, Sep-Oct;18(5):457-61.

Lovell MA, Markesbery WR. (2007a). Oxidative damage in mild cognitive impairment and early Alzheimer's disease. *J Neurosci Res*, Nov 1;85(14):3036-40.

Lovell MA, Markesbery WR. (2007b). Oxidative DNA damage in mild cognitive impairment and late-stage Alzheimer's disease. *Nucleic Acids Res*, 35(22):7497-504.

Lovell MA, Markesbery WR. (2001). Ratio of 8-hydroxyguanine in intact DNA to free 8-hydroxyguanine is increased in Alzheimer disease ventricular cerebrospinal fluid. *Arch Neurol*, Mar;58(3):392-6.

Loy C & Schneider L. (2004). Galantamine for Alzheimer's disease. *Cochrane Database Syst Rev*, (4)CD001747.

Luchsinger JA, Tang MX, Shea S et al. (2003). Antioxidant vitamine intake and risk of Alzheimer disease. *Arch Neurol*, 60:203-208.

Luo Y, Smith JV, Paramasivam V et al. (2002). Inhibition of amyloid beta aggregation and caspase-3 activation by the Gingko biloba extract EGb 761. *Proc Natl Acad Sci USA*, 99-12197-12202.

Mandel SA, Amit T, Kalfon L. (2008). Cell signaling pathways and iron chelation in the neurorestorative activity of green tea polyphenols: special reference to epigallocatechin gallate (EGCG). *J Alzheimer Dis*, 17:681-697.

Mangialasche F, Solomon A, Winblad B et al. (2010). Alzheimer's disease: clinical trials and drug development. *Lancet Neurol* 9:702-716.

Markesbery WR, Lovell MA. (1998). Four-hydroxynonenal, a product of lipid peroxidation, is increased in the brain in Alzheimer's disease. *Neurobiol Aging*, Jan-Feb;19(1):33-6.

Markesbery WR, Carney JM. (1999). Oxidative alterations in Alzheimer's disease. *Brain Pathol*, Jan;9(1):133 46.

Mayurama W, Akao Y, Youdim MB et al. (2000). Transfection-enforced Bcl-2 overexpression and an anti-Parkinson drug, rasagiline, prevent nuclear accumulation of GAPDH induced by an endogenous dopaminergic neurotoxin, N-methyl(R)salsolinol. *J Neurochem*, 78:727-735.

McGrath LT, McGleenon BM, Brennan S, McColl D, McILroy S, Passmore AP. (2001). Increased oxidative stress in Alzheimer's disease as assessed with 4-hydroxynonenal but not malondialdehyde. *QJM*, Sep;94(9):485-90.

McIlroy SP, Dynan KB, Lawson JT et al. (2002). Moderately elevated plasma homocysteine, methylenetetrahydrofolate reductase genotype, and risk for stroke, vascular dementia and Alzheimer disease in Northern Ireland. *Stroke*, 33:2351-2356

Mecocci P, Polidori MC, Cherubini A, Ingegni T, Mattioli P, Catani M, Rinaldi P, Cecchetti R, Stahl W, Senin U, Beal MF. (2002). Lymphocyte oxidative DNA damage and plasma antioxidants in Alzheimer disease. *Arch Neurol*, May;59(5):794-8.

Migliore L, Fontana I, Trippi F, Colognato R, Coppedè F, Tognoni G, Nucciarone B, Siciliano G. (2005). Oxidative DNA damage in peripheral leukocytes of mild cognitive impairment and AD patients. *Neurobiol Aging*, May; 26(5):567-73.

Mishra S & Palanivelu K. (2008). The effect of curcumin (turmeric) on Alzheimer's disease: an overwiew. *Ann Indian Acad Neurol*, 11:13-19.

Montgomery SA, Thal LJ & Amrein R. (2003). Meta-analysis of double-blind randomised controlled clinical trials of acetyl-L-carnitine versus placebo in the treatment of mild conginitive impairment and mild Alzheimer's disease. *Int Clin Psychopharmacol*, 18:61-71.

Montine KS, Kim PJ, Olson SJ, Markesbery WR, Montine TJ. (1997). 4-hydroxy-2-nonenal pyrrole adducts in human neurodegenerative disease. *J Neuropathol Exp Neurol*, 56(8): 866-71.

Montine TJ, Markesbery WR, Morrow JD, Roberts LJ 2nd. (1998). Cerebrospinal fluid F2-isoprostane levels are increased in Alzheimer's disease. *Ann Neurol*, Sep;44(3):410-3.

Montine TJ, Quinn JF, Milatovic D, Silbert LC, Dang T, Sanchez S, Terry E, Roberts LJ 2nd, Kaye JA, Morrow JD. Peripheral F2-isoprostanes and F4-neuroprostanes are not increased in Alzheimer's disease. *Ann Neurol*, 2002 Aug;52(2):175-9.

Montine TJ, Peskind ER, Quinn JF, Wilson AM, Montine KS, Galasko D. Increased Cerebrospinal Fluid F(2)-Isoprostanes are Associated with Aging and Latent Alzheimer's Disease as Identified by Biomarkers. *Neuromolecular Med*, 2011 Mar;13(1):37-43.

Montuschi P, Barnes PJ, Roberts LJ 2nd. Isoprostanes: markers and mediators of oxidative stress. *FASEB J*, 2004 Dec; 18(15):1791-800.

Morris MC, Beckett LA, Scherr PA et al (1998) Vitamin E and vitamin C supplement use and risk of incident Alzheimer disease. *Alzheimer Dis assoc Disord*,12:121-126.

Morris MC, Evans DA, Bienias JL et al (2002) Dietary intake of antioxidant nutrients and the risk of incident Alzheimer disease in a biracial community study. *J Am Med Assoc*, 287:3230-3237.

Morris MC, Evans DA, Bienias JL et al (2003). Consumption of fish and n-3 fatty acids and risk of incident Alzheimer disease. *Arch Neurol*, 60(7):940-946.

Morris MC, Evans DA, Tagney CC (2005) Relation of the tocopherol forms to incident Alzheiemr disese and to cognitive change. *Am J Clin Nutr*, 81:508-514.

Morris MC, Evans DA, Tagney CC et al. (2005). Fish consumption and cognitive decline with age in a large community study. *Arch Neurol,* 62(12):1849-1853.

Morris MS, Jacques PF, Rosenberg IH et al. (2007). Folate and vitamine B12 status in relation to anemia, macrocytosis and cognitive impairment in older Americans in the age of folic acid fortification. *Am J Clin Nutr,* 85:193-200.

Morrow JD, Tapper AR, Zackert WE, Yang J, Sanchez SC, Montine TJ, Roberts LJ. (1999). Formation of novel isoprostane-like compounds from docosahexaenoic acid. *Adv Exp Med Biol,* 469:343-7.

Napryeyenko O, Sonnik G, Tartakovsky I. (2009). Efficacy and tolerability of gingko biloba extract EGb 761 by type of dementia: analyses of a randomised controlled trial. *J Neurol Sci,* 283:224-229.

Nunomura A, Perry G, Aliev G, Hirai K, Takeda A, Balraj EK, Jones PK, Ghanbari H, Wataya T, Shimohama S, Chiba S, Atwood CS, Petersen RB, Smith MA. (2001). Oxidative damage is the earliest event in Alzheimer disease. *J Neuropathol Exp Neurol,* Aug;60(8):759-67.

Oken BS, Storzbach DM, Kaye JA. (1998). The efficacy og Gingko biloba on cognitive function in Alzheimer's disease. *Arch Neurol,* 55:1409-1415.

Okun I, Tkachenko SE, Khvat A et al. (2010). From anti-allergic to anti-Alzheimer's: molecular pharmacology of dimebon. *Curr Alzheimer Res,* 7:97-112.

Olinski R, Siomek A, Rozalski R, Gackowski D, Foksinski M, Guz J, Dziaman T, Szpila A, Tudek B. (2007). Oxidative damage to DNA and antioxidant status in aging and age-related diseases. *Acta Biochim Pol,* 54(1):11-26.

Perry G, Raina AK, Nunomura A, Wataya T, Sayre LM, Smith MA. (2000). How important is oxidative damage? Lessons from Alzheimer's disease. *Free Radic Biol Med,* Mar 1;28(5):831-4.

Perry G, Nunomura A, Cash AD, Taddeo MA, Hirai K, Aliev G, Avila J, Wataya T, Shimohama S, Atwood CS, Smith MA. (2002). *Reactive oxygen: its sources and significance in Alzheimer disease. J Neural Transm Suppl,* (62):69-75.

Petersen RC, Thomas RG, Grudman N et al. (2005). Vitamin E and donepezil for the treatment of mild cognitive impairment. *N Engl J Med* 352:2379-2388,

Pettergrew JW, Klunk WE, Panchalingam K et al, (1995). Clinical and neurochemical effects of acetyl-L-carnitine in Alzheimer's disease. *Neurobiol Aging,* 16:1-4,

Praticò D, Clark CM, Liun F, Rokach J, Lee VY, Troianowski JQ. (2002). Increase of brain oxidative stress in mild cognitive impairment: a possible predictor of Alzheimer disease. *Arch Neurol,* Jun:59(6): 972-6.

Puchades M, Hansson SF, Nilsson CL, Andreasen N, Blennow K, Davidsson P. (2003). Proteomic studies of potential cerebrospinal fluid protein markers for Alzheimer's disease. *Brain Res Mol Brain Res,* Oct 21;118(1-2):140-6.

Quinn JF, Raman R, Thomas RG et al. (2009). A clinical trial of docohexanoic acid (DHA) for the treatment of Alzheimer's disease. *Alzheimers Assoc Int Conf Alzheimer Dis*; July 12.

Riederer P, Danielczyk W, Grünblatt E. (2004). Monoamine oxidase-B inhibition in Alzheimer's disease. *Neurotoxicology,* 25 (1-2):271-277.

Roberts LJ 2nd, Montine TJ, Markesbery WR, Tapper AR, Hardy P, Chemtob S, Dettbarn WD, Morrow JD. (1998). Formation of isoprostane-like compounds (neuroprostanes) in vivo from docosahexaenoic acid. *J Biol Chem,* May 29;273(22):13605-12.

Sahin M, Karauzum SB, Perry G et al. (2005). Retinoic acid isomers protect hippocampal neurons from amyloid-beta induced neurodegeneration. *Neurotox Res,* 7:243-250.

Sano M, Ernesto C, Thomas RG et al. (1997). A controlled trial of selegiline, alpha tocopherol, or both as treatment for Alzheimer's disease. The Alzheimer's disease cooperative study. *N Engl J Med,* 336:1216-1222.

Sanz E, Romera M, Bellik L et al. (2004). Indolalkylamines derivatives as antioxidant and neuroprotective agents in an experimental model of Parkinson's disease. *Med Sci Monit,* 10(12):BR477-484.

Sayre LM, Zelasko DA, Harris PL, Perry G, Salomon RG, Smith MA. (1997). 4-Hydroxynonenal-derived advanced lipid peroxidation end products are increased in Alzheimer's disease. *J Neurochem,* May;68(5):2092-7.

Schneider LS, DeKosky ST, Farlow MR et al. (2005). A randomised, double-bind, placebo controlled trial of two doses of Gongko biloba extract in dementa of the Alzhemier's type. *Curr Alzheimer Res,* 2 541-551.

Senin U, Parnetti L, Barbagallo-Sangiorgi G et al. (1992). Idebenone in senile dementia of Alzheimer type:a multicenter study. *Arch Gerontol Geriatr,* 15:249-260.

Shigenaga MK, Gimeno CJ, Ames BN. (1989). Urinary 8-hydroxy-2'-deoxyguanosine as a biological marker of in vivo oxidative DNA damage. *Proc Natl Acad Sci USA,* Dec;86(24):9697-701.

Shoba G, Joy S, Joseph T et al. (1998). Influence of piperine on the pharmacokinetics of curcumin in animals and human volunteers. *Planta Med,* 64:353-356.

Smith MA, Sayre LM, Monnier VM, Perry G. (1995). Radical AGEing in Alzheimer's disease. Trends Neurosci, Apr;18(4):172-6.

Snitz BE, O'Meara ES, Carlsom MC et al. (2009). Gingko biloba for preventing cognitive decline in older adults: a randomised trial. *JAMA,* 302:2663-2670.

Southern L, Williams J, Esiri MM. (2007). Immunohistochemical study of N-epsilon-carboxymethyl lysine (CML) in human brain: relation to vascular dementia. *BMC Neurol,* Oct 16;7:35.

Sultana R, Butterfield DA. (2011). Identification of the oxidative stress proteome in the brain. *Free Radic Biol Med,* Feb 15;50(4):487-94. Epub 2010 Nov 25.

Tabet N, Birks J, Grimley EF. (2000). Vitamine E for Alhzheimer's disease. *Cochrane database Syst Rev* (4) CD002854.

Tamagno E, Guglielmotto M, Aragno M, Borghi R, Autelli R, Giliberto L, Muraca G, Danni O, Zhu X, Smith MA, Perry G, Jo DG, Mattson MP, Tabaton M. (2008). Oxidative stress activates a positive feedback between the gamma- and beta-secretase cleavages of the beta-amyloid precursor protein. *J Neurochem,* Feb;104(3):683-95.

Thal LJ, Grundman M, Berg J et al. (2003). Idebenone treatment fails to slow cognitive decline in Alzheimer's disease. *Neurology,* 61:1498-1502.

Thal LJ, Calvani M, Amato A et al. (2000). A 1-year controlled trial of acetyl-L-carnitine in early onset AD. *Neurology,* 55:805-810.

Thomas T. (2000). Monoamine oxidase-B inhibitors in the treatment of Alzheimer's disease. *Neurobiol Aging,* 21(2):343-348.

Thome J, Münch G, Muller R, Schinzel R, Kornhuber J, Blum-Degen D et al. (1996). Advanced glycation endproducts-associated parameters in the peripheral blood of patients with Alzheimer's disease. *Neurotox Res*, 4:191-209.

Tucker JM & Townsend DM. (2005). Alpha-tocopherol: roles in prevention and therapy of human disease. *Biomed Pharmacother*, 59 (7):380-387.

Tully AM, Roche HM, Doyle R et al. (2003). Low serum cholesteryl ester-docohexanoic acid levels in Alzheimer's disease: a case-control study. *Br J Nutr*, 89(4):483-489.

Uchida K. (2003). 4-Hydroxy-2-nonenal: a product and mediator of oxidative stress. *Prog Lipid Res*, Jul;42(4):318-43.

Van Gelder BM, Tijhuis M, Kalmijn S et al. (2007). Fish consumption, n-3 fatty acids, and subsequent 5-y cognitive decline in elderly men: the Zutphen Elderly Study. *Am J Clin Nutr*, 85(4):1142-1147.

Vitek MP, Bhattacharya K, Glendening JM, Stopa E, Vlassara H, Bucala R, Manogue K, Cerami A. (1994). Advanced glycation end products contribute to amyloidosis in Alzheimer disease. *Proc Natl Acad Sci USA*, May 24;91(11):4766-70.

Von Arnim CA, Gola U and Biesalski HK. (2010). More than the sumo f its parts? Nutrition in Alzheimer's disease. *Nutrition*, 26(7-8):694-700.

Wadsworth TL, Bishop JA, PAppu AS et al. (2008). Evaluation of Coenzyme Q as an antioxidant strategy for Alzheimer's disease. *J Alzheimer's Dis*, 14:225-234.

Wataya T, Nunomura A, Smith MA, Siedlak SL, Harris PL, Shimohama S, Szweda LI, Kaminski MA, Avila J, Price DL, Cleveland DW, Sayre LM, Perry G. (2002). High molecular weight neurofilament proteins are physiological substrates of adduction by the lipid peroxidation product hydroxynonenal. *J Biol Chem*, Feb 15;277(7):4644-8.

Weyer G, Babej.Dolle RM, Hadler D et al. (1997). A controlled study of 2 doses of idebenone in the treatment of Alzheimer's disease. *Neuropsychobiology*, 36:73-82.

White AR, Barnham KJ, Huang X et al. (2004). Iron inhibits neurotoxicity induced by trace cooper and biological reductants. *J Biol Inorg Chem*, 9:269-280.

Williams TI, Lynn BC, Markesbery WR, Lovell MA. (2006). Increased levels of 4-hydroxynonenal and acrolein, neurotoxic markers of lipid peroxidation, in the brain in Mild Cognitive Impairment and early Alzheimer's disease. *Neurobiol Aging*, Aug;27(8):1094-9.

Yao Z & Drieu V. (2001). Papadopoulos, the Gingko biloba extract Egb 761 rescues the PC12 neuronal cells from beta-amyloid-induced cell death by inhibiting the formation of beta-amyloid-derived diffusible neurotoxic ligands. *Brain Res*, 889:181-190.

Yan SD, Chen X, Schmidt AM, Brett J, Godman G, Zou YS, Scott CW, Caputo C, Frappier T, Smith MA, et al. (1994). Glycated tau protein in Alzheimer disease: a mechanism for induction of oxidant stress. Proc Natl Acad Sci USA, Aug 2;91(16):7787-91.

Youdim BM, Fridkin M and Zheng H. (2005). Bifunctional drug derivates of MAO-B inhibitor rasagiline and iron chelator VK28 as a more effective approach to treatment of brain aging and aging neurodegenerative diseases. *Mech Aging Dev*, 126: 317-326.

Yu HL, Chertkow HM, Bergman H, Schipper HM. (2003). Aberrant profiles of native and oxidized glycoproteins in Alzheimer plasma. *Proteomics*, Nov;3(11):2240-8.

Yurko-Mauro K, McCarthy D, Bailey-Hall E et al. (2009). Results of the MIDAS trial: effects of docohexanoic acid on physiological and safety parameters in age-related cognitive decline. *Alzheimers Assoc Int Conf Alzheimer Dis*; July 12.

# 10

# Advances in MicroRNAs and Alzheimer's Disease Research

Francesca Ruberti[1], Silvia Pezzola[2] and Christian Barbato[3]
[1,3]*CNR, National Research Council of Italy,*
*Cell Biology and Neurobiology Institute (IBCN),*
*IRCCS Fondazione Santa Lucia,*
[2,3]*EBRI - European Brain Research Institute-*
*Fondazione EBRI- Rita Levi-Montalcini*
*Italy*

## 1. Introduction

Molecular and cellular neurobiological studies of the miRNA-mediated gene silencing in Alzheimer's disease represent the exploration of a new frontier of miRNAs biology and the potential development of new diagnostic tests and genetic therapies for this neurodegenerative disease. In few years our understanding of microRNA (miRNA) biogenesis, molecular mechanisms by which miRNAs regulate gene expression, and the functional roles of miRNAs has been expanded. MiRNA are double-stranded RNAs (dsRNAs) ≈22 nucleotides in lenght. These small noncoding RNA molecules operate as guides for RISC (RNA Induced Silencing Complex) to cleave a target mRNA in case of a perfect complementarity (siRNA) or to block the target mRNA translation (miRNA) when there is an imperfect pairing between miRNAs and the targets. In mammalian cells the repression of translation by miRNA is mediated by an imperfect pairing with the 3'UTRs of the mRNA targets. Interestingly, numerous miRNAs are expressed in a spatially and temporally controlled manner in the nervous system, suggesting that mRNA post-transcriptional regulation by microRNAs may be particularly relevant in neural development and function. Individual microRNAs can reduce the production of hundred proteins and miRNAs-mediated post-transcriptional regulation is involved in neuronal differentiation, dendritic spine development and synaptic plasticity. Recently expression profiles of miRNA in Alzheimer's disease brain revealed alterations in many indiviual miRNAs and several in vitro and in vivo studies aimed to the exploration of functional role of miRNA in Alzheimer's disease pathogenesis.

### 1.1 MicroRNA-mediated gene silencing

MicroRNAs are non-coding single stranded RNA molecules, 18- to 25 nucleotides in lenght, encoded in the genomes of invertebrates, plants and vertebrates. MicroRNA genes represent about 1-2% of the known eukaryotic genomes. The first two miRNAs to be discovered were *lin-4* and *let-7* in *Caenorhabditis elegans,* which regulate expression of *lin-14* and *lin-28* mRNAs, respectively, and are required for larval developmental timing (Lee et al., 1993;

Olsen et al., 1999; Reinhart et al., 2000). Since then, miRNAs have been observed in many contexts and their function involved in numerous regulatory pathways, deserving the attention they are now receiving.

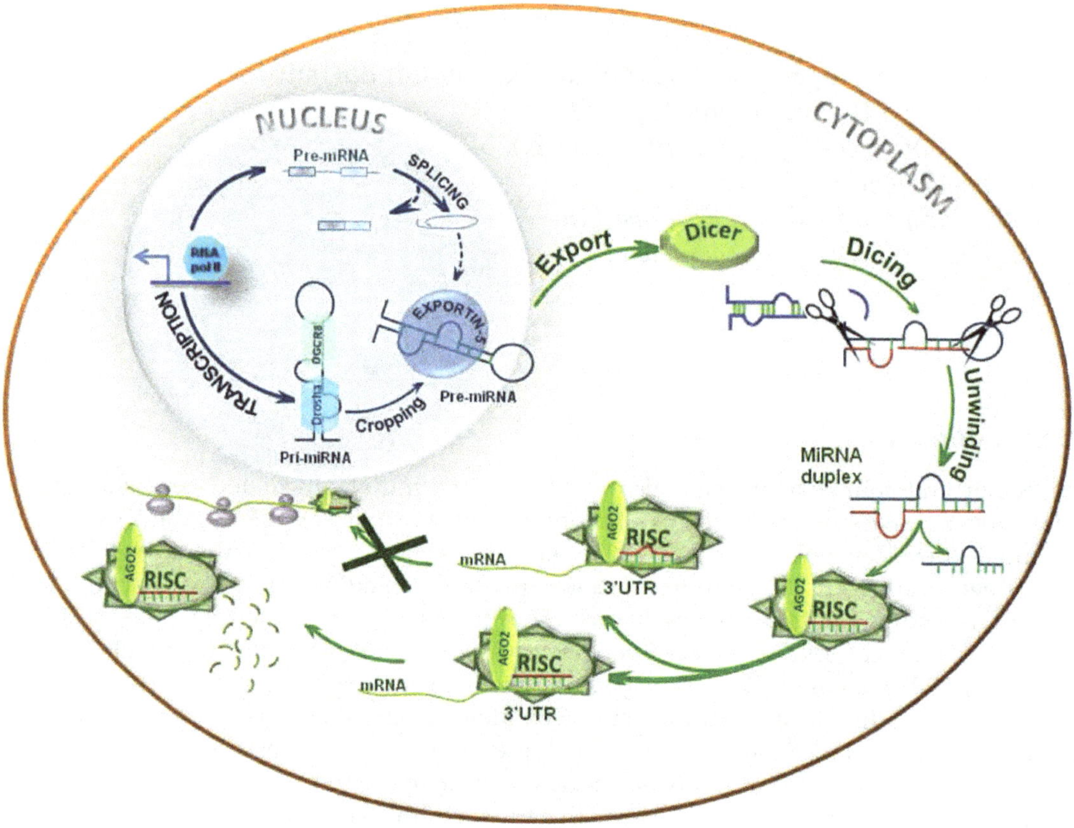


Fig. 1. MicroRNAs biogenesis and activity.

MiRNAs are transcribed by RNA polymerase II (Rodriguez et al., 2004), which mediates the transcription of most miRNA genes to generate an initial transcript, named primary miRNA (pri-miRNA). Pri-miRNAs can be hundreds to thousands nucleotides long, contain several hairpin structures, and undergo capping and polyadenylation (Lee et al., 2003). The first step in miRNA biogenesis occurs in the nucleus and requires the excision of this hairpin structure by a complex containing the RNAse III-endonuclease Drosha enzyme and the RNA binding protein DiGeorge syndrome critical region gene 8 (DGCR8) (Gregory et al., 2004). Apart from canonical intronic miRNAs, a group of intronic miRNAs (named mirtrons), present in the introns of flies and mammals, are derived from small introns that resemble pre-miRNAs and can bypass the Drosha-processing step. The excised hairpin, now called pre-miRNA, is exported to the cytoplasm by a protein heterodimer consisting of the transport factor Exportin-5/RanGTP (Bohnsack et al., 2004), and processed by Dicer, a double-stranded RNA (dsRNA)-specific endonuclease RNaseIII, which removes the loop region of the hairpin, releasing the mature miRNA: miRNA duplex. Dicer interacts with several RNA binding proteins, such as TRBP and PACT, which are not essential for its cleavage activity but are important for miRNA stability and loading of the effector complex RISC (RNA-induced silencing complex) (Chendrimada et al., 2005; Lee et al., 2006). During the assembly of the RISC complex with the miRNA, only one strand of the duplex is loaded, whereas the complementary miRNA* strand is removed and degraded (Kim et al., 2005). The mature miRNA is now ready to direct its activity on a target mRNA, by binding miRNA responsive elements usually located in the 3'UTR of the transcript, which leads to post-transcriptional gene silencing via inhibition of translation initiation or elongation. MicroRNAs associate with Argonaute proteins (Ago1-4, in mammals), which constitute the core of the RISC complex, and mediate post-transcriptional repression of target messenger RNAs. In particular Argonaute proteins are highly basic proteins which contain four domains: the N-terminal, PAZ, Mid and PIWI domains (Hutvagner and Simard, 2008). The PAZ domain binds the single stranded 3'end of miRNAs.

### 1.2 MicroRNAs in nervous system

The bewildering diversity of neurons, including their distribution in specific functional areas and complex synaptic circuitry, is determined during development and differentiation and is achieved by multiple levels of gene regulation. The transcriptional and post-transcriptional gene regulation mechanisms of development, plasticity and networking might participate in the determination and maintenance of such complexity. Recently, microRNAs are emerging as important players in post-transcriptional regulation in the brain. A major advancement in understanding how miRNAs are involved in this phenomenon comes from studies on miRNAs expression profiles. Several analyses have shown spatially and/or temporally restricted distribution of miRNAs, suggesting that they may control the fine-tuning regulation of neuronal gene expression (Cao et al., 2006; Schratt, 2009).

### 1.3 MicroRNAs, synaptic plasticity and memory

This section focuses on more relevant works highlighting the relevance of microRNAs post-transcriptional regulation in cellular pathways and functions such as synaptic plasticity and memory. However pathological implications of miRNAs expression associated to cognitive decline in Alzheimer's disease, are still unknown.

#### 1.3.1 MicroRNAs and the dendritic neuronal compartment

Synaptic loss is the major neurobiological substrate of cognitive decline in Alzheimer's disease. The alteration of synaptic integrity occurs very early in AD, and it can be observed in patients with mild cognitive impairment (MCI) (Scheff et al., 2006). Loss of molecular components of presynaptic and postsynaptic membranes, synaptic vescicles, and proteins contributing to the morphological and architectural characteristic of axons and dendrites, is the main feature associated with an impairment of synaptic plasticity in neuronal cells. Neuronal activity is a critical regulator of several nervous system functions, including long-term memory (Malenka and Nicoll, 1999; Sutton and Schuman, 2006). Beyond the reduction of transcripts related to synaptic vesicle trafficking (Coleman and Yao, 2003), it is questionable if there is a post-transcriptional deregulation of mRNAs functionally associated to axonal and dendritic synaptic remodelling in AD. Little is known about the mechanisms that underlie the regulation of protein synthesis in polarized cells like neurons. The synaptic protein synthesis makes necessary the corresponding mRNAs to be transported in the dendritic compartment and to be translated upon site-specific activation. It is generally thought that dendritic mRNAs are transported in a translationally silenced state within ribonucleoprotein complexes (Kiebler and Bassell, 2006). The recent discovery of the existence of a group of molecules regulating gene expression at post-transcriptional levels, named microRNAs, opened a new window on the research of molecular mechanisms of plasticity in the nervous system. Specific sites of protein synthesis are the dendritic spines. In neurons there are thousand of spines throughout multiple arborizations. Spine structures are dinamically regulated (Hotulainen and Hoogenraad, 2010), and functional and structural changes at spines and synapses are proposed as the basis of learning and memory (Kasai et al., 2010). MiRNAs, that are expressed in spatially and temporally controlled manner in the brain, are ideal candidates as modulators of dendritic protein synthesis. MicroRNAs modulate dendritic morphology by regulating expression of proteins involved in the actin cytoskeleton (Vo et al., 2005; Schratt et al., 2006; Siegel et al., 2009; Wayman et al., 2008) mRNA transport (Fiore et al., 2009) and neurotrasmission (Edbauer et al., 2010). The participation of miRNAs in synaptic expression of mRNAs was first observed in *Drosophila melanogaster.* The *Drosophila* ortholog of mammalian fragile X protein, dFmr1 was described to interact with RISC complex, and in particular with the main component Ago2 (Caudy et al., 2002; Ishizuka et al., 2002). Two years later, Warren and collaborators showed that FMRP associates with endogenous miRNAs and Ago1 (Jin et al., 2004). They performed genetic studies in *Drosophila* to find that Ago1 depletion suppresses dFrm1 overexpression phenotype, and that a trans-heterozygote for both AGO1 and dFmrp1 shows an even more pronounced synaptic overgrowth phenotype than the dFmr1 null mutant. This indicates that AGO1 might be a limiting factor in dFmr1 function in synaptogenesis, and suggests that microRNAs might mediate the FMR1 role in silencing of neuronal mRNAs.

### 1.3.2 RISC, microRNAs and synaptic plasticity

Evidence of miRNAs involvement in synaptic plasticity was first reported by Kunes' laboratory (Ashraf et al., 2006). The regulated disruption of the silencing complex component Armitage, led to the removal of miRNA-mediated repression of CaMKII, an mRNA involved in synaptic plasticity. Putative miRNA binding sites are present within the 3'UTR of CaMKII, as well as within the 3'UTR of the transcripts coding for Staufen and Kinesin-Heavy Chain, two dendritic granule-associated proteins. To test whether these mRNAs are targets of miRNA-silencing activity, their expression levels were assayed in brains from mutants of the RISC pathway. The results indicate that synaptic translation of CaMKII increases in dicer-, armitage-, and aubergine-mutant brains. Indeed, this work suggests an armitage-driven repression of CaMKII expression in drosophila olfactory system. Synaptic activation induces a decrease in the levels of Armitage protein and a correspondent increase in CaMKII abundance. The decrease in Armitage protein is shown to be due to the activity of the proteasome which is known to act at the synaptic level to contribute in modulating synaptic protein content (Bingol and Schuman 2005; 2006). Overall, Ashraf et al. (2006) propose a novel and intriguing regulatory mechanism whereby CaMKII translational repression is driven by miRNAs and in turn is relieved by activity-dependent proteasome-mediated degradation of Armitage (Fig.2)

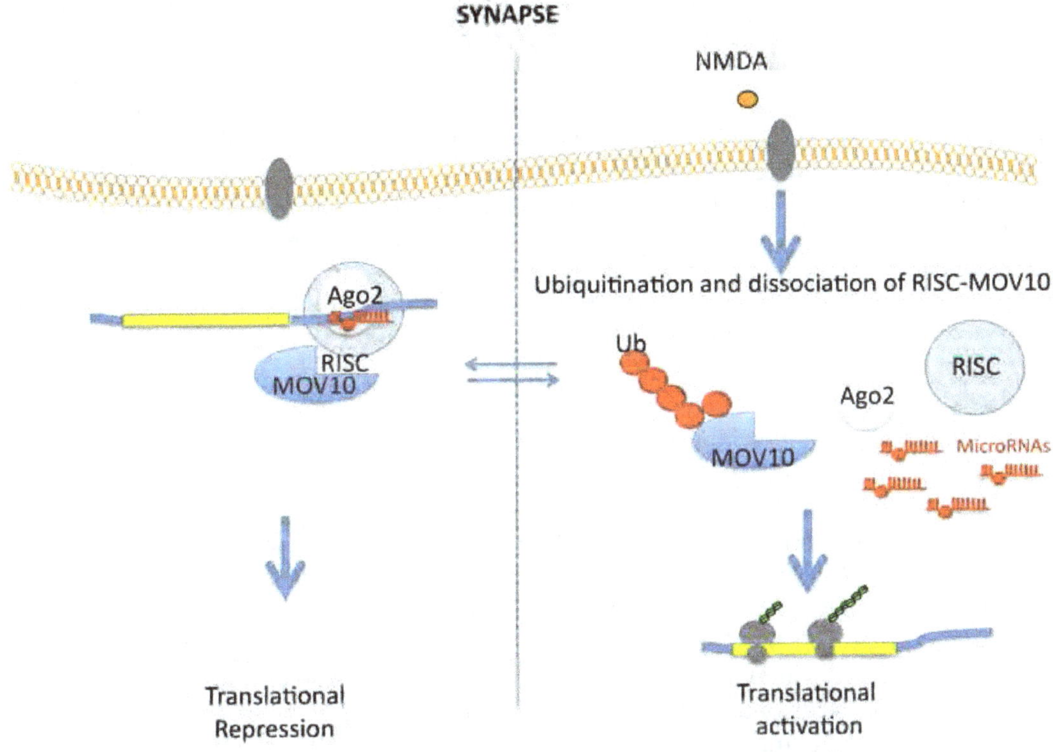


The model depicted here summarizes miRNAs modulation of synaptic protein synthesis and plasticity (Ashraf et al., 2006; Banerjee et al., 2009) MiRNAs are required for the translational silencing of several neuronal mRNAs important for synaptic protein synthesis (see text). Patterns of synaptic activity that induce long-term memory trigger localized proteasome-mediated degradation of MOV10 in mammalian (Armitage in Drosophila RISC) and consequent release of the translational repression guided by miRNAs at synapse.

Fig. 2. RISC regulation in synaptic plasticity.

More recently the silencing of the mammalian ortholog of Armitage, Moloney leukemia virus 10 homolog (MOV10), by RNA interference mediated knockdown, showed the relief of translational repression of miRNA targets. Kosik's group, with the aim to identify dendritic mRNAs under RISC's degradative control, individuated several mRNA localized in the dendrites. They trapped both known RISC-regulated mRNAs, as Limk1 and alfaCaMKII, and novel mRNA Lysophospholipase 1(Lypla1), (also known as acyl protein thioesterase (APT)1), a depalmitoylation enzyme, regulated post-transcriptionally by dendritic miR-138 (Banerjee et al., 2009). Previously Schratt's group showed that in rat hippocampal neurons, miR-138 was enriched at synapses and modulated synaptic development and spine size through the regulation levels of the APT1 (Siegel et al., 2009), followed by depalmitoylation of Ga13, a downstream target of APT1, which is an activator of Rho downstream of G-protein coupled receptor (Kurose et al., 2003). Another finding which associates miRNA function to the synaptic plasticity in mammalian neurons, was made by Schratt and collaborators, with the brain-specific microRNA-134 (Schratt et al., 2006). The overexpression of miR-134 causes a significant reduction in dendritic spine size, whereas its inhibition by 2'-O-methyl antisense oligonucleotides induces a slight increase in spine volume. The mRNA target of miR-134 was identified as Lim-domain containing protein kinase 1 (Limk1). Like to Kunes' laboratory findings (Ashraf et al., 2006), in this case neuronal activation also intervenes to put a brake on miRNA-mediated silencing. MiR-134 repression of Limk1 translation is mitigated upon BDNF stimulation of synaptic activity. In cortical neurons, BDNF induced the translation of the 3'UTR Limk1 mRNA luciferase reporter, but not when neurons were trasfected with a reporter in which miR-134 responsive sequence was mutated. This suggests that the BDNF/miR-134/Limk1 connection plays a role in synaptic plasticity at synaptodendritic compartment of hippocampal neurons (Fig.3). The studies described above, indicate that miRNAs might contribute to fine-tuning regulation of synaptic protein synthesis and plasticity by modulating expression of dendritic mRNAs.

### 1.3.3 Memory

Dysregulation in the enthorinal cortex and dentate gyrus during the acquisition of memory is one of the hallmarks that occurs early during Alzheimer's neurodegeneration. The loss of coordination between different pathways orchestrating protein expression at synapses, consists in a loss of control of plasticity. The assumption that synaptic plasticity is considered to underlie memory formation (Morris et al., 2003), and the evidence that forms of long-lasting synaptic plasticity depend on protein synthesis (Manahan-Vaughan et al., 2000), suggest that microRNAs may indeed be important for this phenomenon. What are the downstream effectors that mediate such activity? Several observations suggest that the induction of long-term potentiation (LTP) and long-term depression (LTD), two forms of synaptic plasticity, requires microRNAs. Park and Tang (2009) performed the temporal expression profile of sixty hippocampal microRNAs following induction of chemical LTP (C-LTP) and metabotropic glutamate receptor-dependent LTD (mGluR-LTD) in hippocampal slices. They observed that C-LTP or mGluR-LTD evokes changes of the expression levels of most hippocampal miRNAs, suggesting a role for miRNA-mediated translational repression. MiRNAs regulated in both experimental paradigma, displayed distinct temporal expression dynamics. Further, many miRNAs were upregulated at specific time points of C-LTP and mGluR-LTD induction, like to provide an active mechanism to restore the dormant state of mRNA translation after a transient activation (Park and Tang, 2009). Recent studies demonstrated finely regulation of primary and mature miRNA expression by mGluR and NMDAR signaling during LTP induction (Wibrand et al., 2010). Transgenic mouse strain that expresses miR-132 in forebrain neurons, showed an increase in dendritic spine density and a deficits in novel object recognition, suggesting that dysregulation of miR-132 could contribute to an array of cognitive disorders (Hansen et al., 2010). The first evidence that miRNA expression is specifically altered during an in vivo learning paradigm in mammals was carried out by Smalheiser's group, demonstrating that olfactory discrimination training, up-regulates and reorganizes expression of microRNAs in adult mouse hippocampus (Smalheiser et al., 2010). How up-regulation of a subset of miRNAs modulates gene expression pathways during several phases of learning and memory? A new work showing miRNAs as key players in the learning and memory process of mammals, was published by (Konopka et al., 2010). In a mouse model with an inducible disruption of the Dicer1 gene in the adult forebrain, after induction of Dicer1 gene deletion, a progressive loss of a whole set of brain-specific miRNAs was observed. Mice were tested in a battery of both aversively and appetitively motivated cognitive tasks, such as Morris water maze, IntelliCage system, or trace fear conditioning. An enhancement of memory was recorded twelwe weeks after the Dicer1 gene mutation. To date, we can't say a "better memory with less microRNA" or the reverse, but only that microRNAs may modulate memory, that components of long-term potentiation (LTP) require local protein translation, which regulate synaptic plasticity, and that microRNAs have been identified as master regulators of protein synthesis.

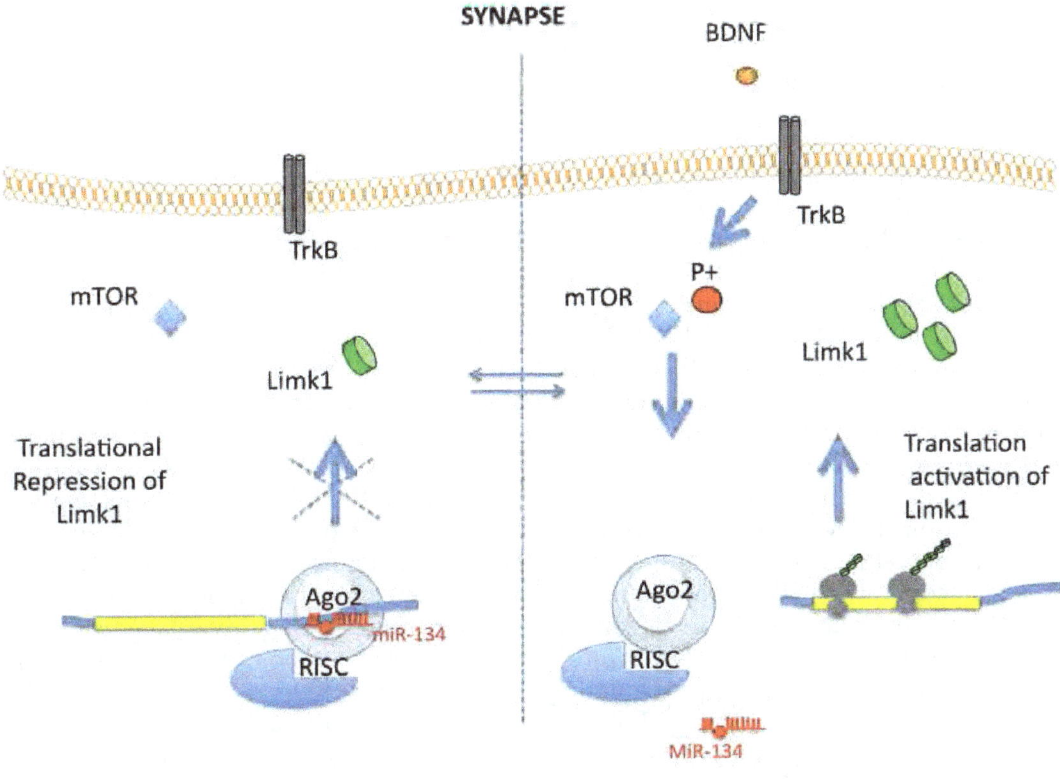


The mechanism unveiled by Schratt et al. (2006) in mammalian neurons is illustrated. Limk1 mRNA is subject to miR-134-mediated repression. Upon synaptic activation, induced by BDNF treatment, the authors observe translational derepression of Limk1 mRNA and an increase in spine size. How synaptic activity might release Limk1 mRNA from miR-134 repression is unclear.

Fig. 3. MicroRNA targets in synaptic plasticity and memory.

## 2. MicroRNA expression profiles in Alzheimer's disease brain

During the last four years, great strides have been made to profile miRNA expression in several regions of the AD brain. To point out whether miRNA expression may be misregulated in AD, Cogswell and coworkers compared the expression of over 300 miRNAs, isolated from hippocampus, medial frontal gyrus and cerebellum from early and late stage AD, to normal age-matched controls (Cogswell et al., 2008). Tissues were grouped by Braak stage and miRNAs were extracted, quantified and amplified by real-time quantitative PCR assay. Experimental data provide a statistically significant number of under- and over-expressed microRNAs. In particular, hippocampus and medial frontal gyrus, which are the earlier regions affected by AD pathology, were characterized by the major modifications. Expression of twenty-one miRNA (miR-200c, -212, -26a, -27a, -30c, -30e-5p, -34a, 381, -422a, -423, -9, -92, 100, -125b, -132, -145, -146b, -148a, -210, -27b, -425) was altered both in early and in end stages of pathology (Cogswell et al., 2008). The pathological cerebrospinal fluids (CSF) were also analyzed. These samples show a different miRNAs expression between AD and non-affected patients. Both miRNA expression profiles represent the first work aimed to identify specific miRNAs as biomarkers of AD (Cogswell et al., 2008). Several efforts have been made to understand whether miRNAs are also altered in sporadic AD. A microRNA expression profile shows that many miRNAs are potentially involved in the regulation of APP and BACE1 (Hebert et al., 2008). In this study the expression of 328 human miRNAs in the anterior temporal cortex and the cerebellum from five AD patients was monitored and compared with age-matched controls. Among all miRNAs analyzed, 13 were significantly altered and at least 7 were predicted to target the 3′ UTR of BACE1 (miR-15a, 29b-1, -9, and -19b) or APP (let-7, miR101, miR15a, and miR106b) (Hebert et al., 2008). Nunez-Iglesias (2010) used microarrays for the first joint profiling and analysis of miRNAs and mRNAs expression in brain cortex from AD and age-matched control subjects. These data provided the unique opportunity to study the relationship between miRNA and mRNA expression in normal and AD brains. Starting from genome-wide miRNA and mRNA data expression, analysis was carried out to determine the correlation between levels of miRNAs and their target mRNAs (Nunez-Iglesias et al., 2010). The results reveal that most miRNA-mRNA pairs are actually uncorrelated making more difficult to understand the correlation level between miRNAs with their targets. By an elegant analysis performed taking advantage from gene ontology biological processes, RNAs were grouped together. Among the processes most positively correlated with their regulating miRNA, the authors found some specific processes, including metabolism of both carbohydrates and fatty acid, as well as protein refolding which indicate the importance of these processes in the brain. Among the processes most negatively correlated are oxygen transport, cell adhesion, inflammatory response, cytoskeletal organization and dendrite development (Nunez-Iglesias et al., 2010). The method depicted can find active miRNA-mRNA relationships dependent from the tissue context. These authors demonstrate a relationship between the levels of miRNAs and those of their targets in the brain, identyfing a large set of miRNA-mRNA associations that are changed in AD versus control, and AD-specific changes in the miRNA regulatory system. Microarray techniques, based on correlation methods, are proving to be powerful tools for investigation on miRNAs deregulation in AD. The expression of 5-6% of miRNAs was affected by AD at statistical significant level in the studies described above (Hebert et al., 2008; Cogswell et al., 2008; Nunez-Iglesias et al., 2010) suggesting that a substantial number of miRNAs are deregulated in this pathology.

| BRAIN AREA | EXPRESSION IN ALZHEIMER'S DISEASE | miRNA | Reference |
|---|---|---|---|
| Gray matter | Upregulated | miR-519e, miR-574-5p, miR-498, miR-518a-5p/miR-527, miR-525-5p, miR-300, miR-576-3p, miR-583, miR-146b-3p, miR-490-3p, miR-549, miR-516a-5p, miR-510, miR-184, miR-516b, miR-298, miR-214, miR-198, miR-451, miR-144, miR-424, let-7e | (Wang et al., 2011) |
| Gray matter | Downregulated | miR-485-3p, miR-381, miR-124, miR-34a, miR-129-5p, miR-29a, miR-143, miR-36, miR-145, miR-138, miR-129-3p, miR-128, miR-143, miR-136, miR-145, miR-138, miR-129-3p, miR-128, miR-126, miR-411, miR-335, miR-9, miR-378, miR-488, miR-32, miR-127-5p, miR-127-3p, miR-491-5p, miR-376c, miR-377, miR-95, miR-222, miR-29b, miR-329, miR-495, miR-551b, miR-195, miR-125b, miR-30b, miR-221, miR-139-5p, miR-487a, miR-487b, miR-107, miR-146b-5p, miR-29c, miR-30a, miR-582-5p, miR-103, miR-342-3p, miR-331-3p, miR-30c, miR-30d, miR-382, miR-22, miR-125a-5p, miR-425, miR-191, miR-519d, let-7g, miR-98, miR-99a, miR-30e | (Wang et al., 2011) |
| White matter | Upregulated | miR-509-5p, miR-574-3p, miR-576-5p, miR-302e, miR-220b, miR-208a, miR-215 | (Wang et al., 2011) |
| White matter | Downregulated | miR-491-3p, miR-423-5p, miR-34b, miR-422a, miR-34c-5p, miR-584, miR-219-5p, miR-338-3p, miR-219-2-3p, miR-338-5p, miR-181a, miR-181b, let-7b, miR-151-3p, miR-197, miR-19a, miR-20a, miR-17, miR-106a, miR-32, miR-340, miR-19b, miR-21, miR-151-5p, miR-194, let-7c, miR-330-3p, miR-27b, miR-93, miR-15a, miR-339-5p, miR-193b, miR-106b, miR-16, miR-23b, miR-15b, miR-320d, miR-320b, miR-320c, miR-320a, miR-557, miR-33a, let-7a, miR-374b, miR-140-3p, miR-374a, miR-24, miR-140-5p, miR-26a, miR-513a-5p, miR-212, miR-142-5p, miR-142-3p, miR-26b, miR-520d-5p, miR-193a-3p, miR-92b, miR-330-5p, miR-186, let-7f, miR-223, miR-412, miR-185, miR-148b, miR-101, miR-99b, miR-27a, miR-589, let-7i, miR-361-3p, miR-361-5p, miR-423-3p, miR-190, miR-301a, miR-365, miR-23a, miR-363, miR-326 | (Wang et al., 2011) |
| Hippocampus | Upregulated | miR-26a,miR-27a, miR-30e-5p, miR-34a, miR-92, miR-381, miR-422a, miR-423, miR-27b, miR-125b, miR-145, miR200c | (Cogswell et al., 2008) |
| | | mR-146a | (Cui et al., 2010) |
| Hippocampus | Downregulated | miR-9,miR-128, miR-125b | (Lukiw, 2007) |
| | | miR-30c, miR-212, miR-132, miR-146b, miR-210, miR-425, miR-9 | (Cogswell et al., 2008) |
| Medial frontal gyrus | Upregulated | miR-27a, miR-30c, miR-30e-5p, miR-34a, miR-92, miR-381, miR-422a, mir-423,miR-27b, miR-100, miR-125b, miR-145, miR-148a, miR-29a, miR-29b, miR-423, miR-145 | (Cogswell et al., 2008) |
| Medial frontal gyrus | Downregulated | miR-26a, miR-200c, miR-212,miR-132, miR-146b, miR-210, miR-425 | (Cogswell et al., 2008) |

| Parietal lobe cortex | Upregulated | miR-30184, miR-617,miR-188,miR-06383, miR-10912,miR-601,miR-23974, miR-10939, miR-19790, miR-35456, miR-134, miR-671, miR-320, miR-575, miR572, miR-45605, miR-765, miR-18895, miR-432, miR-382, miR-185, miR-486, miR-28648 | (Nunez-Iglesias et al., 2010) |
|---|---|---|---|
| Parietal lobe cortex | Downregulated | miR-101,miR-20546,miR-29b, miR-181c, miR-08570, miR-42448, miR-44608, miR-02532, miR-12497, miR-582, miR-15a, miR-374, miR-95, miR-05109, miR-30e-5p, miR-148b, miR-130a, miR-598, miR-376a, miR-29c, miR-12504, miR-494, miR-20b, miR-368 | (Nunez-Iglesias et al., 2010) |
| Temporal lobe cortex (Sporadic AD) | Upregulated | miR-197, miR-511, miR-320 | (Hebert et al., 2008) |
| Temporal lobe cortex (Sporadic AD) | Downregulated | miR-210, miR-181c, miR-15a, miR-9, miR-22, miR-101, miR-29b-1, miR-19b, let-7i, miR-106b, miR-26b, miR-363, miR-93 | (Hebert et al., 2008) |
| Temporal lobe cortex | Upregulated | miR-9, miR-125b, miR-146a | (Sethi & Lukiw, 2009) |

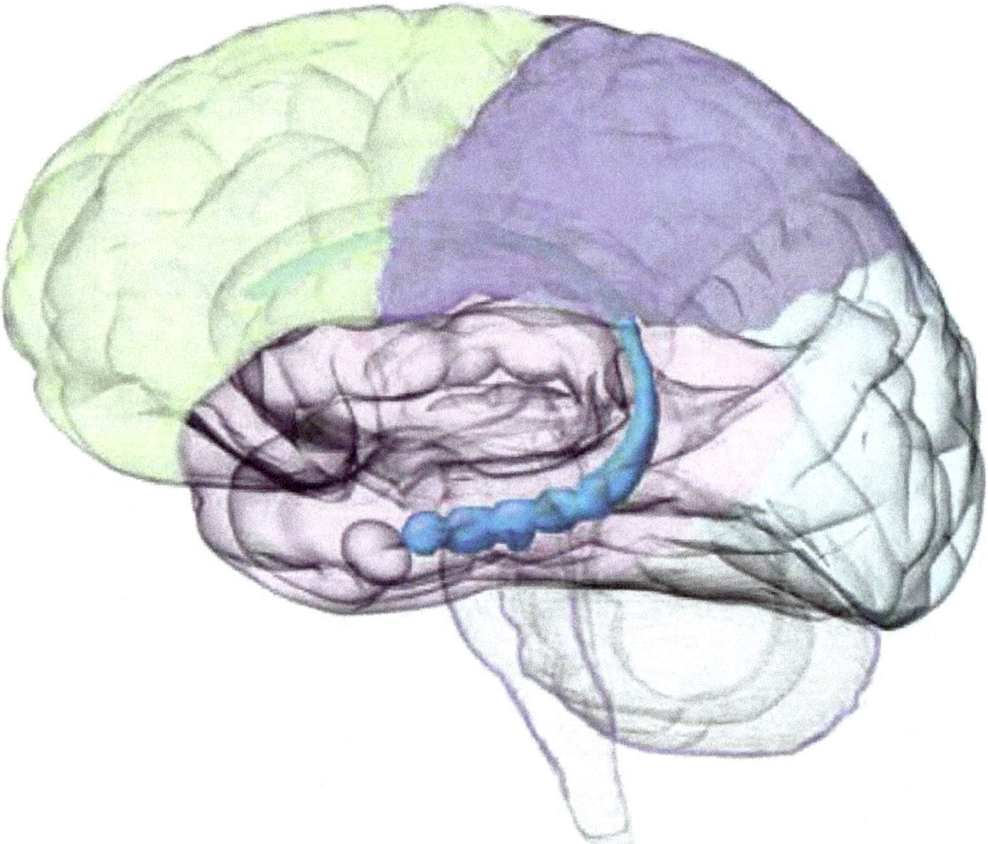

Table 1. Studies reporting changes of miRNAs expression profiles in Alzheimer's disease and in different brain areas.

### 2.1 Addressing brain tissue complexity

In gene expression studies the heterogeneity of the human cerebral cortex should be considered. For example, former tissue sampling protocols did not segregate white matter from gray matter, increasing variability that reflects differently sample cell population rather than a disease condition (Wang et al., 2011) (Table 1). Nelson's laboratory deals with this question either analyzing different miRNAs expression in human cerebral cortical white matter and gray matter in normal and early AD pathology and using different experimental techniques. MiRNA profiling experiments were performed using a locked nucleic-acid-microarray (LNA-microarray) which highlights a subset of miRNAs that appeared to be strongly expressed and did not appear to be conventional miRNAs (Wang et al., 2011). Using clustering analysis they demonstrated a different miRNA expression pattern between white matter and gray matter and between normal and pathological condition. Further, they found that there was an apparent clustering between samples derived from gray matter relative to those derived from white matter, and also cases with more AD pathology tended to cluster together relative to control cases. Moreover, miRNA expression may be correlated to neuropathological hallmarks in AD: amyloid plaques (with or without degenerating neuritis) and neurofibrillary tangles. Because of the major pathological changes affected gray matter, it is not surprising that a number of miRNAs altered in AD was higher in gray matter than white matter, but a handful of miRNAs was altered specifically in white matter. These data indicate an emerging need: while the expression of individual miRNA may be impactful alone, it is necessary to assess the aggregate impact of multiple miRNAs and the connection between AD pathological features and miRNA alteration (Wang et al., 2011). In fact, miRNA expression profiles highlight almost two altered pathways in AD, which involve inflammatory alteration response and $A\beta_{1-42}$ production and physiology. However, bioinformatic tools and miRNA expression profile offer a data set that have to be validate in cellular system in order to understand which are the mRNA targets and, eventually the physiopathological implications. Variation in tissue sampling may contribute to heterogeneus results. Banked tissue is essential to the study of neurological diseases but the use of postmortem tissue introduces a number of possible confounds. A variety of antemortem factors may influence the quality of harvested tissue including fever, hypoxia-ischemia and acidosis, while critical postmortem variables include postmortem interval (PMI), brain or cerebrospinal fluid pH, ambient temperature in the postmortem period, harvesting procedures, storage temperature and accidental or systematic thawing and freezing. Interindividual differences in postmortem tissue studies are typically large and often prevent the attainment of statistical significance. Much of interindividual variability may be due to highly variable agonal condition; RNA yield and quality may be affected by the extraction method employed. Many report that global measures of total RNA quality are relatively stable over a wide range of PMIs while some others report a definite loss with increasing time (Birdsill et al., 2010). However, in all extraction techniques employed a negative correlation between PMI and RNA quality-yield is point out. Furthermore, miRNA half-life appears significantly correlated with content of AU and UA dinucleotides in the RNA sequence. MiRNA-9, for example, which has 26.1% of AU in the sequence, has a half-life shorter (c.a 1 h) than miRNA-125b, 9.5% AU rich and 3.5h half-life. These data suggest the importance to compare normal and pathological tissue with similar PMI. In fact, analysis of miRNAs in autopsied brain tissue with post-mortem intervals many-fold greater than the half-lives of miRNAs may lead to inaccurate conclusions concerning their absolute abundance and hence the contribution of miRNAs to gene regulation in the brain during development, aging and in disease processes (Sethi et al., 2009). Studies performed in brain tissues with short PMI indicate that miR-9, miR-146 and miR-125 were significantly upregulated in AD-affected temporal lobe. Importantly comparative expression analysis showed no change of these microRNAs in tissues derived from patients affected with amyotropic lateral sclerosis, Parkinson's disease, schizophrenia. These data suggest that these miRNAs may contribute to the pathogenesis characteristic of AD. Microarray system is suitable to perform miRNA expression profiling but it did not show specific cellular distribution. Instead in situ hybridation (ISH) should be a method to directly understand the specific roles of miRNAs in the human brain at the cellular and sub-cellular levels. ISH is more labor-intensive and "low-throughput" compared to other RNA expression profiling techniques, but allows far greater resolution of given RNA's expression (Nelson et al., 2009). For example, ISH shows important cerebral cortical lamina-specific patterns of miRNA expression that would be lost on most tissue level expression studies, and these lamina-specific patterns may be relevant to human brain disease.

## 3. Exploring microRNA function in Alzheimer's disease

MiRNA target prediction programs, cell-based functional assays and studies in mouse models have been used to identify some of the molecular and biological functions of microRNAs dysregulated in AD brain tissues.

### 3.1 miRNAs dysregulated in AD modulate BACE and other targets

The amyloid precursor protein (APP), its proteolytic product amyloid beta (Aβ), generated by beta secretase (BACE) and gamma secretase, are all associated with both familial and sporadic forms of Alzheimer disease (AD) (Fig.4). BACE1 gene was shown post-transcriptionally regulated by miR-107 (Wang et al 2008) and miR-29a/b-1 (Hebert et al 2008). Interstingly miR-107 expression levels decreased during AD pathology progression (Wang et al 2008). On the other hand miR-29 was downregulated in anterior temporal cortex from sporadic AD patients in which BACE 1 protein was abnormally upregulated while BACE 1 mRNA levels were unchanged (Hebert et al 2008). Using BACE1 3'UTR luciferase reporter carrying wild type or mutated miRNA responsive sites BACE1 post-transcriptional regulation by those microRNA was demonstrated. Moreover, upon either overexpression or downregulation of miR-29a/b-1 in human cell culture both BACE1 protein levels and APP cleavage product $A\beta$ were, respectively, reduced and increased (Hebert et al 2008) (Fig.4).
Although these studies clearly indicate a relationship of both miR-29 and miR-107 with a gene associated to AD pathology identification of all mRNA targets affected by each microRNA deregulated in AD is the real challenge of future investigations. Indeed other studies indicate that miR-29 may play a more complex role in neurons during AD neurodegeneration. Neuron navigator 3 (NAV3), a regulator of axon guidance, was validated as miR-29 target and by immunohistochemistry NAV3 expression was found enhanced in degenerating pyramidal neurons in the cerebral cortex of AD (Shyoia et al., 2010). Moreover studies in sympathetic neurons have shown that miR-29b function as an inhibitor of neuronal apoptosis (Kole et al., 2011) by inhibition of multiple redundant BH3 only proteins (Bim, Bmf, Hrk, Puma and N-Bak) that are key iniziators of apoptosis. Therefore loss of miR-29 expression may lead to neuron vulnerability and neurodegeneration. Additional roles for miR-107 in AD pathogenesis are demonstrated by studies in a transgenic mouse model of AD which over-expresses human APP carrying familial AD mutations (Yao et al., 2010). In particular reduced levels of miR-103 or miR-107 are associated with elevated cofilin protein levels and formation of rod-like structures in this

AD mouse model. Rod-like structures composed of actin and the actin-binding protein cofilin are also found in Alzheimer's disease (AD) patients (Whiteman et al., 2009).

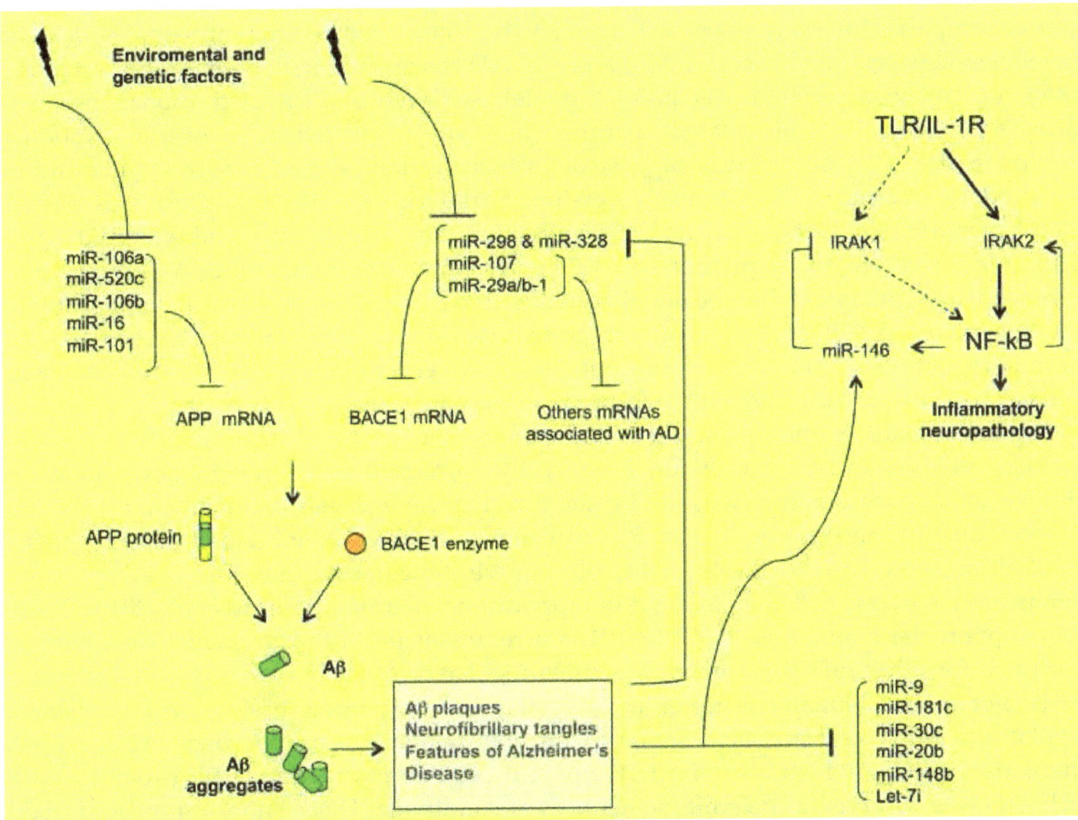


Fig. 4. MiRNAs deregulation in Alzheimer's disease pathology.

### 3.2 Several miRNAs regulate APP

Among mutations causing familial AD, duplication of the APP gene has also been detected (Rovelet-Lecrux et al., 2006). In addition, individuals with trisomy 21 (the APP gene is located on chromosome 21) are at increased risk of developing AD late in life (Podlisny et al., 1987). Several studies have reported that APP expression is post-transcriptionally regulated by microRNAs. A list of microRNAs: miR-106a and miR-520c, miR-20a family members (including miR-20a, miR-106b and miR-17-5p), miR-16 and miR-101, was demonstrated to downregulate APP expression (Patel et al., 2008; Hebert et al., 2009; Liu et al., 2010; Vilardo et al., 2010). The expression levels of these miRNAs were reduced in AD tissues (Fig. 4). When overexpressed in human cell lines, both miR-106a and miR-520c reduced endogenous APP levels by 50% compared to cells transfected with a non-targeting miRNA (Patel et al., 2008). However, only miR-106a is expressed in neuronal context. Overexpression of miR-20a (and miR-17-5p/106b) post-transcriptionally reduced endogenous APP expression in both non-neuronal and neuronal cells. Moreover, reduction of miR-20a, miR-17-5p and miR-106b levels was correlated with an increase in APP protein levels in developing mouse brain and in primary cultured neurons. Although two putative miR-20 family responsive elements (REs) are predicted within the APP 3'UTR only one RE functionally interacted with miR-20 family miRNAs. When miRNA expression levels in human AD brains were analyzed, miR-106b was significantly reduced with respect to control samples. However, since APP levels varied among the different samples, a tight correlation between miR-106b and APP levels in AD tissues was not obtained (Hebert et al., 2009). In an age-associated AD animal model, senescence-accelerated mouse prone 8 (SAMP8), which has age-related learning and memory deficits post-transcriptional regulation of APP by miR-16 was suggested. Overexpression of miR-16, both in vitro and in vivo, led to reduced APP protein expression. Furthermore, miR-16 and APP displayed complementary expression patterns in SAMP8 mice and BALb/c mice embryos (Liu et al., 2010). More recently, the regulation of APP expression by the RISC/miRNA pathway was examined in primary rat hippocampal neurons. First, silencing of Ago2 in hippocampal neurons increased APP protein levels, suggesting that APP translation may be regulated by an miRNA pathway. Among miRNAs potentially targeting the APP 3'UTR, miR- 101 was selected for further study because two putative miR-101 target sites, which are conserved among the human, rat and murine APP genes, are present in the 3'UTR. MiR-101 is a brain-enriched miRNA and its expression is inversely correlated with APP in developing rat hippocampal neurons and tissues. Using site directed mutagenesis, a functional interaction between miR-101 and one of the two REs was demonstrated. The inhibition of endogenous miR-101 increased APP levels, whereas lentiviral-mediated miR-101 overexpression significantly reduced APP and Aβ load in hippocampal neurons (Vilardo et al., 2010). These data support the hypothesis that miR-101 is a repressor of APP expression. Moreover, as described for other miRNAs, miR-101 is downregulated in the human AD cerebral cortex (Hebert et al 2008; Nunez-Iglesias et al., 2010) (Fig.4). Interestingly besides APP expression regulation, miRNAs were also involved in the regulation of neuronal APP mRNA alternative splicing which also affects β-amyloid peptide production. APP exons 7 and 8 inclusion was observed in postmitotic neurons of conditional Dicer knock-out mice (Hebert et al., 2010), while over-expression of miR-124, an abundant neuronal-specific miRNA, reversed these effects in cultured neurons. Similar results were obtained by depletion of endogenous polypyrimidine tract binding protein 1 (PTBP1) in cells, a recognized miR-124 target gene. Furthermore, PTBP1 levels correlate with the presence of APP exons 7 and 8, while PTBP2 levels correlate with the skipping of these exons during neuronal differentiation. Expression studies in AD brain showed that miR-124 expression was down-regulated (Smith et al., 2011).

### 3.3 Changes of miRNA in AD are implicated in inflammation, aging and oxidative stress

Inflammatory signaling plays determinant roles in brain homeostasis and neuroprotection however, altered or excessive signaling in these injury defense systems contributes to the irreversible degeneration of brain cells, in neurodegenerative disorders such as Alzheimer disease (AD). The inflammatory processes are involved during progression of AD pathogenesis, and Aβ42 peptides , cytokine IL-1β upregulation and oxidative stress are inflammatory mediators (Lukiw, 2004). A mouse and human brain abundant miRNA-146 was upregulated in AD brain and associated with the down-regulation of complement factor H, an important repressor of inflammatory signaling in the complement cascade, in

AD brain (Lukiw et al 2008). Furthermore in the hippocampus and neocortex of Alzheimer disease (AD) brain as well as in stressed human astroglial (HAG) cells in primary culture, increased expression of an NF-kB-regulated miRNA-146 down-regulates expression of the interleukin-1 receptor-associated kinase-1 (IRAK-1), an essential component of Toll-like/IL-1 receptor signaling (Cui et al 2010). Family of interleukin-1 receptor-associated kinases (IRAKs) in the human genome, including IRAK-1, IRAK-2, IRAK-4, and IRAK-M, are key mediators in the immune pathways utilized by TLR/IL-1R (TIR) signaling. By means of their integral kinase IRAKs initiate diverse downstream signaling processes that can eventually lead to the induction of pro-inflammatory transcription factors such as NF-kB. In control and AD samples a significant up-regulation of miRNA-146a coupled to down-regulation of IRAK-1 and a parallel up-regulation of IRAK-2 was noted. Finally independent regulation of IRAK-1 and IRAK-2 in IL-1β+Aβ42 peptide-stressed HAG cells and inducible, NF-kB-sensitive, miRNA-146a-mediated downregulation of IRAK-1 coupled to an NF-kB-induced up-regulation of IRAK-2 expression was demonstrated (Cui et al., 2010). This regulatory network provides an important basis for a self-perpetuating inflammatory signaling loop (Fig.4). For sporadic Alzheimer's disease, which accounts for the majority of Alzheimer's disease cases, the most important risk factor is aging. Several miRNAs that are modulated in various aging model system, might contribute to AD. It was proposed that an alteration of miRNAs expression control in mid-life may be the putative force inducing molecular frailty in individual cell signaling, and in time leading to tissue-wide dysfunction (Wang, 2007). For example, miR-34a is increased in AD, peripheral blood mononuclear cell, aging mouse liver and *C. elegans* (Cogswell et al., 2008; Schipper et al., 2007; Maes et al., 2008; Ibanez-Ventoso et al., 2006). MiRNA lin-4 has been elegantly shown to influence lifespan and healthspan via its lin-14 mRNA target and the insulin signaling pathway, and several *C. elegans* age-regulated miRNAs have sequence similarity with both fly and human miRNAs (Ibanez-Ventoso & Driscoll, 2009). The question is whether there are evolutionary-conserved homologs of lin-4 and lin-14 that control human longevity and if miRNAs are implicated in many age-associated pathologies. Other miRNAs are upregulated during aging as let-7f, miR-30d, miR -432, miR-517 and downregulated as let-7i and miR-451 (Maes et al., 2009). Are they involved in gene regulation of aging related mechanism in AD? There is a great deal of evidence that suggests that oxidative stress plays a crucial role in the initiation and progression of Alzheimer's disease. In AD peripheral blood mononuclear cells, an impairment in DNA repair and antioxidant gene responses was observed and correlated to the up-regulation of miR-181b, miR-200a, miR-517* and miR-520, that may repress DNA repair and the response to oxidative stress (Shipper et al., 2007).

### 3.4 Studies in mouse models exploring microRNAs function in Alzheimer's disease

Mouse models have been recently used to investigate microRNA function in AD pathology. Specific deletion of Dicer in the adult forebrain leading to loss of microRNAs, was accompanied by a mixed neurodegenerative phenotype (Hebert et al., 2010). Although neuronal loss was observed in the hippocampus, cellular shrinkage was predominant in the cortex. Interestingly, neuronal degeneration coincides with the hyperphosphorylation of endogenous tau at several epitopes previously associated with neurofibrillary pathology.

Changes of miRNA expression might trigger molecular events inducing AD pathology or generate a feed-forward mechanism during AD progression. Two recent studies performed on mouse models of AD suggest that progression of AD pathology may produce alteration of microRNAs expression (Fig. 4). In APPswe/Psen1 transgenic mice, an AD mouse model which recapitulates some features of the disease, it was observed that BACE1 mRNA decreased and protein levels increased in the hippocampus at 19 months of age (Boissonneault et al., 2009). Two microRNAs, miR-298 and miR- 328, were found to regulate BACE 1 protein expression in mouse cultured neuronal cells. In transgenic mice, the expression of miR- 298 and miR-328 decreased in the granular neurons of the hippocampus during aging. However, while the miR-328 sequence is perfectly conserved between mouse and human, that of miR-298 is only 72% identical. More recently the hypothesis that Aβ itself causes neuronal miRNA deregulation which could contribute to the pathology associated with AD was explored (Schonrock et al 2010). A list of miRNAs, miR-9, miR-181c, miR-30c, miR-20b, miR-148b and Let-7i, was also downregulated in primary hippocampal cell cultures treated with Aβ. The miRNAs changes overlap with those occuring in the hippocampus of APP 23 mice (expressing human APP751 cDNA containing the Swedish double mutation (K651M and N652L) at 7 months of age At this age, mice reach the critical period of Aβ plaque formation where insoluble Aβ42 peptides increase five-fold compared to younger animals and small plaques can be seen in hippocampus and neocortex. In addition, the mice display major cognitive deficits affecting visuo-spatial learning abilities. These deregulated miRNAs overlap also with those found in sporadic human AD brain and potentially affect important biological pathways essential for proper brain function relevant to AD. The overlap between human AD brain and in vitro/in vivo AD models indicates that among the complex AD pathology, downregulation of miR-9, miR-181c, miR-30c, miR-20b, miR-148b and Let-7i could be attributed at least in part to the presence of Aβ (Fig.4).

## 4. Conclusion

Until now altered expression of miRNAs in Alzheimer's Disease brain tissues was demonstrated, however different studies identified various microRNAs. Increasing the numbers of miRNA expression profiles using large cohort of sporadic AD patients may allow us to better understand whether the variability among different profiles may be due to disease specific interindividual differences. It is difficult to determine if the changes in miRNA expression detected in the brains or CSF of patients are primary or secondary events, or both. Nevertheless early or late in the evolution of the disease, they could contribute to the pathogenesis of the observed lesions and neuronal loss. Unique patterns of miRNA expression profile in the CSF of AD could be useful as molecular biomarkers for disease diagnosis and eventually prediction of therapeutic responses. Target prediction analysis and cell-based assay linked miRNAs dysregulated in AD to APP and BACE1 genes which are associated with the pathology. Now the effort is to identify all targets of individual microRNA and to evaluate the impact that more than one microRNA may play on a specific target. In this regard computational prediction programs may be complemented by experiments in which the changes in transcripts and protein levels due to miRNA induction or knockdown are analysed using microarray platforms and SILAC (stable-isotope labelling with aminoacid in cell culture) and mass spectrometry (Selbach et al 2008). Also the co-immunoprecipitation of mRNA targets with Ago2 combined with microarray analysis of RNA (RIP-Chip assay) represents an alternative approach (Tan et al 2009). As demonstrated for the upregulation of miR-146 by the transcription factor NFkB the charachterization of promoters as well as transcriptional activators and repressors regulating microRNAs expression will be instrumental to delineate the relationship of microRNAs with networks involved in AD pathology. The use of transgenic animal models, manipulated in putative brain-expressed microRNAs associated to high-throughput methodologies, integrating transcriptomic, mirnomic and proteomics, will help to evaluate the potential association between RNA-mediated gene regulation and the pathogenesis of Alzheimer Disease and might indicate unexpected gene networks underlying Alzheimer's Disease.

## 5. Acknowledgment

This work was supported by Compagnia di San Paolo, Programma Neuroscienze, grant 'MicroRNAs in Neurodegenerative Diseases' (to C.B.), and by CNR grant DG.RSTL.059.012 (to F.R). We thank for graphical assistance -Studio 2CV idee e paesaggi- (www.studio2cv.it).

## 6. References

Ashraf, SI.; McLoon, AL.; Sclarsic, SM. & Kunes, S. (2006). *Synaptic protein synthesis associated with memory is regulated by the RISC pathway in Drosophila.* Cell 124:191–205

Banerjee, S.; Neveu, P. & Kosik, KS. (2009) *A coordinated local translational control point at the synapse involving relief from silencing and MOV10 degradation.* Neuron. 64(6):871-84

Bingol, B. & Schuman, EM. (2005) *Synaptic protein degradation by the ubiquitin proteasome system.* Curr Opin Neurobiol 15:536- 541

Bingol, B. & Schuman, EM. (2006) *Activity-dependent dynamics and sequestration of proteasomes in dendritic spines.* Nature 441:1144–1148

Birdsill, A.C.; Walker, D. G.; Lue, L.F.; Sue, LI. & Beach, TG. (2010) *Postmortem interval effect on RNA and gene expression in human brain tissue.* Cell Tissue Bank. DOI: 10.1007/s10561-010-9210-8

Bohnsack, M.T; Czaplinski, K. & Gorlich, D. (2004) *Exportin 5 is a RanGTP-dependent dsRNA-binding protein that mediates nuclear export of pre-miRNAs.* RNA 10(2):185–191

Boissonneault, V.; Plante, I.; Rivest, S. & Provost, P. (2009) *MicroRNA-298 and microRNA-328 regulate expression of mouse beta-amyloid precursor protein-converting enzyme 1.* J Biol Chem 284(4):1971-81

Caudy, AA.; Myers, M.; Hannon, GJ. & Hammond, SM. (2002) *Fragile Xrelated protein and VIG associate with the RNA interference machinery.* Genes Dev 16:2491–2496

Cao, X.; Yeo, G.; Muotri, AR., Kuwabara, T. & Gage, FH. (2006) *Noncoding RNAs in the mammalian central nervous system.* Annu Rev Neurosci. 29:77-103.

Chendrimada, TP.; Gregory, RI.; Kumaraswamy, E.; Norman, J. & Cooch, N. et al. (2005) *TRBP recruits the Dicer complex to Ago2 for microRNA processing and gene silencing.* Nature 436(7051): 740–744

Cogswell, J.P.; Ward, J.; Taylor, I.A.; Waters, M.; Shi, Y.; Cannon, B.; Kelnar, K.; Kemppainen, J.; Brown, D.; Chen, C.; Prinjha, C.; Richardson, J.; Saunders, A.M.; Roses, A.D. & Ricards, C.A. (2008). *Identification of miRNA changes in Alzheimerr's Disease brain and CSF yields putative biomarkers insights into disease pathways*. J. Alzheimer's Disease 14: 27-41

Coleman, PD.; & Yao, PJ. (2003) *Synaptic slaughter in Alzheimer's disease*. Neurobiol Aging 24(8):1023-7.

Cui, J.G.; Li, YY., Zhao, Y., Battacharjee, S. & Lukiw, W. (2010). *Differential regulation of interleukin-1 receptor-associated kinase-1 (IRAK-1) and IRAK-2 by microRNA-146a and NF-kB in stressed human astroglial cells and Alzheimer disease*. J. Biol. Chem. 285 (50): 38951-38960

Edbauer, D.; Neilson, JR., Foster, KA., Wang, CF., Seeburg, DP., Batterton, MN., Tada, T., Dolan, BM., Sharp, PA. & Sheng, M. (2010) *Regulation of synaptic structure and function by FMRP-associated microRNAs miR-125b and miR-132*. Neuron 65:373–384

Fiore, R.; Khudayberdiev, S., Christensen, M., Siegel, G., Flavell, SW., Kim, T., Greenberg, ME. & Schratt, G. (2009) *Mef2-mediated transcription of the miR379–410 cluster regulates activity-dependent dendritogenesis by fine-tuning Pumilio2 protein levels*. EMBO J 28:697–710

Gregory, RI.; Yan, KP., Amuthan, G., Chendrimada, TP., Doratotaj, B. et al. (2004) *The microprocessor complex mediates the genesis of microRNAs*. Nature 432(7014):235–240

Hansen, KF; Sakamoto, K., Wayman, GA., Impey, S. & Obrietan, K. (2010) *Transgenic miR132 alters neuronal spine density and impairs novel object recognition memory*. PLoS One. 5(11):e15497.

Hébert, S.; Horré, K., Nicolai, L., Papadopoulou, A., Mandemakers, A. N., Kauppinen, S., Delacourte, A., De Stropper, B. (2008) *Loss of microRNA cluster miR29a/b in sporadic Alzheimer's disease correlates with increased Bace1/β-secretase expression*. PNAS 105(17): 6415-6420

Hébert, S.; Horré, K., Nicolai, L., Bergmans, B., Papadopoulou, A. S., Delacourte, A., De Stropper, B. (2009) *MicroRNA regulation of Alzheimer's amyloid precursor protein expression*. Neurobiol Dis. 33:422-428

Hébert, S.; Papadopoulou, AS., Smith, P., Galas, MC., Planel, E., Silahtaroglu, AN., Sergeant, N., Buée, L. & De Strooper, B. (2010) *Genetic ablation of Dicer in adult forebrain neurons results in abnormal tau hyperphosphorylation and neurodegeneration*. Hum Mol Genet. 19(20):3959-69

Hotulainen, P.; & Hoogenraad, CC. (2010) *Actin in dendritic spines: connecting dynamics to function*. J Cell Biol. 189(4):619-29

Hutvagner, G.; & Simard, MJ. (2008) *Argonaute proteins: key players in RNA silencing*. Nat Rev Mol Cell Biol 9(1):22–32

Ibanez-Ventoso, C.; Yang, M., Guo, S., Robins, H., Padgett, RW. & Driscoll, M. (2006) *Modulated microRNA expression during adult lifespan in Caenorhabditis elegans*. Aging Cell 5:235–246

Ibáñez-Ventoso, C.; & Driscoll, M. (2009) *MicroRNAs in C. elegans Aging: Molecular Insurance for Robustness?* Curr Genomics. 10(3):144-53

Ishizuka, A.; Siomi, MC. & Siomi, H. (2002) *A Drosophila fragile X protein interacts with components of RNAi and ribosomal proteins.* Genes Dev 16:2497–2508

Jin, P.; Zarnescu, DC., Ceman, S., Nakamoto, M., Mowrey, J. et al. (2004) *Biochemical and genetic interaction between the fragile X mental retardation protein and the microRNA pathway.* Nat Neurosci 7:113–117

Kasai, H.; Fukuda M, Watanabe S, Hayashi-Takagi A, Noguchi J. (2010) *Structural dynamics of dendritic spines in memory and cognition.* Trends Neurosci. 33(3):121-9

Kiebler, MA.; & Bassel, GJ. (2006) *Neuronal RNA granules: movers and makers* Neuron. 51(6):685-90

Kim, VN.; (2005) *MicroRNA biogenesis: coordinated cropping and dicing.* Nat Rev Mol Cell Biol 6(5):376–385

Kole, A.; Swhari, V., Hammomnd, S. & Deshmukh, M. (2011) *miR-29b is activated during neuronal maturation and targets BH3-only genes to restrict apoptosis.* Genes Dev 15;25(2):125-30

Konopka, W.; Kiryk, A., Novak, M., Herwerth, M., Parkitna, JR., Wawrzyniak, M., Kowarsch, A. Michaluk, P., Dzwonek, J., Arnsperger, T., Wilczynski, G., Merkenschlager, M., Theis, FJ., Köhr, G., Kaczmarek, L. & Schütz, G. (2010) *MicroRNA loss enhances learning and memory in mice.* J Neurosci. 30(44):14835-42

Kurose, H.; (2003) *Galpha12 and Galpha13 as key regulatory mediator in signal transduction.* Life Sci. 74(2-3):155-61

Lee, RC.; Feinbaum, RL. & Ambros, V. (1993) *The C. elegans heterochronic gene lin-4 encodes small RNAs with antisense complementarity to lin-14.* Cell 75(5):843–854

Lee, Y.; Ahn, C., Han, J., Choi, H., Kim. J et al., (2003) The nuclear Rnase III Drosha initiates microRNA processing. Nature 425(6956): 415–419

Lee, Y.; Hur, I., Park, SY., Kim, YK., Suh, MR. et al. (2006) *The role of PACT in the RNA silencing pathway.* EMBO J 25(3):522–532

Liu, W.; Liu C, Zhu J, Shu P, Yin B, Gong Y, Qiang B, Yuan J, Peng X. (2010) *MicroRNA-16 targets amyloid precursor protein to potentially modulate Alzheimer's-associated pathogenesis in SAMP8 mice.* DOI:10.1016/neurobiolaging.2010.04.034 Neurobiol Aging

Lukiw, WJ.; (2004) *Gene expression profiling in fetal, aged, and Alzheimer hippocampus: a continuum of stress-related signaling.* Neurochem Res 29(6):1287-97

Lukiw, WJ.; (2007) *Micro-RNA speciation in fetal, adult and Alzheimer's disease hippocampus.Neuroreport.* 18(3):297-300

Lukiw, WJ.; Zhao, Y. & Cui, JG. (2008) *An NF-kappaB-sensitive micro RNA-146a-mediated inflammatory circuit in Alzheimer disease and in stressed human brain cells.* J Biol Chem. 283(46):31315-22

Malenka, RC.; & Nicoll, RA. (1999) *Long-term potentiation--a decade of progress?* Science 285(5435):1870-4

Manahan-Vaughan, D.; Kulla, A., & Frey, JU. (2000) *Requirement of translation but not transcription for the maintenance of long-term depression in the CA1 region of freely moving rats.* J Neurosci. 20(22):8572-6

Maes, OC.; An, J., Sarojini, H. & Wang, E. (2008) *Murine microRNAs implicated in liver functions and aging process.* Mech. Ageing Dev 129:534–541

Maes, OC.; Chertkow, HM., Wang, E. & Schipper, HM. (2009) *MicroRNA: Implications for Alzheimer Disease and other Human CNS Disorders.* Curr Genomics. 10(3):154-68

Morris, RG.; (2003) *Long-term potentiation and memory.* Philos Trans R Soc Lond B Biol Sci. 358(1432):643-7

Nelson, PT.; & Wilfred, BN.(2009) *In situ hybridization is a necessary experimental complement to microRNA (miRNA) expression profiling in the human brain.* Neurosci Lett. 4466(2):69-72

Nunez-Iglesias, C.; Lui, C., Morgan, T.E. & Zhou, X.J. (2010) *Joint genome-wide profiling of miRNA and mRNA expression in Alzheimer's disease cortex reveals altered miRNA regulation.* PLoS One 5(2): e8898

Olsen, PH.; & Ambros, V. (1999) *The lin-4 regulatory RNA controls developmental timing in Caenorhabditis elegans by blocking LIN-14 protein synthesis after the initiation of translation.* Dev Biol 216(2):671–680

Park, CS.; & Tang, SJ. (2009) *Regulation of microRNA expression by induction of bidirectional synaptic plasticity.* J Mol Neurosci. 38(1):50-6

Patel, N.; Hoang, D., Miller, N., Ansaloni, S., Huang, Q., Rogers, J. T., Lee, J. C., Saunders, A. J. (2008) *MicroRNA can regulate human APP levels.* Mol Neurodegener 3:10

Podlisny, M.; Lee, G. & Selkoe, DJ. (1987) *Gene dosage of the amyloid beta precursor protein in Alzheimer's disease.* Science 238:669-71.

Reinhart, BJ.; Slack, FJ., Basson, M., Pasquinelli, AE., Bettinger, JC. et al. (2000) *The 21-nucleotide let-7 RNA regulates developmental timing in Caenorhabditis elegans.* Nature 403(6772):901–906

Rodriguez, A.; Griffiths-Jones, S., Ashurst, JL., & Bradley, A. (2004) *Identification of mammalian microRNA host genes and transcription units.* Genome Res 14(10A):1902–1910

Rovelet-Lecrux, A.; Hannequin, D., Raux, G., Le Meur, N., Laquerrie're, A., Vital, A., et al. (2006) *APP locus duplication causes autosomal dominant early-onset Alzheimer disease with cerebral amyloid angiopathy.* Nat Genet 38:24-6

Scheff, S.; & Price, DA.(2006) *Alzheimer's disease-related alterations in synaptic density: neocortex and hippocampus.* J Alzheimers Dis 9(3 Suppl):101-15

Schipper, HM.; Maes, OC., Chertkow, HM. & Wang, E. (2007) *MicroRNA expression in Alzheimer blood mononuclear cells.* Gene Regul. Syst. Bio. 1:263–274

Schonrock, N.; Ke, YD., Humphreys, D., Staufenbiel, M., Ittner, LM., Preiss, T. & Götz, J. (2010) Neuronal microRNA deregulation in response to Alzheimer's disease amyloid-beta. PLoS One. 5(6):e11070

Schratt, GM.; Tuebing, F., Nigh, EA., Kane, CG., Sabatini, ME. et al. (2006) *A brain-specific microRNA regulates dendritic spine development.* Nature 439(7074):283–289

Schratt, G.; (2009) *Fine-tuning neural gene expression with microRNAs.* Curr Opin Neurobiol 19(2):213-9

Selbach, M.; Schwanhäusser, B., Thierfelder, N., Fang, Z., Khanin, R. & Rajewsky, N. (2008) *Widespread changes in protein synthesis induced by microRNAs.* Nature 455(7209):58-63.

Sethi, P.; & Lukiw, WJ. (2009) *Micro-RNA abundance and stability in human brain: specific alterations in Alzheimer's disease temporal lobe neocortex.* Neurosci. Letters 459:100-104.

Shioya, M.; Obayashi, S., Tabunoki, H., Arima, K., Saito, Y., Ishida, T. & Satoh, J. (2010) *Aberrant microRNA expression in the brains of neurodegenerative diseases: miR-29a decreased in Alzheimer disease brains targets neurone navigator 3.* Neuropathology and Applied Neurobiology 36: 320-330

Siegel, G.; Obernosterer, G., Fiore, R., Oehmen, M., Bicker, S., et al.(2009) *A functional screen implicates microRNA-138-dependent regulation of the depalmitoylation enzyme APT1 in dendritic spine morphogenesis.* Nat Cell Biol 11:705–716

Smalheiser, NR.; Lugli, G., Lenon, AL., Davis, JM., Torvik, V. & Larson J. (2010) *Olfactory discrimination training up-regulates and reorganizes expression of microRNAs in adult mouse hippocampus.* ASN Neuro. 2(1):e00028.

Smith, P.; Al Hashimi, A., Girard, J., Delay, C. & Hébert, SS. (2011) *In vivo regulation of amyloid precursor protein neuronal splicing by microRNAs.* 116(2):240-7

Sutton, MA.; & Schuman, EM. (2006) *Dendritic protein synthesis, synaptic plasticity, and memory.* Cell. 2006 Oct 6;127(1):49-58

Tan, LP.; Seinen, E., Duns, G., de Jong, D., Sibon, OC., Poppema, S., Kroesen, BJ., Kok, K., & van den Berg, A. (2009) *A high throughput experimental approach to identify miRNA targets in human cells.*Nucleic Acids Res. 37(20):e137

Vilardo, E.; Barbato, C., Ciotti, MT., Cogoni, C. & Ruberti, F. (2010) *MicroRNA-101 regulates amyloid precursor protein expression in hippocampal neurons.* J Biol Chem 285:18344-51

Vo, N.; Klein, ME., Varlamova, O., Keller, DM., Yamamoto, T. et al. (2005) *A cAMP-response element binding protein-induced microRNA regulates neuronal morphogenesis.* Proc Natl Acad Sci USA 102(45):16426–16431

Wang, E.; (2007) *MicroRNA, the putative molecular control for mid-life decline.* Ageing Res. Rev. 6:1–11

Wang, W.; Rajeev, B., Stromberg, A., Ren, N., Tang., G., Huang, Q., Rigoutsos, I. & Nelson, P.T. (2008). *The Expression of MicroRNA miR-107 Decreases Early in Alzheimer's Disease and may Accelerate Disease Progression through Regulation of β-Site Amyloid Precursor Protein-Cleaving Enzyme 1. J. Neurosci.* 28(5): 1213-1223

Wang, X.; Huang, Q., Hu, Y., Stromberg, A.J. &Nelson, P.T. (2011) *Patterns of microRNA expression in normal and early Alzheimer'disease human temporal cortex: white matter versus gray matter.* Acta Neuropathol 121:193-205

Wayman, GA.; Davare, M., Ando, H., Fortin, D., Varlamova, O., et al. (2008) *An activity-regulated microRNA controls dendritic plasticity by down-regulating p250GAP.* Proc Natl Acad Sci 105:9093–9098

Wibrand, K.; Panja, D., Tiron, A., Ofte, ML., Skaftnesmo, KO., et al. (2010) *Differential regulation of mature and precursor microRNA expression by NMDA and metabotropic glutamate receptor activation during LTP in the adult dentate gyrus in vivo. Eur J Neurosci.* 31(4):636-45

Whiteman, IT.; Gervasio, OL., Cullen, KM., Guillemin, GJ., Jeong, EV., et al. (2009) *Activated actin-depolymerizing factor/cofilin sequesters phosphorylated microtubule- associated protein during the assembly of alzheimer-like neuritic cytoskeletal striations.* J Neurosci 29: 12994–13005

Yao, J.; Hennessey, T., Flynt, A., Lai, E., Beal, MF., et al. (2010) *MicroRNA-related cofilin abnormality in Alzheimer's disease.* PLoS One 5(12):e15546

# 11

# Expression and Cerebral Function of Amyloid Precursor Protein After Rat Traumatic Brain Injury

Tatsuki Itoh[1], Motohiro Imano[2], Shozo Nishida[3], Masahiro Tsubaki[3], Shigeo Hashimoto[4], Akihiko Ito[1] and Takao Satou[1,5,6]
[1]*Department of Pathology, Kinki University Faculty of Medicine,*
[2]*Department of Surgery, Kinki University Faculty of Medicine,*
[3]*Kinki University Faculty of Pharmaceutical Sciences,*
[4]*Department of Pathology, PL Hospital,*
[5]*Division of Hospital Pathology, Hospital of Kinki University Faculty of Medicine,*
*Division of Sports Medicine, Institute of Life Science, Kinki University,*
*Japan*

## 1. Introduction

The β-amyloid protein derived from amyloid precursor protein (APP) (Goldgaber et al., 1987; Robakis et al., 1987) is a major component of senile plaque, and β-amyloid protein deposits in Alzheimer disease (AD) (Masters et al., 1985; Selkoe et al., 1986) are thought to be produced by alternative processing of APP (Golde et al., 1992). Therefore, the overexpression of APP is an important factor in the neuronal degeneration of AD (Murakami et al., 1998). The expression of APP has also been shown to increase in swollen axons and neuronal perikarya after neuronal injury, including ischemia (Stephenson et al., 1992) and stab injury (Otsuka et al., 1991). As the pathological findings in dementia pugilistica mimic those in AD (Roberts et al., 1990), it has been posited that traumatic brain injury (TBI) is an epidemiological risk factor for AD (Schofield et al., 1997; DeKosky et al., 2007), although other genetic factors, which include the apoE genotype, might act additively (Nicoll et al., 1995; DeKosky et al., 2007). These findings suggest that the overexpression of APP after TBI may potentiate Alzheimer disease pathology. However, the chronological changes in APP expression have not been evaluated after TBI. Furthermore, the function of APP has not been evaluated after TBI.

In this study,

1. we immunohistochemically investigated chronogical changes in cellular sources and levels of APP production compared to that of mRNA for APP as assessed by RT-PCR in the rat brain following traumatic brain injury.
2. In addition, we investigated the function of APP by assessing water maze and morphological changes following direct infusion of the anti-APP antibody into the damaged brain region following TBI.

## 2. Materials and methods

### 2.1 Surgical procedure

Male Wistar rats (8–9 weeks old, 200–250g in weight) were anesthetized by intraperitoneal pentobarbital (50mg/kg) injection. The scalp was incised on the midline and the skull was exposed. A 2–2.5mm hole was drilled (1 mm posterior, + 1 mm right lateral to bregma) in the right parietal calvaria. Brain injury above the dura mater was then induced with a pneumatic control injury device (Itoh et al., 2005; Itoh et al., 2007; Itoh et al., 2009) at an impact velocity of 4m/sec (impact tip diameter of 1mm; fixed impact deformation of 2mm depth from the cerebral surface) (Itoh et al., 2005; Itoh et al., 2007; Itoh et al., 2009). Control rats were subjected to a sham operation, but no cortical penetration injury was inflicted. The contralateral hemisphere was not used as a control, since that area may have been affected by the impact. Rats were placed in a heated cage to maintain their body temperature at 37°C during the recovery from anesthesia.

### 2.2 Anti-APP antibody infusion

The drug infusion protocol was as previously described (Green-Sadan et al., 2003). Immediately, after TBI, the animals were placed in a stereotactic frame and fitted with a brain infusion cannula (Alzet brain infusion kit 3, 1mm, Alzet, San Diego, CA, USA). The cannula was implanted with the tip inserted into the damaged brain region (1 mm posterior, + 1 mm right lateral to bregma). The cannula was secured with dental cement. A micro-osmotic pump (Model 2001; rate of 1µl/h, Alzet), filled with 300 µl infusion volume kept 37°C, was implanted subcutaneously in the neck and connected to the infusion cannula. Rats received an infusion of either anti-APP antibody (IgG2a isoform, 1µg/ml; anti-APP antibody group; Chemicon, Temecula, CA, USA) diluted in sterilized phosphate buffer saline (0.1M PBS, pH 7.4–7.5; n=20) or sterilized PBS only (PBS group; n=20) for seven days immediately after TBI. For the control of the Morris water maze experiments, ten animals with no operation (sham operation group, no injury) were also collected. In sham operation group, a micro-osmotic pump was implanted subcutaneously in the neck without infusion cannula. Moreover, sham operation group was used only the behavioural experiments. As probe and the extent of APP antibody infusion test, although data not shown in this study, we investigated that the extent of APP antibody diffusion with Evans blue using the osmotic pump and confirmed Evans blue extended whole brain from center of infusion area.

### 2.3 Morris water maze experiments

A circular, thermostatically regulated, dark gray PVC-plastic water tank (180cm wide, 45cm deep, filled with tap water at 22±1°C), located in the center of the testing room and surrounded by extra-maze cues, was used in the spatial learning task. A constant asymmetrical array of lamps and pictures served as cues for spatial orientation. A circular dark gray platform (15cm wide) submerged 1cm below the water surface served as a platform. The platform was placed in the center of one of the quadrants, i.e., the target quadrant, of the water maze (Elvander et al., 2004). The experiments were monitored using a digital TV system connected to a computer (Elvander et al., 2004). Training took place between 8:00a.m. and 3:00p.m. during seven consecutive days. Each daily training session consisted of four trials with a 120s cutoff time, followed by 30s rest on the platform. Memory was tested in fifteen animals from each of the anti-APP antibody group and the PBS group, and in ten sham operation group animals, starting at day one and continued up to seven days after TBI/sham operation.

## 2.4 Immunohistochemistry

1, 3, 7, 30 and 90 days after TBI and after the last the Morris water maze test at seven days, rats from each group were perfused intracardially with 300ml of PBS followed by 300ml of 4% paraformaldehyde (PFA; pH 7.4–7.5) in PBS. The brains were then removed and stored in PFA for three days, before the maximum size of the lesion was sliced into serial coronal sections (50μm thick) using a microslicer (Dousaka EM, Kyoto, Japan).

Sections were treated with 3% $H_2O_2$ in Tris-buffered saline (TBS; 0.1M Tris-HCl, pH 7.5, 0.15M NaCl) containing 0.1% Triton X-100 (TBS-T) for 30min. Next, the sections were washed three times with TBS-T, blocked with 3% bovine serum albumin (BSA; Sigma-Aldrich, St. Louis, MO, USA) in TBS-T for 30min, and incubated with a mouse monoclonal anti- microtubule associate protein-2 (MAP-2) antibody as a marker of neuronal cell (1:10000 dilution; Sigma-Aldrich), a mouse monoclonal anti-neurofilament (NF) antibody as a marker of neuronal cell (1:10000 dilution; DAKO, Glostrup, Denmark), a rabbit polyclonal anti-Glial Fibrillary Acidic Protein (GFAP) antibody (1:10000 dilution; DAKO, Glostrup, Denmark), a mouse monoclonal anti-APP antibody (1:1000 dilution; Chemicon, Temecula, CA, USA) or a mouse monoclonal anti-CD11b antibody as a marker of microglia/macrophage (1:1000 dilution; Chemicon, Temecula, CA, USA) overnight at room temperature. Following extensive washing, the sections were further incubated with a HISTIFINE Rat-PO (multi)-kit (Nichirei, Osaka, Japan), consisting of a mixed solution of peroxidase-conjugated anti-mouse and rabbit IgG as the secondary antibody, for 60min at room temperature. The HISTIFINE Rat-PO kits contained preabsorbed rat serum, and showed very minimal non-specific binding by rat serum in injured rat tissues. Labeling was visualized using diaminobenzidine (DAB; Vector Peroxidase Substrate Kit; Vector Laboratories, Burlingame, CA, USA) for 5min, and the sections were counterstained with hematoxylin.

For TUNEL-staining at three days after TBI, the brains from five rats in each of the anti-APP antibody group and the PBS group were collected as above. Sections were used for TUNEL-staining, a marker of apoptosis. TUNEL-staining was performed using an *in situ* Apoptosis Detection Kit (TaKaRa Biochemicals Co., Kyoto, Japan) according to the manufacturer's instructions. Sections were treated with Proteinase K for 10min, followed by treatment with 3% $H_2O_2$ in TBS-T for 30min. Next, the sections were washed three times with TBS-T, and incubated with a TdT Enzyme Labeling solution for 90min at room temperature. Labeling was visualized using DAB. The controls for the TUNEL stains were performed without enzyme. Furthermore, to investigate TUNEL-positive cells phenotype, MAP-2 or GFAP immunofluorescence staining was performed following TUNEL-staining. Sections were treated with Proteinase K for 10min. Next, the sections incubated with a fluorescein isothiocyanate (FITC)-conjugated TdT Enzyme Labeling solution for 90min at room temperature. Next, the sections were washed extensively and incubated with an anti-MAP-2 antibody (1:300 dilution; Sigma) or anti-GFAP antibody (1:300 dilution; DAKO) overnight at room temperature. Following extensive washing, the sections were further incubated with Alexa Flour 555 anti-mouse IgG (for anti-MAP-2 antibody) or rabbit IgG (for anti-GFAP antibody, 1:300 dilution; BD Biosciences Pharmingen, San Diego, CA) for 80 min at room temperature. Subsequently, the sections were observed using a confocal laser-scanning microscope (LSM5 PASCAL; Carl Zeiss Jena GmbH, Jena, Germany).

## 2.5 Quantification

To determined the number of APP -positive neurites and cells, MAP-2-, GFAP-, or TUNEL-positive cells, each DAB-positive cells around the damaged area (cortex) without white matter after TBI were observed and DAB-labeled cells were counted in three serial sections (each section was 50 μm in thickness) under a Nikon E 1000M microscope (Nikon Corporation, Tokyo, Japan) using a 20x objective. To determine the measured area of DAB-positive cells, an image of the measured area was captured under the Nikon E 1000M microscope at 1x magnification using a CCD camera (ACT-2U; Nikon Corporation). The measured area in each image was traced and measured using a computer (Power Macintosh G3; Apple Computers, Cupertino, CA) and the NIH Image 1.6 software (NIH, Bethesda, MD). The number of DAB-positive cells was expressed as positive cell number/100$\mu m^3$.

### 2.6 Double-immunofluorescence staining

Each serial section was washed with TBS-T, blocked with 3% BSA in TBS-T for 30 min, and incubated with a polyclonal rabbit anti-APP antibody (1:300 dilution; Chemicon) overnight at room temperature. Following extensive washing, the sections were further incubated with a polyclonal rhodamine-conjugated anti-rabbit IgG antibody (1:300 dilution; DAKO) for 80 min at room temperature. Next, the APP-stained sections were washed extensively and incubated with a monoclonal mouse anti-NF antibody (1:300 dilution; DAKO), a marker for neurons and nerve fiver; a monoclonal mouse anti-MAP-2 antibody (1:300 dilution; Sigma), a marker for neurons; a monoclonal mouse anti-CD11b antibody (1:300 dilution; AbD Serotec, Raleigh, NC), a marker for macrophages/microglia or a monoclonal mouse anti-GFAP antibody (1:300 dilution; DAKO), a marker for astroglia overnight at room temperature. Following extensive washing, the sections were further incubated with a polyclonal fluorescein isothiocyanate (FITC)-conjugated anti-mouse IgG antibody (1:300 dilution; DAKO) for 80 min at room temperature. Subsequently, the sections were observed by fluorescence microscopy (Nikon E-800; Nikon, Tokyo, Japan).

### 2.7 Reverse transcription-polymerase chain reaction (RT-PCR)

The mRNA expression levels were investigated by RT-PCR at 1 to 90 days after TBI. Five rats were used for each time point. Briefly, total RNA was isolated from an area of the cerebral cortex (without the corpus callosum and hippocampus) with a diameter of 2 mm from the center of the lesion using RNA-Bee (Tel-Test Inc., Friendswood, TX) and redissolved in water, before the concentration was determined photometrically using the wavelength ratio of 260 nm/280 nm. The two oligonucleotide primers used for APP mRNA were: (accession No X07648): sense primer: 5 ′-GGA TGC GGA GTT CGG ACA TG -3 ′antisense primer: 5 ′-GTT CTG CAT CTG CTC AAA G -3 ′Rat glyceraldehyde-3-phosphate dehydrogenase (GAPDH) (CLONTECH, No5507, BD Biosciences Pharmingen, San Diego, CA) was used as an internal control.

RT-PCR was performed using an mRNA PCR Kit (TaKaRa Biochemicals Co., Kyoto, Japan) according to the manufacturer's instructions. RT was performed at 42°C for 25 min, followed by heat inactivation at 99°C for 5 min. PCR amplification was carried out in a PCR EXPRESS (Hybaid US, Franklin, MA) for 30 cycles of 2 min at 94°C, 30 s at 94°C, 30 s at 55°C and 1.5 min at 72°C. The final step was extended to 5 min at 72°C. After separation by electrophoresis in 1.5% agarose gels, the products were stained with ethidium bromide and located by fluorescence using UV light (3UV Transilluminator; UVP, Upland, CA). Bio Max 1D TM1.5.1 (Kodak, Tokyo, Japan) was used to evaluate the band intensities of the PCR bands. The signals were normalized to the corresponding GAPDH signal in the same RNA sample.

### 2.8 Enzyme-linked immunosorbent assay (ELISA) for APP

The APP protein levels after TBI were investigated by ELISA using extracts of the TBI area. Five rats were used for each time point. Briefly, brain tissue from the above-described TBI area was isolated at each time point, and homogenized (10% w/v) in homogenizing buffer (PBS containing 0.25 mol/L sucrose, 5 mmol/L ethylene glycol bis(2-aminoethyl ether)-tetraacetic acid (EGTA), 25 μg/ml leupeptin, 25 μg/ml aprotinin) at 4°C using a hand homogenizer. After treatment of the homogenates with ultrasonic waves at 4°C for 100 s and centrifugation at 20,000 *g* for 30 min at 4°C, the resulting supernatants were collected. The protein concentrations of the supernatants were determined using a DC Protein Assay Kit (Bio-Rad Laboratories, Hercules, CA) according to the manufacturer's instructions, and then adjusted to 1 μg/μl. The brain tissue samples were stored at -80°C until analysis by ELISA. ELISAs were performed as previously described. Briefly, flat-bottomed microtiter plates (type H for ELISA; Sumitomo Bakelite Co., Tokyo, Japan) were coated with a rabbit polyclonal anti-APP antibody (diluted to 0.5 μg/ml in PBS containing 3% BSA (PBS-B); Chemicon) and blocked with 300 μl of PBS containing 3% BSA, 1% sucrose and 0.05% Tween 20 for 120 min at room temperature. The plates were then washed three times with PBS containing 0.05% Tween 20 (PBS-T). Recombinant APP (Chemicon) was serially diluted with PBS-B (0.001-12 ng/ml) and used to construct a standard curve. Aliquots (100 μl) of the diluted samples were incubated in the wells at 4°C overnight. After washing, 100 μl of a mouse monoclonal anti-APP antibody (1:10000 dilution in PBS-B; Chemicon) was added to each well and incubated for 2 h at room temperature. After washing, 100 μl of simple-stain MAX-PO (mouse)-kit (Nichirei) consisting of a peroxidase-conjugated anti-mouse IgG was added to each well. Color development was carried out using an Enzyme Reaction Kit Type T (Sumitomo Bakelite Co., Tokyo, Japan), and the absorbances at 490 nm were measured using a microplate reader (Model 3550UV; Bio-Rad Laboratories). The detection limit of the assay for APP was 0.005 ng/ml. The measurements were made in duplicate.

### 2.9 Area measurement of damaged brain region

To determine the area of the damage region at seven days after TBI, after the last the Morris water maze five rats per group were collected as above, and the anteroposterior of the maximum size of the lesion was sliced into forty serial coronal sections (50μm thick). Anteroposterior sections 1–40 were stained with hematoxylin and eosin (HE). Images of the HE stain in the forty anteroposterior serial sections were captured using a Nikon E 1000M microscope at 1X magnification and a CCD camera. The area of the damaged region in each image was traced and measured by computer, and the average area of the damaged region calculated over the forty serial sections.

### 2.10 Statistical analysis

Water maze data were expressed as mean±SE. Data were analyzed using ANOVA and Fisher's PLSD-test (Stat View®; SAS Institute Inc, Cary, NC. USA). Other data were expressed as mean±SD and analyzed using ANOVA. $p<0.05$ was considered statistically significant.

## 3. Results

### 3.1 Double-immunofluorescence of amyloid precursor protein (APP) and neurofilament (NF), microtubule-associated protein-2 (MAP-2), glial fibrillary acidic protein (GFAP) or CD11b

The neuronal or microglial localizations of APP protein in the cortical traumatic injured rats at 1 day, 3 days and 7 days post-lesion are illustrated (Fig.1-3). Neurons, astroglia or microglia were identified by immunohistochemical staining using anti-NF, anti-MAP-2, and anti-GFAP or anti-CD11b, respectively. Double labeling immunohistochemistry with anti-

NF (Fig. 1A) and anti-APP (Fig. 1B) antibodies clearly demonstrated the co-localization of NF and APP proteins in swollen and dystrophic nerve fibers at 1day after TBI (Fig. 1C). At 7 days after cortical traumatic injury, MAP-2-positive nerve cell cytoplasm (Fig. 1D) was positive for APP (Fig. 1E&F).
Anti-GFAP (Fig. 2A) or anti-CD11b (Fig. 2D) and anti-APP (Fig. 2B&E) antibodies did not demonstrate co-localization in the same cells at 3 days after cortical traumatic injury (Fig. 2C&F). At 7 days after traumatic injury, a few CD11b-positive cells (Fig. 2G) expressed weakly positive APP immunoreactivity (Fig. 2H&I).

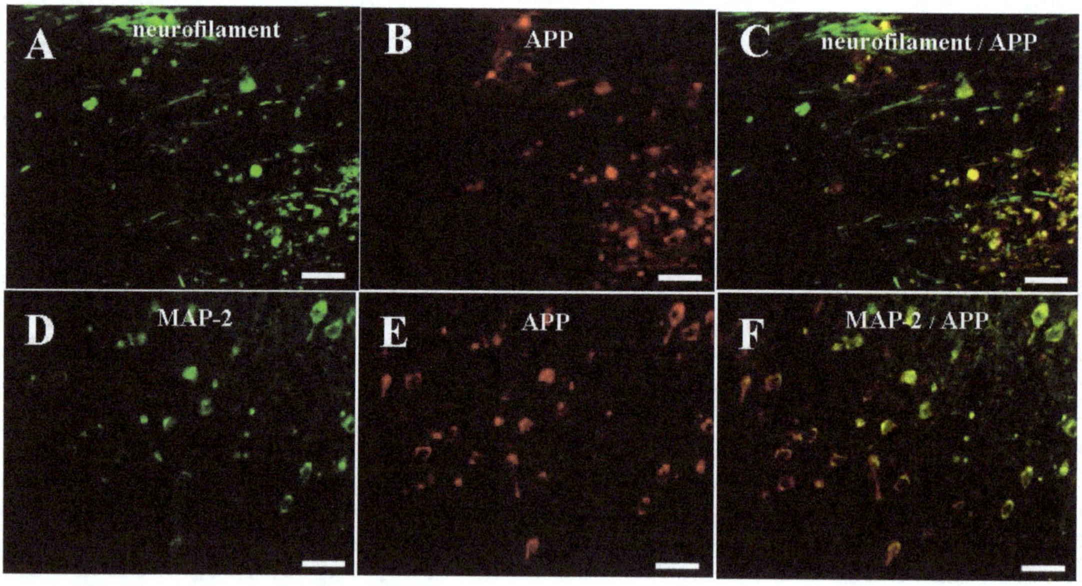


Fig. 1. Double-immunofluorescence staining of localized neurofilaments (A) or MAP-2 (D) and APP (B, E) around the damaged area after traumatic brain injury. At 1 day after injury, damaged dystrophic and swollen neurites (A, green) in the cortex were APP-positive (B, red). The merged image (C) of panels (A) and (B) reveals colocalization of these proteins (yellow). At 7 days after injury, neurons near the injured portion were positive for MAP-2 (D, green) and APP (E, red). The merged image (F) of panels (D) and (E) reveals colocalization of these proteins (yellow). Scale bar = 50 μm.

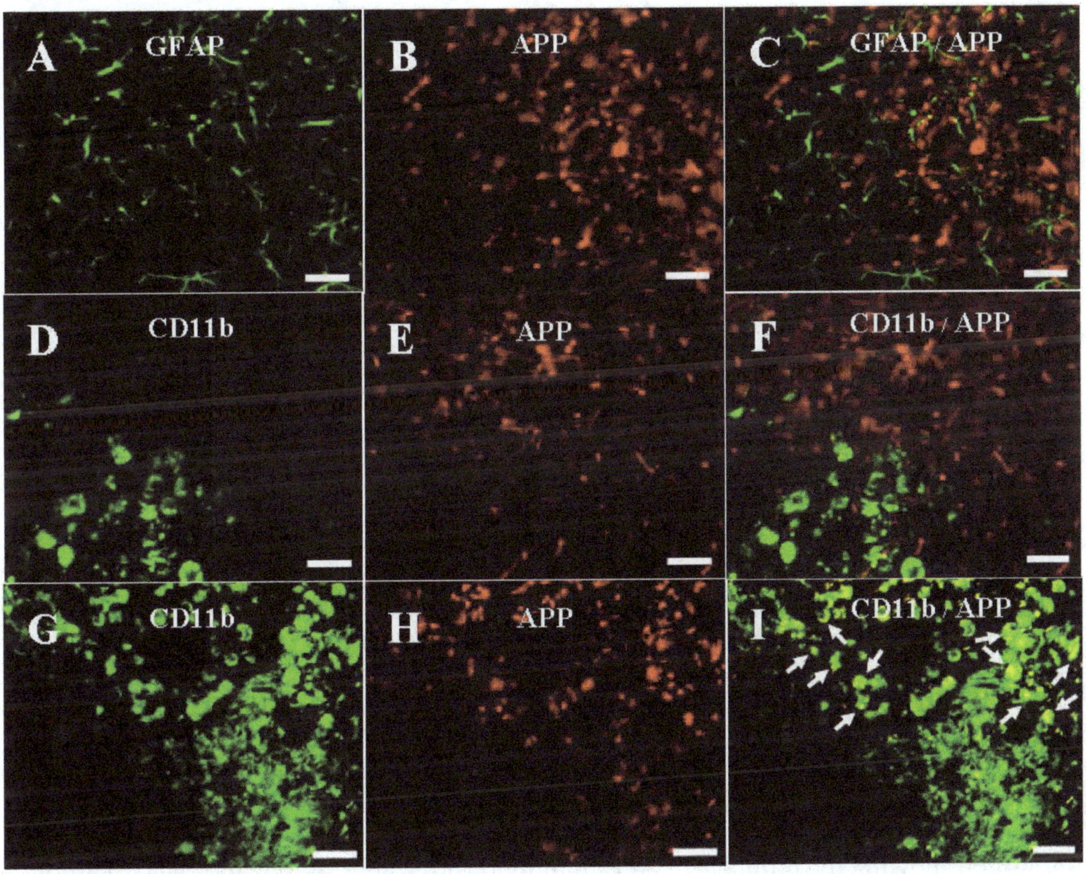


Fig. 2. Double-immunofluorescence staining for GFAP (A) or CD11b (D, G) and APP (B, E, H) around the damaged area after traumatic brain injury. At 3 days after the injury, GFAP-immunopositive (A, green) and APP-immunopositive (B, red) cells are observed. The merged image (C) of panels (A) and (B) does not show any colocalization. At 3 days after the injury, CD11b-immunopositive (D, green) and APP-immunopositive (E, red) cells are observed. The merged image (F) of panels (D) and (E) does not show any colocalization. However, at 7 days after the injury, CD11b-immunopositive (G, green) and APP-immunopositive (H, red) cells are colocalization (I, arrows). Scale bar = 50 μm.

### 3.2 Immunostaining and APP-immunopositive cell and neurites count after TBI

There were many APP-positive damaged swollen and dystrophic neurites at 1 day after TBI (Fig. 3A). At 7 days after TBI, there were many APP-positive neurons and a few APP-positive damaged swollen and dystrophic neurites (Fig. 3B). However, there were no APP-immunopositive cells and fivers in the sham-operated cerebral cortex (Fig. 3C). The number of APP-positive neurites ($p<0.001$, Fig. 3D) and cells ($p<0.001$, Fig. 3E) was increased in the cortex as early as 1 day following injury, with the elevation becoming significant from 1 day to 90 days($p<0.001$, Fig. 3E). There were no such changes in the sham group (Fig. 3D&E).

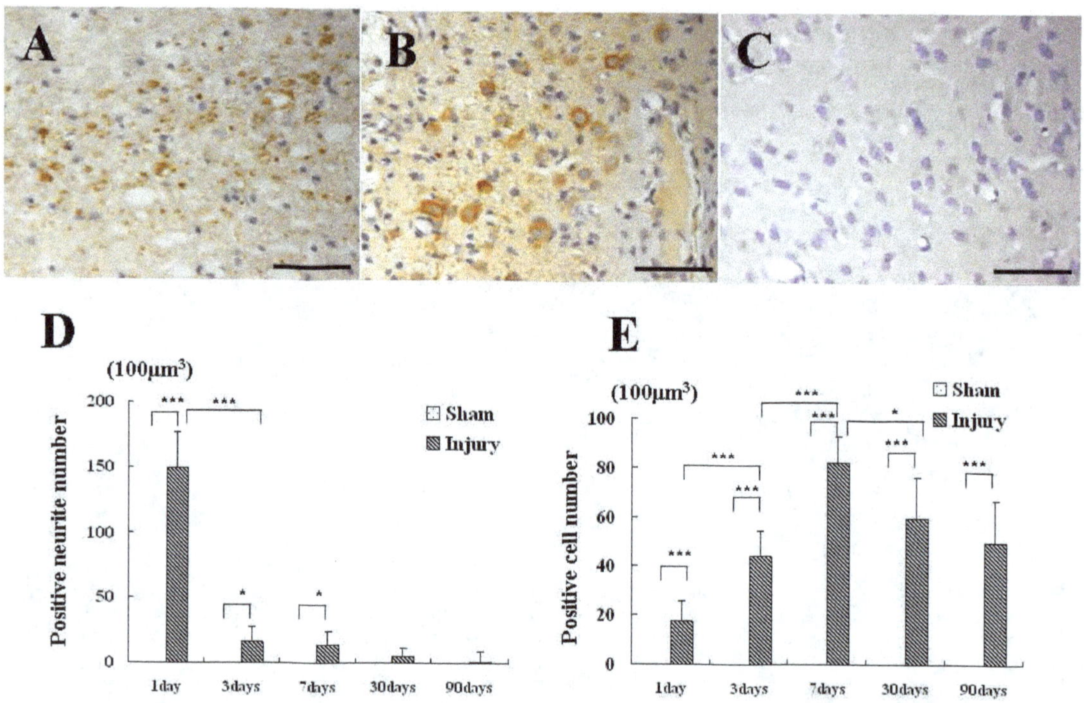


Fig. 3. Immunostaining for APP around the damaged cerebral cortex after traumatic brain injury. At 1 day after injury, there are many APP-positive damaged dystrophic and swollen neurites (A). At 7 days after injury, there are many APP-positive neurons and a few APP-positive damaged dystrophic and swollen neurites (B). However, the sham-operated control cortex does not contain any APP staining or APP-immunopositive cells (C). Scale bar = 50 μm. Graph showing the numbers of APP-immunopositive neurites (D) and cells (E) around the damaged cerebral cortex after traumatic rat brain injury. The results are shown as the mean ± SD. $^{*}P < 0.05$, $^{***}P < 0.001$, $n = 5$.

### 3.3 RT-PCR analysis of APP

As determined by RT-PCR, the mRNA levels for APP were elevated after cortical injury. The APP transcript level displayed an increase in the cortex as early as 1 day following injury, with the elevation becoming significant between 1 day and 30 days and returning to the control level by 90 days ($p<0.05$, Fig. 4A) . One peak of elevation was determined between 1 day and 30 days after injury. There were no such changes in the sham group (Fig. 4A).

### 3.4 APP protein in brain tissue after TBI

As determined by ELISA, the levels of APP were elevated after cortical injury. ELISA demonstrated a pattern similar to that showing by RT-PCR. APP levels displayed an increase in the injured side as early as 1 day following injury, with the elevation becoming significant between 1 day and 90 days ($p<0.001$, Fig. 4B). One peak of elevation was determined between 1 day and 90 days after injury (Fig. 4B). There were no such changes in the sham group (Fig. 4B).

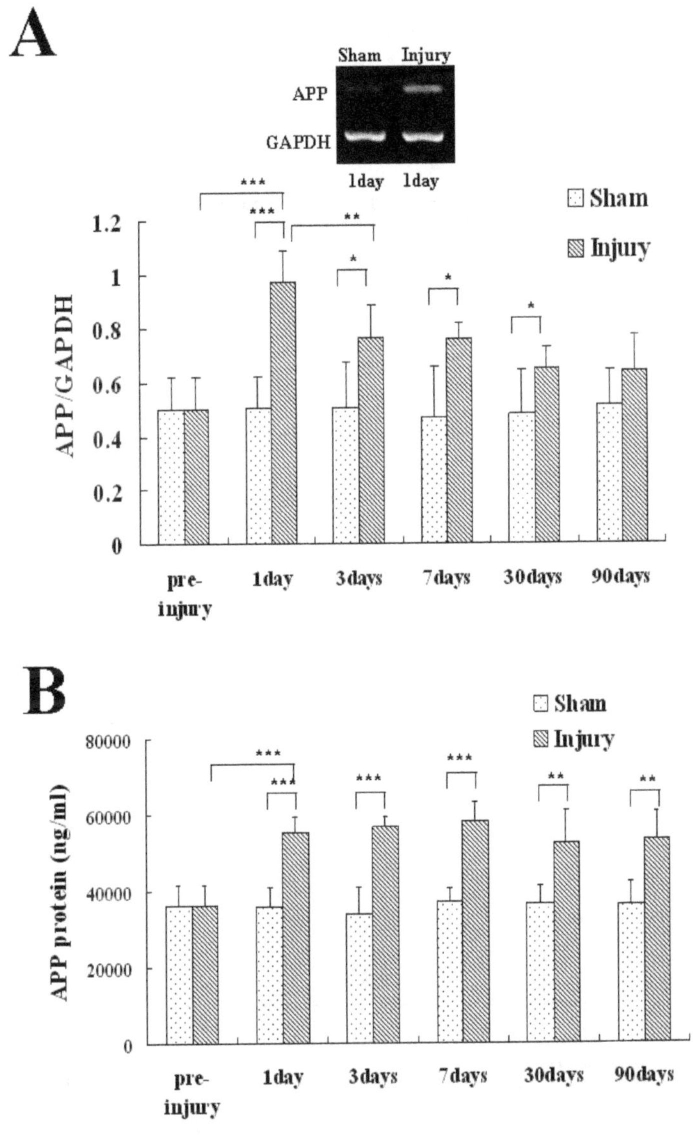


Fig. 4. Graphs show the optical density units of ethidium bromide-stained RT-PCR products for APPmRNA expression (A) and the level of APP protein (B) after traumatic brain injury. The results are shown as the mean ± SD. $^{*}P < 0.05$, $^{**}P < 0.01$, $^{***}P < 0.001$, $n = 5$.

### 3.5 Water maze experiments

When compared with the sham operation group, the arrival time to platform was significantly increased at seven days after TBI in the PBS group ($p$<0.001, Fig. 5). However, at seven days after TBI, the arrival time to platform was significantly decreased in the anti-APP antibody group versus the PBS group ($p<0.001$, Fig. 5), and was not different from the sham operation group at seven days after TBI (Fig. 5).

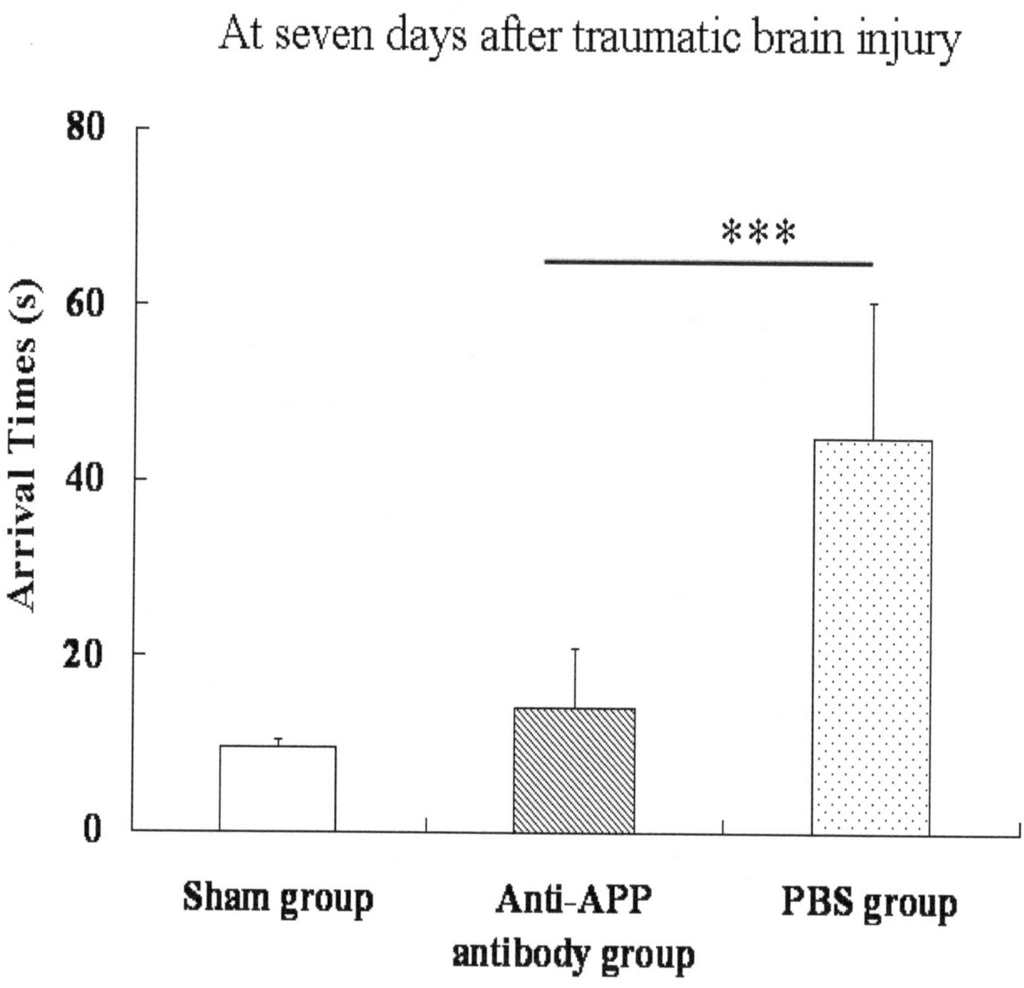


Fig. 5. The effect of anti-APP antibody on cerebral function at seven days after TBI. Anti-APP antibody (1μg/ml) or PBS was infused over seven days by osmotic pump (1μl/hr). The sham operation group had no injury. The effects of treatment group on arrival time to platform are shown. Values represent mean±SE (n=10/group). PBS group *vs*. anti-APP antibody group *vs*. sham operation group. ***$p<0.001$

### 3.6 Area of the damaged brain region after TBI

HE images of the damaged brain region at seven days after TBI can be seen in Figure 6A-B. The area of the damaged brain region was significantly decreased in the anti-APP antibody group versus the PBS group ($p<0.001$, Fig. 6C).

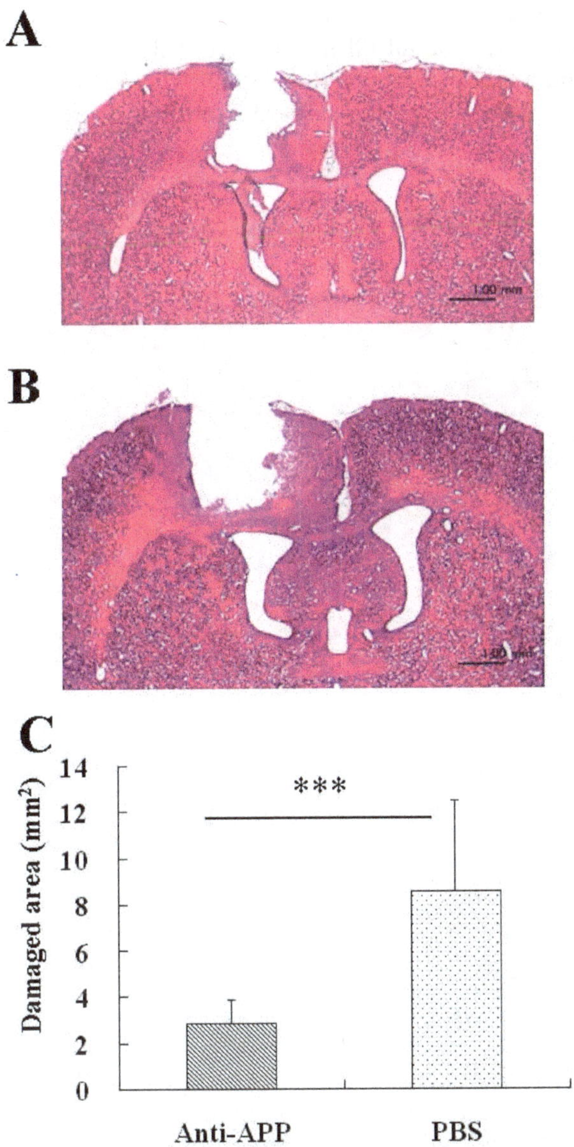


Fig. 6. The size of the damaged brain region at seven days after TBI. HE stains show the anti-APP antibody group (1μg/ml) (A) and the PBS group (B). Scale bar = 1mm. (C) Measurement results of each group (n=5/group). Anti-APP antibody group *vs.* PBS group. ***$p<0.001$.

### 3.7 Immunostaining and GFAP-immunopositive cell counts after TBI

Immunostaining results for GFAP expression and the numbers of GFAP-positive cells around the damaged brain region at seven days after TBI can be seen in Figure 7A-E. In the anti-APP antibody group there were many larger GFAP-positive cells with GFAP staining in their cytoplasm and long elongated projections around the damaged region (Fig 7. A-B). Furthermore, there were many GFAP-positive fibers that formed glial scars after TBI, and these fibers were enriched at the damaged brain region (Fig. 7A). In contrast, in the PBS group there were only a few small GFAP-positive cells which possessed a small GFAP-positive cytoplasm and a few projections (Fig. 7C-D). There was a significant increase in the number of GFAP-positive cells in the anti-APP antibody group versus the PBS group ($p<0.001$, Fig. 7E).

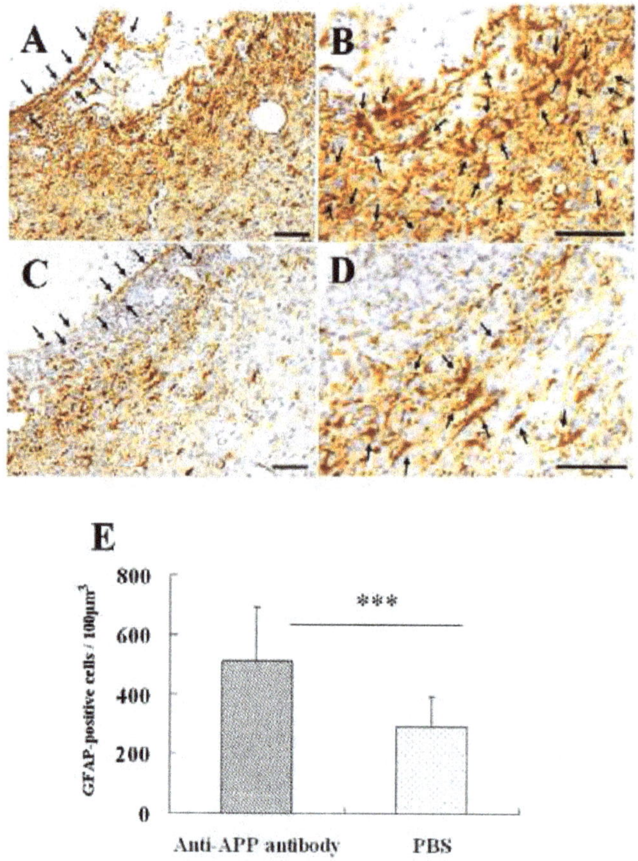


Fig. 7. GFAP expression around the damaged region at seven days after TBI. Note that there were many glial scars (A, arrows) and many large GFAP-positive cells and projections (B, arrows) in the anti-APP antibody group (1μg/ml; A: low power, B: high power), while glial scars (C, arrows), only a few small GFAP-positive cells, and a few projections (D, arrows) were observed in the PBS group (C: low power, D: high power). Scale bar = 50μm. (E) Number of GFAP-positive cells in each group (n=10/group). Anti-APP antibody group *vs.* PBS group. ***$p<0.001$.

### 3.8 Immunostaining and MAP-2-immunopositive cell counts after TBI

Immunostaining results for MAP-2 expression and the numbers of MAP-2-positive cells around the damaged region at seven days after TBI can be seen in Figure 8A-C. In the anti-APP antibody group there were many large MAP-2-positive nerve cells (cytoplasm stained) and MAP-2-positive fibers (Fig. 8A). In contrast, in the PBS group there were only a few small MAP-2-positive cells which possessed a small MAP-2-immunopositive cytoplasm and a few MAP-2-positive fibers (Fig. 8B). There was a significant increase in the number of MAP-2-positive cells in the anti-APP antibody group versus the PBS group ($p$<0.001, Fig. 8C).

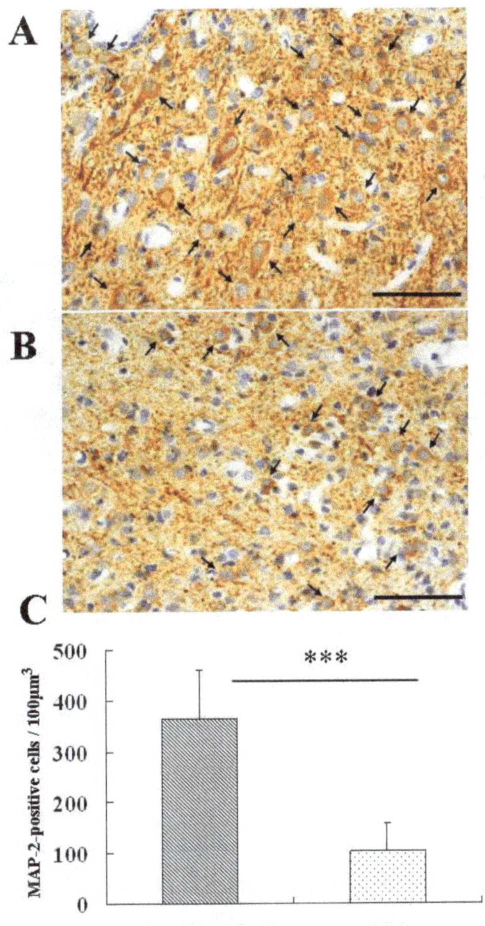


Fig. 8. MAP-2 expression around the damaged region at seven days after TBI. Note that numerous large MAP-2-positive cells and fibers were observed in the anti-APP antibody group (1μg/ml; A, arrows), while only a few small MAP-2-positive cells and a few fibers were observed in the PBS group (B, arrows). Scale bar = 50μm. (C) The number of MAP-2-positive cells in each group (n=10/group). Anti-APP antibody group *vs.* PBS group. ***$p$<0.001.

### 3.9 TUNEL-staining and TUNEL-positive cells counts after TBI

TUNEL-staining results and the numbers of TUNEL-positive cells around the damaged region at three days after TBI can be seen in Figure 9A-E. In the anti-APP antibody group there were only a few TUNEL-positive cells which possessed a small cytoplasm, such as glial cells, or a large cytoplasm, such as neural cells (Fig. 9A). In contrast, in the PBS group there were many TUNEL-positive cells which possessed small or large cytoplasm's (Fig. 9B). Furthermore, Almost TUNEL-positive cells in PBS group colocalize with the MAP-2 staining (Fig. 9C). A few TUNEL-positive cells in PBS group colocalize with the GFAP staining (Fig. 9D). In addition, the number of TUNEL-positive cells in the anti-APP antibody group was significantly decreased versus the PBS group ($p<0.001$, Fig. 9E).

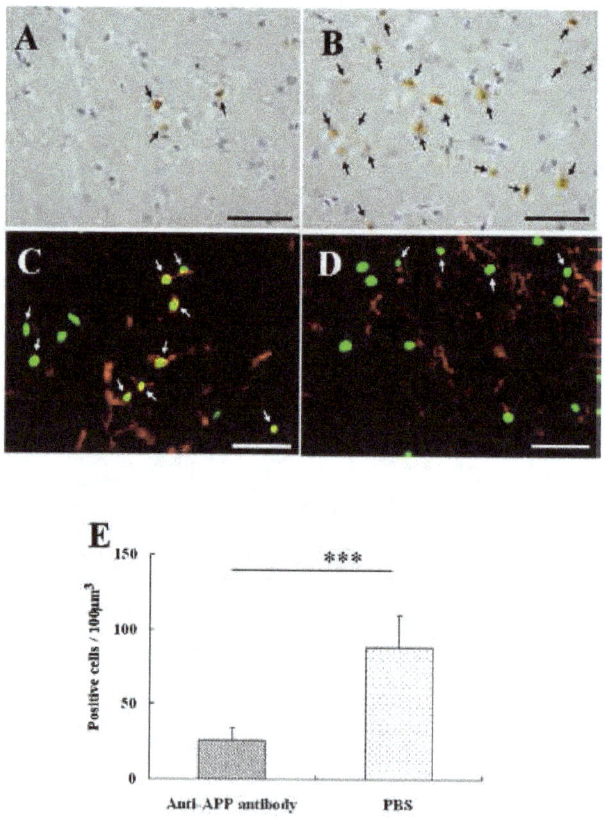


Fig. 9. TUNEL-staining around the damaged region at three days after TBI. Note that there were only a few TUNEL-positive cells, which possessed small or large cytoplasms, in the anti-APP antibody group (1μg/ml; A, arrows), while many small or large cytoplasm TUNEL-positive cells were observed in the PBS group (B, arrows). (C) and (D) were indicated TUNEL-staining (green) and MAP-2 (C, red) or GFAP (D, red) immunofluorescence staining in PBS group. Many TUNEL-positive (C, green) cells showed MAP-2-immunopositive (C, red). A few TUNEL-positive (D, green) cells showed GFAP-immunopositive (D, red). The merged image of TUNEL- and MAP-2- or GFAP-positive cells showed arrows (C&D). Scale bar = 50μm. (E) Number of TUNEL-positive cells in each group (n=5/group). Anti-APP antibody group *vs.* PBS group. ***$p<0.001$.

## 4. Discussion

The hypothesis that head trauma is a risk factor associated with subsequent development of Alzheimer disease is based on the neuropathology of dementia (Roberts 1988; Roberts et al., 1994). Some reports have shown that the expression of APP is enhanced by various forms of brain injury, including traumatic (Otsuka et al., 1991), chemical (Nakamura et al., 1992) , and ischemic injury (Stephenson et al., 1992). Further, the overexpression of APP suggests the possibility of an Alzheimer disease-like pathology after traumatic brain injury (Rumble et al., 1989). Previously, the appearance of APP in the brain during pathological events was usually attributed to its synthesis by neurons, macrophages, microglia or astrocytes (Otsuka et al., 1991). However, APP was synthesized by neurons, as showing by immunohistochemical, ELISA and RT-PCR obtained performed in this study. In the present report, double labeling immunohistochemistry with anti-NF or anti-MAP-2 and anti-APP antibodies demonstrated the co-localization. Furthermore, we showed that the expression of APP in neurons and neurites was significantly increased in the cerebral cortex after traumatic brain injury. It has been pointed out that increased APP immunoreactivity occurrs in damaged axons due to disturbance of fast anterograde axonal transport (Koo et al., 1990)by destroyed cytoskeletal proteins, including neurofilaments (Posmantur et al., 1994) and MAP-2 (Taft et al., 1992). These results suggested that APP synthesis was increased from the early phase after brain injury and it lasted for a long period during the experiment.

In the present study, the mRNA and protein levels for APP were elevated after TBI. It was previously reported that APP mRNA and protein levels were increased in neurons after TBI (Van den Heuvel et al., 1999; Ciallella et al., 2002). Furthermore, expression of APP was increased in neurons after ischemia and axonal injury (Stephenson et al., 1992; Xie et al., 2003). Taken together, these results suggest that APP is synthesized by neurons, rather than glial cells and macrophages/microglia, after TBI. In future studies, it will be necessary to further clarify the cell type producing APP after TBI.

TBI occurs as the result of a direct mechanical insult to the brain, and induces degeneration and death in the central nervous system (CNS) (Chirumamilla et al., 2002; Rice et al., 2003). Following the initial mechanical insult, secondary pathways are activated that contribute to the ischemic damage induced by circulatory disturbance, blood-brain barrier disruption and excitotoxic damage (Kawamata et al., 1995; Azbill et al., 1997; Xiong et al., 1997). The expression of APP has also been shown to increase in swollen axons and neuronal perikarya after neuronal injuries, including ischemia (Stephenson et al., 1992) and stab injuries (Otsuka et al., 1991). CNS disorders can be caused by the widespread neuronal and axonal degeneration induced by TBI (Chirumamilla et al., 2002; Rice et al., 2003). Taken together, these results suggest that APP leaks out from damaged and necrotic axons and neuronal cytoplasm after TBI. In the present study, CD11b-positive cells were colocalized with APP protein at 7 days after TBI. It appeared that macrophages/microglia engulfed and digested the APP that leaked from axons and neurons during this phase. Therefore, at 7 days after TBI, both neurons and macrophages/microglia expressed APP.

The overexpression of APP suggests the possibility of an Alzheimer disease-like pathology after TBI (Rumble et al., 1989; Itoh et al., 2009). Previously, the appearance of APP in the brain during pathological events was usually attributed to its synthesis by neurons, macrophages, microglia, or astrocytes (Otsuka et al., 1991). Sun *et al.* reported that overproduction of APP induced expression of the apoptosis-related Fas antigen in cultured neural, astrocytes, and microglia (Sun et al., 2004). Furthermore, APP induced nitric oxide synthetase (iNOS) and nitric oxide (NOS) production, and induced neural and glial cell apoptosis(Sun et al., 2004). In the present study, a continuous infusion of the anti-APP antibody infusion inhibited neural and glial apoptotic cell death at three days after TBI. This neuroprotection was associated with numerous GFAP-positive cells and glial scars, suggesting that the anti-APP antibody inhibited APP-induced glial cell apoptosis.

It was previously reported that APP which was expressed on the cell membrane of cultured cortical neural cells controlled intracellular $Ca^{2+}$ entry (Bouron et al., 2004). Intracellular entry of $Ca^{2+}$ activates $Ca^{2+}$-dependent signal pathways and can induce neural cell death. Additionally, choline acetyltransferase (ChAT) activity was decreased in the frontal cortex and hippocampus of APP 695 transgenic mice, an Alzheimer model overexpressing APP, and increased the number of apoptotic neurons(Feng et al., 2004). These APP 695 transgenic mice exhibit increased learning and memory impairment (Feng et al., 2004). In the present study, in the anti-APP antibody group there was an increase in the number of MAP-2-positive cells and a reduction in the arrival time to platform versus the PBS group. These data suggested that the anti-APP antibody increased ChAT activity and inhibited neural degeneration induced by overproduced APP in the frontal cortex and hippocampus after TBI, while cerebral function may be improved. As such, measurement of ChAT activity in the anti-APP antibody and the PBS groups after TBI will form the basis of future research.

Recent evidence suggests that APP, a ubiquitously expressed, highly conserved integral membrane glycoprotein, is not only a sensitive marker of axonal injury (Gentleman et al., 1993; Blumbergs et al., 1995), but may also have an important functional role following TBI. APP is upregulated acutely in injured neurons and reactive astrocytes following TBI (Pierce et al., 1996; Van den Heuvel et al., 1999), and this upregulation has been associated with increase hippocampal cell death (Murakami et al., 1998). Although the mechanisms leading to cell death are unknown, as the precursor to the neurotoxic Aβ protein, the conversion of APP to Aβ may have detrimental effects including an increased risk for development of Alzheimer's disease (Chen et al., 2004). Indeed, there are numerous clinical studies demonstrating substantial Aβ deposition and the formation of amyloid plaques (Smith et al., 2003; Ikonomovic et al., 2004). Furthermore, following TBI in the rat there is an increased β-secretase enzyme expression (BACE 11) that could potentially facilitate Aβ production (Blasko et al., 2004), a direct link between increase APP levels and increased Aβ deposition and toxicity (Stone et al., 2002).

In contrast to the potential deleterious effects of APP, an early acute rise in APP during the reparative phase of injury has resulted in the hypothesis that APP may actually serve a neuroprotective function (Van Den Heuvel et al., 2004). APP has been shown to be both beneficial and detrimental depending on its method of posttranslational processing within cells. The beneficial, secreted α form of APP (sAPPα) is generated by α-secretase cleavage, whereas the secreted APPβ (sAPPβ) and deleterious Aβ are generated from cleavage by β- and γ-secretases (Hardy 1997). sAPPα has been reported to have many neuroprotective and neurotrophic functions within the central nervous system (CNS) (Mattson et al., 1993); for instance, sAPPα administration reduced neuronal injury and improved functional outcome following rat TBI (Thornton et al., 2006). The α-secretase pathway is a non-amyloidogenic pathway in which the majority of APP is normally processed (Suh and Checler 2002), while after brain injury the β- and γ-secretase pathways are activated and are responsible for producing the toxic sAPPβ (Matrone et al., 2008; Sola Vigo et al., 2008) and Aβ (Mills and

Reiner 1999; Stone et al., 2002; Blasko et al., 2004). For instance, sAPPβ was shown to induce apoptotic cell death in PC 12 cells and neuronal degeneration in rat hippocampal neurons (Matrone et al., 2008; Sola Vigo et al., 2008). Nakagawa et al. reported that the APP overexpression of ST6Gal-1 in Neuro2 enhanced producing sAPP and the level of the extracellular sAPP β form is increased the level of sAPPα form(Nakagawa et al., 2006). In AD brain, increase of the extracellular sAPP beta level could affect the pathology of AD(Nakagawa et al., 2006). In the present study, anti-APP antibody treatment resulted in a reduction of neuronal and glial apoptotic cell death and recovery of memory and learning function to sham operation group levels, after TBI. These data suggest that toxic sAPPβ is produced more than sAPPα after TBI, and that toxic sAPPβ may be responsible for the neuronal and glial cell degeneration and death. Additionally, overproduction of sAPPβ after brain injury may facilitate Aβ production and deposition.

In the adult CNS, TBI results in a rapid response from resident astrocytes, a process often referred to as reactive astrocytosis or glial scarring (Davies et al., 1999; Jurynec et al., 2003). Glial scars have been reported to inhibit neurite elongation of damaged neurons and axonal regeneration, and thus prevent functional recovery (Davies et al., 1999; Jurynec et al., 2003). Furthermore, neurite outgrowth of cultured rat hippocampal neurons was found to be inhibited by glial scars *in vitro* (Rudge and Silver 1990). However, gliosis and glial scars protect against secondary insults that contribute to the ischemic damage induced by circulatory disturbance, blood-brain barrier disruption, excitotoxic damage, and free radicals (Pekny and Nilsson 2005). Moreover, reactive astrocytes secrete neurotrophic factor (NTF), nerve growth factor (NGF), and extracellular matrix which induce axonal outgrowth and regeneration of the neural network (Bechmann and Nitsch 2000; Deller et al., 2000). In addition, the formation of glial scars prevents leakage of secreted factors, and separates non-damaged areas from damaged areas, thereby maintaining normal CNS homeostasis (Silver et al., 1997; Gallo and Chittajallu 2001). Therefore, although the role of gliosis and glial scars in neuronal regeneration after brain injury remains controversial, the results from the present study suggest that gliosis and glial scars after TBI might be beneficial.

The results from the present study also demonstrated that infusion of the anti-APP antibody into the damaged region following TBI inhibited degeneration of neuronal and glial cells induced by overproduced APP after brain injury, with a significant reduction in injury size. This may be attributed a protective effect of the anti-APP antibody against neural and glial cell death induced by overproduced APP after TBI.

## 5. Conclusion

In conclusion, the results of the present study have demonstrated that TBI induces long-term increases in APP overexpression in the neuronal perikarya and neurites. In addition, endogenous overproduced APP after TBI inhibited astrocyte activity around the damaged brain region and induced neural cell degeneration. On the basis of these findings, we speculate that overexpression of APP after TBI is related to Alzheimer type dementia, and is an important risk factor for this disease.

## 6. Acknowledgments

The authors thank Mari Yachi and Emi Watanabe for technical assistance.

## 7. References


Azbill, R. D., Mu, X., Bruce-Keller, A. J., et al. (1997). Impaired mitochondrial function, oxidative stress and altered antioxidant enzyme activities following traumatic spinal cord injury. *Brain Res*, Vol.765, No.2, (September 2007), pp.283-290, ISSN 0006-8993.

Bechmann, I., & Nitsch, R. (2000). Involvement of non-neuronal cells in entorhinal-hippocampal reorganization following lesions. *Ann N Y Acad Sci*, Vol.911, (September 2007), pp.192-206, ISSN1749-6632.

Blasko, I., Beer, R., Bigl, M., et al. (2004). Experimental traumatic brain injury in rats stimulates the expression, production and activity of Alzheimer's disease beta-secretase (BACE-1). *J Neural Transm*, Vol.111, No.4, (September 2007), pp.523-536, ISSN 1435-1463.

Blumbergs, P. C., Scott, G., Manavis, J., et al. (1995). Topography of axonal injury as defined by amyloid precursor protein and the sector scoring method in mild and severe closed head injury. *J Neurotrauma*, Vol.12, No.4, (September 2007), pp.565-572, ISSN 1557-9042.

Bouron, A., Mbebi, C., Loeffler, J. P., et al. (2004). The beta-amyloid precursor protein controls a store-operated Ca2+ entry in cortical neurons. *Eur J Neurosci*, Vol.20, No.8, (September 2007), 2071-2078, ISSN 1460-9568.

Chen, X. H., Siman, R., Iwata, A., et al. (2004). Long-term accumulation of amyloid-beta, beta-secretase, presenilin-1, and caspase-3 in damaged axons following brain trauma. *Am J Pathol*, Vol.165,No. 2, (September 2007), pp.357-371, ISSN 0002-9440.

Chirumamilla, S., Sun, D., Bullock, M. R., et al. (2002). Traumatic brain injury induced cell proliferation in the adult mammalian central nervous system. *J Neurotrauma*, Vol.19, No. 6, (September 2007), pp.693-703, ISSN 1557-9042.

Ciallella, J. R., Ikonomovic, M. D., Paljug, W. R., et al. (2002). Changes in expression of amyloid precursor protein and interleukin-1beta after experimental traumatic brain injury in rats. *J Neurotrauma*, Vol.19, No.12, (September 2007), pp.1555-1567, ISSN 1557-9042.

Davies, S. J., Goucher, D. R., Doller, C., et al. (1999). Robust regeneration of adult sensory axons in degenerating white matter of the adult rat spinal cord. *J Neurosci*, Vol.19, No.14, (September 2007), pp.5810-5822, ISSN 1529-2401.

DeKosky, S. T., Abrahamson, E. E., Ciallella, J. R., et al. (2007). Association of increased cortical soluble abeta42 levels with diffuse plaques after severe brain injury in humans. *Arch Neurol*, Vol.64, No.4, (March 2008), pp.541-544, ISSN 0003-9942.

Deller, T., Haas, C. A., & Frotscher, M. (2000). Reorganization of the rat fascia dentata after a unilateral entorhinal cortex lesion. Role of the extracellular matrix. *Ann N Y Acad Sci*, Vol.911, (September 2007), pp.207-220, ISSN 0077-8923.

Elvander, E., Schott, P. A., Sandin, J., et al. (2004). Intraseptal muscarinic ligands and galanin: influence on hippocampal acetylcholine and cognition. *Neuroscience*, Vol.126, No.3, (September 2007), pp.541-557, ISSN 0306-4522.

Feng, Z., Chang, Y., Cheng, Y., et al. (2004). Melatonin alleviates behavioral deficits associated with apoptosis and cholinergic system dysfunction in the APP 695 transgenic mouse model of Alzheimer's disease. *J Pineal Res*, Vol.37, No.2, (September 2007), pp.129-136, ISSN 0742-3098.

Gallo, V., & Chittajallu, R. (2001). Neuroscience. Unwrapping glial cells from the synapse: what lies inside? *Science*, Vol.292, No.5518, (September 2007), pp.872-873, ISSN 0036-8075.

Gentleman, S. M., Nash, M. J., Sweeting, C. J., et al. (1993). Beta-amyloid precursor protein (beta APP) as a marker for axonal injury after head injury. *Neurosci Lett*, Vol.160, No.2, (September 2007), pp.139-144, ISSN 0304-3940.

Golde, T. E., Estus, S., Younkin, L. H., et al. (1992). Processing of the amyloid protein precursor to potentially amyloidogenic derivatives. *Science*, Vol.255, No.5045, (September 2007), pp.728-730, ISSN 0036-8075.

Goldgaber, D., Lerman, M. I., McBride, O. W., et al. (1987). Characterization and chromosomal localization of a cDNA encoding brain amyloid of Alzheimer's disease. *Science*, Vol.235, No.4791, (September 2007), pp.877-880, ISSN 0036-8075.

Green-Sadan, T., Kinor, N., Roth-Deri, I., et al. (2003). Transplantation of glial cell line-derived neurotrophic factor-expressing cells into the striatum and nucleus accumbens attenuates acquisition of cocaine self-administration in rats. *Eur J Neurosci*, Vol.18, No.7, (September 2007), pp2093-2098, ISSN 1460-9568.

Hardy, J. (1997). Amyloid, the presenilins and Alzheimer's disease. *Trends Neurosci*, Vol.20, No.4, (September 2007), pp.154-159, ISSN 0166-2236.

Ikonomovic, M. D., Uryu, K., Abrahamson, E. E., et al. (2004). Alzheimer's pathology in human temporal cortex surgically excised after severe brain injury. *Exp Neurol*, Vol.190, No.1, (September 2007), pp.192-203, ISSN 0041-4886.

Itoh, T., Satou, T., Hashimoto, S., et al. (2005). Isolation of neural stem cells from damaged rat cerebral cortex after TBI. *Neuroreport*, Vol.16, No.15, (September 2007), pp.1687-1691, ISSN 0959-4965.

Itoh, T., Satou, T., Nishida, S., et al. (2007). Immature and mature neurons coexist among glial scars after rat traumatic brain injury. *Neurol Res*, Vol.29, No.7, (December 2010), pp.734-742, ISSN 0161-6412.

Itoh, T., Satou, T., Nishida, S., et al. (2009). Expression of amyloid precursor protein after rat traumatic brain injury. *Neurol Res*, Vol.31, No.1, (December 2010), pp.103-109, ISSN 0161-6412.

Jurynec, M. J., Riley, C. P., Gupta, D. K., et al. (2003). TIGR is upregulated in the chronic glial scar in response to central nervous system injury and inhibits neurite outgrowth. *Mol Cell Neurosci*, Vol.23, No.1, (September 2007), pp.69-80, ISSN 1044-7431.

Kawamata, T., Katayama, Y., Hovda, D. A., et al. (1995). Lactate accumulation following concussive brain injury: the role of ionic fluxes induced by excitatory amino acids. *Brain Res*, Vol.674, No.2, (September 2007), pp.196-204, ISSN 0006-8993.

Koo, E. H., Sisodia, S. S., Archer, D. R., et al. (1990). Precursor of amyloid protein in Alzheimer disease undergoes fast anterograde axonal transport. *Proc Natl Acad Sci U S A*, Vol.87, No.4, (September 2007), pp.1561-1565, ISSN 0027-8424.

Lewen, A., Li, G. L., Olsson, Y., et al. (1996). Changes in microtubule-associated protein 2 and amyloid precursor protein immunoreactivity following traumatic brain injury in rat: influence of MK-801 treatment. *Brain Res*, Vol.719, No.1-2, (September 2007), pp.161-171, ISSN 0006-8993.

Masters, C. L., Multhaup, G., Simms, G., et al. (1985). Neuronal origin of a cerebral amyloid: neurofibrillary tangles of Alzheimer's disease contain the same protein as the amyloid of plaque cores and blood vessels. *Embo J*, Vol.4, No.11, (September 2007), pp.2757-2763, ISSN 0261-4189.

Matrone, C., Di Luzio, A., Meli, G., et al. (2008). Activation of the amyloidogenic route by NGF deprivation induces apoptotic death in PC12 cells. *J Alzheimers Dis*, Vol.13, No.1, (September 2007), pp.81-96, ISSN 1387-2877.

Mattson, M. P., Cheng, B., Culwell, A. R., et al. (1993). Evidence for excitoprotective and intraneuronal calcium-regulating roles for secreted forms of the beta-amyloid precursor protein. *Neuron*, Vol.10, No.2, (September 2007), pp.243-254, ISSN 0896-6273.

Mills, J., & Reiner, P. B. (1999). Regulation of amyloid precursor protein cleavage. *J Neurochem*, Vol.72, No.2, (September 2007), pp.443-460, ISSN 0022-3042.

Murakami, N., Yamaki, T., Iwamoto, Y., et al. (1998). Experimental brain injury induces expression of amyloid precursor protein, which may be related to neuronal loss in the hippocampus. *J Neurotrauma*, Vol.15, No.11, (September 2007), pp.993-1003, ISSN 1557-9042.

Nakagawa, K., Kitazume, S., Oka, R., et al. (2006). Sialylation enhances the secretion of neurotoxic amyloid-beta peptides. *J Neurochem*, Vol.96, No.4, (December 2010), pp.924-933, ISSN 0022-3042.

Nakamura, Y., Takeda, M., Niigawa, H., et al. (1992). Amyloid beta-protein precursor deposition in rat hippocampus lesioned by ibotenic acid injection. *Neurosci Lett*, Vol.136, No.1, (September 2007), pp.95-98, ISSN 0304-3940.

Nicoll, J. A., Roberts, G. W., & Graham, D. I. (1995). Apolipoprotein E epsilon 4 allele is associated with deposition of amyloid beta-protein following head injury. *Nat Med*, Vol.1, No.2, (September 2007), pp.135-137, ISSN 0065-1311.

Otsuka, N., Tomonaga, M., & Ikeda, K. (1991). Rapid appearance of beta-amyloid precursor protein immunoreactivity in damaged axons and reactive glial cells in rat brain following needle stab injury. *Brain Res*, Vol.568, No.1-2, (September 2007), pp.335-338, ISSN 0006-8993.

Pekny, M., & Nilsson, M. (2005). Astrocyte activation and reactive gliosis. *Glia*, Vol.50, No.4, (September 2007), pp.427-434.

Pierce, J. E., Trojanowski, J. Q., Graham, D. I., et al. (1996). Immunohistochemical characterization of alterations in the distribution of amyloid precursor proteins and beta-amyloid peptide after experimental brain injury in the rat. *J Neurosci*, Vol.16, No.3, (September 2007), pp.1083-1090, ISSN 1529-2401.

Posmantur, R., Hayes, R. L., Dixon, C. E., et al. (1994). Neurofilament 68 and neurofilament 200 protein levels decrease after traumatic brain injury. *J Neurotrauma*, Vol.11, No.5, (September 2007), pp.533-545, ISSN 1557-9042.

Rice, A. C., Khaldi, A., Harvey, H. B., et al. (2003). Proliferation and neuronal differentiation of mitotically active cells following traumatic brain injury. *Exp Neurol*, Vol.183, No2, (September 2007), pp.406-417, ISSN 0014-4886.

Robakis, N. K., Ramakrishna, N., Wolfe, G., et al. (1987). Molecular cloning and characterization of a cDNA encoding the cerebrovascular and the neuritic plaque amyloid peptides. *Proc Natl Acad Sci U S A*, Vol.84, No.12, (September 2007), pp.4190-4194, ISSN 0027-8424.

Roberts, G. W. (1988). Immunocytochemistry of neurofibrillary tangles in dementia pugilistica and Alzheimer's disease: evidence for common genesis. *Lancet*, Vol.2, No.8626-8627, (September 2007), pp.1456-1458, ISSN 0140-6736.

Roberts, G. W., Allsop, D., & Bruton, C. (1990). The occult aftermath of boxing. *J Neurol Neurosurg Psychiatry*, Vol.53, No.5, (September 2007), pp.373-378, ISSN 0027-8424.

Roberts, G. W., Gentleman, S. M., Lynch, A., et al. (1994). Beta amyloid protein deposition in the brain after severe head injury: implications for the pathogenesis of Alzheimer's disease. *J Neurol Neurosurg Psychiatry*, Vol.57, No.4, (September 2007), pp.419-425, ISSN 0027-8424.

Rudge, J. S., & Silver, J. (1990). Inhibition of neurite outgrowth on astroglial scars in vitro. *J Neurosci*, Vol.10, No.11, (September 2007), pp.3594-3603, ISSN 1529-2401.

Rumble, B., Retallack, R., Hilbich, C., et al. (1989). Amyloid A4 protein and its precursor in Down's syndrome and Alzheimer's disease. *N Engl J Med*, Vol.320, No.22, (September 2007), pp.1446-1452, ISSN 1553-4406.

Schofield, P. W., Tang, M., Marder, K., et al. (1997). Alzheimer's disease after remote head injury: an incidence study. *J Neurol Neurosurg Psychiatry*, Vol.62, No.2, (September 2007), pp.119-124, ISSN 0022-3050.

Selkoe, D. J., Abraham, C. R., Podlisny, M. B., et al. (1986). Isolation of low-molecular-weight proteins from amyloid plaque fibers in Alzheimer's disease. *J Neurochem*, Vol.46, No.6, (September 2007), pp.1820-1834, ISSN 0022-3042.

Silver, I. A., Deas, J., & Erecinska, M. (1997). Ion homeostasis in brain cells: differences in intracellular ion responses to energy limitation between cultured neurons and glial cells. *Neuroscience*, Vol.78, No.2, (September 2007), pp.589-601, ISSN 0077-8923.

Smith, D. H., Uryu, K., Saatman, K. E., et al. (2003). Protein accumulation in traumatic brain injury. *Neuromolecular Med*, Vol.4, No.1-2, (September 2007), pp.59-72, ISSN 1535-1084.

Sola Vigo, F., Kedikian, G., Heredia, L., et al. (2008). Amyloid-beta precursor protein mediates neuronal toxicity of amyloid beta through Go protein activation. *Neurobiol Aging*, Vol.30, No.9, (September 2007), pp.1379-1392, ISSN 0197-4587.

Stephenson, D. T., Rash, K., & Clemens, J. A. (1992). Amyloid precursor protein accumulates in regions of neurodegeneration following focal cerebral ischemia in the rat. *Brain Res*, Vol.593, No.1, (September 2007), pp.128-135, ISSN 0006-8993.

Stone, J. R., Okonkwo, D. O., Singleton, R. H., et al. (2002). Caspase-3-mediated cleavage of amyloid precursor protein and formation of amyloid Beta peptide in traumatic axonal injury. *J Neurotrauma*, Vol.19, No.5, (September 2007), pp.601-614, ISSN 1557-9402.

Suh, Y. H., & Checler, F. (2002). Amyloid precursor protein, presenilins, and alpha-synuclein: molecular pathogenesis and pharmacological applications in Alzheimer's disease. *Pharmacol Rev*, Vol.54, No.3, (September 2007), pp.469-525, ISSN 0362-1642.

Sun, K. H., Sun, G. H., Su, Y., et al. (2004). Acidic-rich region of amyloid precursor protein induces glial cell apoptosis. *Apoptosis*, Vol.9, No.6, (September 2007), pp.833-841, ISSN 1360-8185.

Taft, W. C., Yang, K., Dixon, C. E., et al. (1992). Microtubule-associated protein 2 levels decrease in hippocampus following traumatic brain injury. *J Neurotrauma*, Vol.9, No.3, (September 2007), pp.281-290, ISSN 1557-9042.

Thornton, E., Vink, R., Blumbergs, P. C., et al. (2006). Soluble amyloid precursor protein alpha reduces neuronal injury and improves functional outcome following diffuse traumatic brain injury in rats. *Brain Res*, Vol.1094, No.1, (September 2007), pp.38-46, ISSN 0006-8993.

Van den Heuvel, C., Blumbergs, P. C., Finnie, J. W., et al. (1999). Upregulation of amyloid precursor protein messenger RNA in response to traumatic brain injury: an ovine head impact model. *Exp Neurol*, Vol.159, No.2, (September 2007), pp.441-450, ISSN 0014-4886.

Van Den Heuvel, C., Donkin, J. J., Finnie, J. W., et al. (2004). Downregulation of amyloid precursor protein (APP) expression following post-traumatic cyclosporin-A administration. *J Neurotrauma*, Vol.21, No.11, (September 2007), pp.1562-1572, ISSN 1557-9042.

Xie, Y., Yao, Z., Chai, H., et al. (2003). Potential roles of Alzheimer precursor protein A4 and beta-amyloid in survival and function of aged spinal motor neurons after axonal injury. *J Neurosci Res*, Vol.73, No.4, (September 2007), pp.557-564, ISSN 1097-4547.

Xiong, Y., Gu, Q., Peterson, P. L., et al. (1997). Mitochondrial dysfunction and calcium perturbation induced by traumatic brain injury. *J Neurotrauma*, Vol.14, No.1, (September 2007), pp.23-34, ISSN 1557-9042.

# Permissions

All chapters in this book were first published in ADPCCSPTT, by InTech Open; hereby published with permission under the Creative Commons Attribution License or equivalent. Every chapter published in this book has been scrutinized by our experts. Their significance has been extensively debated. The topics covered herein carry significant findings which will fuel the growth of the discipline. They may even be implemented as practical applications or may be referred to as a beginning point for another development.

The contributors of this book come from diverse backgrounds, making this book a truly international effort. This book will bring forth new frontiers with its revolutionizing research information and detailed analysis of the nascent developments around the world.

We would like to thank all the contributing authors for lending their expertise to make the book truly unique. They have played a crucial role in the development of this book. Without their invaluable contributions this book wouldn't have been possible. They have made vital efforts to compile up to date information on the varied aspects of this subject to make this book a valuable addition to the collection of many professionals and students.

This book was conceptualized with the vision of imparting up-to-date information and advanced data in this field. To ensure the same, a matchless editorial board was set up. Every individual on the board went through rigorous rounds of assessment to prove their worth. After which they invested a large part of their time researching and compiling the most relevant data for our readers.

The editorial board has been involved in producing this book since its inception. They have spent rigorous hours researching and exploring the diverse topics which have resulted in the successful publishing of this book. They have passed on their knowledge of decades through this book. To expedite this challenging task, the publisher supported the team at every step. A small team of assistant editors was also appointed to further simplify the editing procedure and attain best results for the readers.

Apart from the editorial board, the designing team has also invested a significant amount of their time in understanding the subject and creating the most relevant covers. They scrutinized every image to scout for the most suitable representation of the subject and create an appropriate cover for the book.

The publishing team has been an ardent support to the editorial, designing and production team. Their endless efforts to recruit the best for this project, has resulted in the accomplishment of this book. They are a veteran in the field of academics and their pool of knowledge is as vast as their experience in printing. Their expertise and guidance has proved useful at every step. Their uncompromising quality standards have made this book an exceptional effort. Their encouragement from time to time has been an inspiration for everyone.

The publisher and the editorial board hope that this book will prove to be a valuable piece of knowledge for researchers, students, practitioners and scholars across the globe.

# List of Contributors

**Ahmet Turan Isik**
Bezmialem Vakif University, Faculty of Medicine, Department of Geriatric Medicine, Istanbul, Turkey

**M. Refik Mas**
9Eylul University, Faculty of Medicine, Department of Internal Medicine, Izmir, Turkey

**Genaro Genaro Gabriel Ortiz et al.**
Lab. Estrés Oxidativo-Mitocondria & Enfermedad. Centro de Investigación Biomédica de Occidente (CIBO). Instituto mexicano del seguro Social (IMSS). Guadalajara, Jalisco, México
División de Ciencias de la Salud-Escuela de Medicina, Tecnológico de Monterrey, Campus Guadalajara. Zapopan, Jalisco,México

**Jesús Avila**
Centro de Biología Molecular "Severo Ochoa" CSIC-UAM, Cantoblanco, Spain

**Kazuhiro Nakamura, Suk Ling Ma and Kun Ping Lu**
Department of Medicine, Beth Israel Deaconess Medical Center Harvard Medical School, Boston, USA

**Cecília R A Santos and Isabel Gonçalves**
University of Beira Interior- Health Sciences Research Centre, Covilhã Portugal

**Isabel Cardoso**
Escola Superior de Tecnologia da Saúde do Porto, Instituto Politécnico do Porto, Vila Nova de Gaia, Portugal
Molecular Neurobiology Unit, IBMC-Instituto de Biologia Molecular e Celular, Porto, Portugal

**Motohiro Imano**
Department of Surgery, Kinki University Faculty of Medicine, Japan

**Lei Wang and Silvia Campioni**
Swiss Federal Institute of Technology (ETH) Zurich Switzerland

**Mario Álvarez Sánchez, Carlos A. Sánchez Catasús, Ivonne Pedroso Ibañez, Maria L. Bringas and Arnoldo Padrón Sánchez**
International Center of Neurological Restoration, Cuba

**Kenneth E. Neet**
Department of Biochemistry and Molecular Biology, The Chicago Medical School, Rosalind Franklin University of Medicine and Science, North Chicago,USA

**Sidharth Mahapatra**
Department of Pediatrics, School of Medicine, USA, Stanford University, Palo Alto, USA

**Hrishikesh M. Mehta**
Department of Pediatrics, Division of Hematology/Oncology/Stem Cell Transplantation Children's, USA
Memorial Hospital, Northwestern Feinberg School of Medicine,Lurie Comprehensive Cancer Center, Chicago, Northwestern University, Chicago, USA

**Alejandro Gella and Irene Bolea**
Universitat Internacional de Catalunya Universitat Autònoma de Barcelona, Spain

**Francesca Ruberti**
CNR, National Research Council of Italy, Cell Biology and Neurobiology Institute (IBCN), IRCCS Fondazione Santa Lucia, Italy

**Silvia Pezzola**
EBRI - European Brain Research Institute-Fondazione EBRI- Rita Levi-Montalcini, Italy

**Christian Barbato**
CNR, National Research Council of Italy, Cell Biology and Neurobiology Institute (IBCN), IRCCS Fondazione Santa Lucia, Italy

**Tatsuki Itoh and Akihiko Ito**
Department of Pathology, Kinki University Faculty of Medicine, Japan

**Shozo Nishida and Masahiro Tsubaki**
Kinki University Faculty of Pharmaceutical Sciences, Japan

**Shigeo Hashimoto**
Department of Pathology, PL Hospital, Japan

**Miguel Medina**
Noscira S.A., Tres Cantos, Spain

**Takao Satou**
Department of Pathology, Kinki University Faculty of Medicine, Japan
Division of Hospital Pathology, Hospital of Kinki University Faculty of Medicine, Japan
Division of Sports Medicine, Institute of Life Science, Kinki University, Japan

# Index

www.ingramcontent.com/pod-product-compliance
Lightning Source LLC
LaVergne TN
LVHW080639210926
848485LV00003B/296